Polycystic Ovary Syndrome

Polycystic ovary syndrome is one of the most common reproductive health problems of women. Despite this, its effective treatment remains a significant challenge to the medical profession. This new publication provides an essential guide to the diagnosis of the syndrome, its aetiology, pathology and effective medical management. An important theme running through the book is the role of polycystic ovary syndrome as a major cause of infertility, and the use of new assisted reproductive technologies to overcome this problem. In addition, this comprehensive account summarizes the most recent advances in the molecular basis of the syndrome, its genetic basis and long-term health effects. Given the significant new developments in all these areas, this up-to-date volume is the definitive guide to effective clinical practice in an area where consensus has previously been lacking. It will appeal to all doctors with an interest in reproductive endocrinology, including gynaecologists, in-vitro fertilization specialists and obstetricians.

Professor Gabor T. Kovacs is Professor of Obstetrics and Gynaecology, at Box Hill Medical School, Monash University, Melbourne, Australia. He is a reproductive gynaecologist, and Medical Director of Monash IVF. He has 25 years of experience with the treatment of women with polycystic ovaries through the Ovulation Induction Program of The Prince Henry's Institute of Medical Research. He is very interested in teaching and education at all levels, undergraduate, postgraduate and public education, having written four books on reproductive topics for the lay public. He is the Chairman of the Continuing Education Committee of the Royal Australian and New Zealand College of Obstetricians and Gynaecologists.

Polycystic Ovary Syndrome

Edited by

Gabor T. Kovacs

Monash Medical School
Box Hill Hospital
Melbourne, Australia

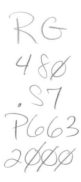

RG
480
.S7
P663
2000

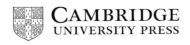

PUBLISHED BY THE PRESS SYNDICATE OF THE UNIVERSITY OF CAMBRIDGE
The Pitt Building, Trumpington Street, Cambridge, United Kingdom

CAMBRIDGE UNIVERSITY PRESS
The Edinburgh Building, Cambridge CB2 2RU, UK   http://www.cup.cam.ac.uk
40 West 20th Street, New York, NY 10011–4211, USA   http://www.cup.org
10 Stamford Road, Oakleigh, Melbourne 3166, Australia
Ruiz de Alarcón 13, 28014 Madrid, Spain

© Cambridge University Press 2000

This book is in copyright. Subject to statutory exception
and to the provisions of relevant collective licensing agreements,
no reproduction of any part may take place without
the written permission of Cambridge University Press.

IPFW
JUN 19 2003
HELMKE LIBRARY
WITHDRAWN

First published 2000

Printed in the United Kingdom

Typeface Minion (Adobe) 10.5/14pt.   *System* QuarkXPress®   [SE]

A catalogue record for this book is available from the British Library

Library of Congress Cataloguing in Publication data

Polycystic ovary syndrome / edited by Gabor T. Kovacs.
      p.   cm.
Includes index.
ISBN 0 521 66073 4 (hb)
1. Stein-Leventhal syndrome. I. Kovacs, Gabor, MRCOG, FRACOG.
[DNLM: 1. Polycystic Ovary Syndrome. WP 320 P7823 2000]
RG480.S7 P663 2000
618.1′1–dc21   99-052561

ISBN 0 521 66073 4 hardback

Every effort has been made in preparing this book to provide accurate and up-to-date
information which is in accord with accepted standards and practice at the time of
publication. Nevertheless, the authors, editors and publisher can make no warranties
that the information contained herein is totally free from error, not least because clinical
standards are constantly changing through research and regulation. The authors, editors
and publisher therefore disclaim all liability for direct or consequential damages
resulting from the use of material contained in this book. Readers are strongly advised
to pay careful attention to information provided by the manufacturer of any drugs or
equipment that they plan to use.

Contents

v

Contributors

Yves Ardaens
Department of Radiology
Hôpital Jeanne de Flandre, Centre Hospitalier et
Universitaire de Lille, Lille, France

Adam Balen
Department of Obstetrics and Gynaecology
The General Infirmary at Leeds, Belmont Grove,
Leeds LS14 3BZ, UK

Alice Benjamin
Department of Obstetrics and Gynaecology
McGill University, Royal Victoria Hospital,
Women's Pavilion, 687 Pine Avenue West,
Montreal, Québec H3A 1A1, Canada

Willam M. Buckett
Department of Obstetrics and Gynaecology
McGill University, Royal Victoria Hospital,
Women's Pavilion, 687 Pine Avenue West,
Montreal, Québec H3A 1A1, Canada

Henry G. Burger
Prince Henry's Institute of Medical Research
PO Box 5152, Clayton, Victoria, Australia 3168

Ester Cela
Department of Reproductive Science and Medicine
and Section of Endocrinology and Metabolism
Imperial College School of Medicine, St Mary's
Hospital, London W2 1PG, UK

Anne M. Clark
Fertility First
Hurstville, NSW, Australia 2220

Jean Cohen
8 rue de Marignan, 75008 Paris, France

Eva Dahlgren
Department of Obstetrics and Gynaecology
Sahlgrenska University Hospital, SE 413 45
Göteborg, Sweden

Didier Dewailly
Department of Endocrinology and Reproductive
Medicine
Marc Linquette, Centre Hospitalier et Universitaire
de Lille, Lille, France

Deborah Driscoll
Center for Research on Reproduction and
Women's Health
University of Pennsylvania Medical Center,
Philadelphia, PA 19104, USA

Andrea Dunaif
Division of Women's Health
Department of Medicine and Department of
Obstetrics and Gynecology
Brigham and Women's Hospital, Boston, MA
02115, USA

Cindy Farquhar
Department of Obstetrics and Gynaecology
National Women's Hospital, Private Bag 92 189,
Auckland 3, New Zealand

Stephen Franks
Department of Reproductive Science and Medicine
and Section of Endocrinology and Metabolism
Imperial College School of Medicine, St Mary's
Hospital, London W2 1PG, UK

Neda Gharani
Department of Reproductive Science and Medicine
and Section of Endocrinology and Metabolism
Imperial College School of Medicine, St Mary's
Hospital, London W2 1PG, UK

Jack Green
Department of Dermatology
St Vincent's Hospital, Melbourne, Australia 3000

Howard Jacobs
Department of Endrocrinology
The Middlesex Hospital, London W1N 8AA, UK

Per Olof Janson
Department of Obstetrics and Gynaecology
Sahlgrenska University Hospital, SE 413 45
Göteborg, Sweden

Lee-Chuan Kao
Center for Research on Reproduction and
Women's Health
University of Pennsylvania Medical Center,
Philadelphia, PA 19104, USA

Gabor T. Kovacs
Department of Obstetrics and Gynaecology
Monash Medical School
Box Hill Hospital, PO Box 94, Box Hill, Victoria,
Australia 3128

Richard S. Legro
Department of Obstetrics and Gynecology
Pennsylvania State University College of Medicine,
Hershey, PA 17033, USA

Mark McCarthy
Department of Reproductive Science and Medicine
and Section of Endocrinology and Metabolism
Imperial College School of Medicine, St Mary's
Hospital, London W2 1PG, UK

Robert J. Norman
Department of Obstetrics and Gynaecology
Queen Elizabeth Hospital, University of Adelaide,
Woodville, South Australia, Australia 5011

Andrew G. Östör
48 Anderson Road, Hawthorn East, Victoria,
Australia 3143

Yann Robert
Department of Radiology
Hôpital Jeanne de Flandre, Centre Hospitalier et
Universitaire de Lille, Lille, France

Seang Lin Tan
Department of Obstetrics and Gynaecology
McGill University, Royal Victoria Hospital,
Women's Pavilion, 687 Pine Avenue West,
Montreal, Québec H3A 1A1, Canada

Julia Shelley
Centre for the Study of Mothers' and Children's
Health
La Trobe University, Locked Bag 6, Post Office
Carlton South, Victoria, Australia 3053

Dr Rodney Sinclair
Department of Dermatology
St Vincents Hospital, Melbourne, Australia 3000

Richard S. Spielman
Department of Genetics
University of Pennsylvania Medical Center,
Philadelphia, PA 19104, USA

Jerome F. Strauss III
Center for Research on Reproduction and
Women's Health
Department of Obstetrics and Gynecology
University of Pennsylvania Medical Center,
Philadelphia, PA 19104, USA

Alan Trounson
Monash University Institute of Reproduction and
Development
Monash Medical Centre, 246 Clayton Road,
Clayton, Victoria, Australia 3168

Margrit Urbanek
Department of Genetics
University of Pennsylvania Medical Center,
Philadelphia, PA 19104, USA

Alison Venn
Centre for the Study of Mothers' and Children's
Health
La Trobe University, Locked Bag 6, Post Office
Carlton South, Victoria, Australia 3053

Dawn Waterworth
Department of Reproductive Science and Medicine
and Section of Endocrinology and Metabolism
Imperial College School of Medicine, St Mary's
Hospital, London W2 1PG, UK

Carl Wood
Monash IVF
89 Bridge Road, Richmond, Victoria,
Australia 3128

Foreword

In recent years we have witnessed an expansion of our knowledge and understanding of the polycystic ovary syndrome (PCOS). Researchers have continued to investigate the pathophysiology and genesis of this fascinating syndrome and clinicians continue to be challenged by new approaches in diagnosis and treatment. The editor of this timely volume, Dr Gabor T. Kovacs, has had a long-term keen interest in PCOS. He has carefully selected a superb group of highly qualified scientists and clinicians as the contributing authors. The book is skillfully organized into chapters that deal with all the relevant issues. It provides the reader with a critical review and update of our current understanding of this clinical endocrinopathy.

Not only is PCOS an endocrinopathy, but it is also an important metabolic disorder – pancreatic b-cell dysfunction. This can occur even in the absence of obesity and glucose intolerance. During my years as editor of *Fertility and Sterility*, it was my privilege to review and publish many of the articles referenced in the pages of this textbook. I am grateful for having had that opportunity to see so quickly many of the fine studies unravelling some of the mysteries of this disorder.

Genetic studies of PCOS suggest that the mode of inheritance within affected families is autosomal dominant. Dr Stephen Franks and collaborators hypothesize that PCOS is an oligogenic disorder with a small number of key genes interacting with each other and with environmental factors. Current investigation is directed towards identifying, on the basis of biochemical criteria, so-called candidate genes. Initial searches have implicated a locus on the insulin gene and the gene encoding P450scc (*CYP 11a*). Dr Jerome F. Strauss III and co-workers focus on follistatin as the primary candidate gene for PCOS, having identified several rare transmitted variants in the follistatin gene. They draw attention to the fact that increased levels of functional activity of follistatin neutralize activin, which in turn leads to increased levels of androgens as are seen in PCOS.

The sometimes controversial use of diagnostic ultrasound in defining the PCOS phenotype is addressed in Chapter 6. While it can be argued that it is not necessary for diagnosis in the majority of women with typical clinical and biochemical features of PCOS, it is helpful in those who do not have characteristic signs of the syndrome such as anovulatory infertility and hyperandrogenicity. Long-term health implications in PCOS patients are examined in Chapter 7. Among these is the controversial potential link between PCOS and cardiovascular disease.

The comprehensive chapters addressing fertility issues in PCOS will be of particular interest to readers who are clinicians. Ovulation induction is carefully reviewed in Chapter 10. Details are provided of management plans, success rates for various treatments and an evaluation of the value of adjuvant treatment for ovulation induction. Chapter 11 revisits the role of laparoscopic surgery for the treatment of infertility in these patients. In chapter 12, special attention is devoted to the PCOS patient in the in-vitro fertilization setting. These patients are some of the most challenging, because they exhibit exaggerated responses to exogenous gonadotrophins.

Particularly challenging and exciting is the chapter written by Carl Wood and Alan Trounson, addressing the issues that surround possible future treatment of PCOS – immature oocytes, their collection and in-vitro maturation. Appropriately, the final chapter answers the question 'Should there be long-term monitoring of women with PCOS?'.

This is a much-welcomed text which will be valued by all those interested in reproductive medicine. It will grace the libraries of basic scientists, clinicians, physicians-in-training, allied health professionals and students alike.

Roger D. Kempers, MD

Professor of Obstetrics and Gynecology, Emeritus
Mayo Medical School and Mayo Graduate School of Medicine
Rochester, Minnesota

Acknowledgements

A special thank you to Penny Heath, my secretary, for her efforts in getting the manuscript together for *Polycystic Ovary Syndrome*, and to Rob Norman for his assistance with selecting the authors. I also would like to thank my wife, Rosie, and daughters, Katie, Georgie and Rebecca, for their support during this project.

1

Introduction: polycystic ovary syndrome is not just a reproductive problem

Gabor T. Kovacs and Henry G. Burger

The polycystic ovary (PCO) was recognized as a relatively frequent cause of irregular ovulation or anovulation in women seeking treatment for subfertility. Although first described as early as 1935 by Stein and Leventhal, who offered surgical treatment, it became easily treatable with the availability of clomiphene citrate in 1961 (Greenblatt, 1961). There was also a group of women who presented, either in association with subfertility or as their main complaint, with symptoms of androgen excess, especially hirsutism, greasy skin and acne, who were found to have PCO. With the availability of radioimmunoassay, it was recognized that many of these women had an increased ratio of luteinizing hormone (LH) to follicle stimulating hormone (FSH) and this became a biochemical diagnostic criterion for the condition. This excess of LH was thought to be the cause of excessive androgen production, resulting in the symptoms of hirsutism and acne.

It was with the availability of ultrasound (Swanson, Sauerbrei and Cooperberg, 1981) that many women were found to have the characteristic appearance of PCO, with or without the biochemical changes or clinical symptoms. It therefore became apparent that PCO were not associated with a single syndrome, but with a range of conditions, the most severe of which was that described by Stein and Leventhal comprising anovulatory infertility, hirsutism and obesity. On the other hand, the ultrasound appearances could be an incidental finding in about 20% of apparently normal women in the community. It is now accepted that 'polycystic ovaries' is an ultrasonic diagnosis (the criteria for diagnosis are discussed in detail in Chapter 6). Women who also have the clinical manifestations of menstrual irregularity and/or hyperandrogenism are said to have the 'polycystic ovary syndrome' (PCOS). This is simply explained by a Venn diagram, where the three circles for ultrasonic appearance, clinical features and biochemical changes are represented by three overlapping circles. This highlights that a small proportion will have all three criteria, whereas others have one or two out of the three (Fig. 1.1).

Gynaecologists have been treating women for anovulation using clomiphene

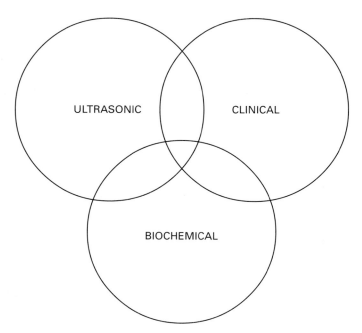

Fig. 1.1   Polycystic ovary syndrome.

citrate in the first instance followed by gonadotrophins with great success for the last 30 years (this is covered in detail in Chapter 10).

Surgical treatment, using the laparoscopic approach, has recently become the preferred option after clomiphene failure (Kovacs, 1996) before embarking on gonadotrophins (this is discussed in detail in Chapter 11). Apart from this new interest in the surgical approach, there has been little change in the management of PCOS to achieve fertility. There has, however, been an interest in PCOS from physicians and dermatologists to whom women were referred because of the symptoms of hirsutism and acne. Many of these women did not wish to conceive, but were concerned by their physical appearance. The approach to these women was often to exclude an endocrinological cause for their increased androgenization, and then to advise cosmetic treatment. In addition, the use of an oral contraceptive, usually oestrogen dominant, was recommended (Kovacs and Marks, 1987). Subsequently, anti-androgens such as cyproterone acetate became available, either as part of a contraceptive pill or in conjunction with sequential oestrogens. As physicians became involved with women with PCOS, more detailed investigations were undertaken, and it was recognized that this disorder is often associated with abnormal carbohydrate metabolism (insulin resistance) (Burghen, Givens and Kitabchi, 1980) and also with disturbance of lipid profile resulting in an unfavourable picture (Givens, 1988; Kidson, 1998). Thus, it appears that PCOS is not just a reproductive disease, easily remedied by the use of ovulation induction, but a systemic condition, the molecular biology (Chapter 4) of which is still being classified. It seems to have a complex inheritance, as discussed in Chapter 3. PCOS is therefore a condition which is of interest to the wider medical community.

With the change of emphasis in medical care for the twenty-first century from disease treatment to illness prevention and health promotion, PCOS is an excellent example of a syndrome for which early recognition and intervention, such as weight control, diet modification and lifestyle changes (as discussed in Chapter 9), may prevent or delay the development of further problems, in this case diabetes or atherosclerosis. We may also need to implement some ongoing surveillance, and take a more long-term holistic interest in affected women (this is considered further in Chapter 15).

This was the reason to collate the currently held views from the leading experts around the world, and to publish them as a single manuscript in *Polycystic Ovary Syndrome*.

We are grateful to our colleagues for their prompt and extensive contributions, and hope that this book will be of interest to those practitioners who treat women with PCOS.

REFERENCES

Burghen, G.A., Givens, G.R. and Kitabchi. A.E. (1980). Correlation of hyperandrogenism with hyperinsulinism in polycystic ovarian disease. *Journal of Clinical Endocrinology and Metabolism* **50**, 113–16.

Givens, J.R. (1988). Familial polycystic ovarian disease. *Endocrinology and Metabolism Clinics of North America* **17**, 771–83.

Greenblatt, R.B. (1961). Chemical induction of ovulation. *Fertility and Sterility* **12**, 402.

Kidson, W. (1998). Polycystic ovary syndrome: a new direction in treatment. *The Medical Journal of Australia* **169**, 537–40.

Kovacs, G. (1996). Polycystic ovary syndrome and contemporary management. *Royal Australian College of Obstetricians and Gynaecologists Resource Unit 136* **5**, 37–42.

Kovacs, G.T. and Marks, R. (1987). Contraception and the skin. *The Australian Journal of Dermatology* **28**, 86–92.

Stein, I.F. and Leventhal (1935). Amenorrhoea associated with bilateral polycystic ovaries. *American Journal of Obstetrics and Gynecology* **29**, 181–91.

Swanson, M., Sauerbrei, E.E. and Cooperberg, P.L. (1981). Medical implications of ultrasonically detected polycystic ovaries. *Journal of Clinical Ultrasound* **9**, 219–22.

History of polycystic ovary syndrome

Cindy Farquhar

Introduction

Clinicians and scientists have been challenged by the polycystic ovary syndrome (PCOS) for several decades. Since the classical observation of Stein and Leventhal more than 60 years ago (Stein and Leventhal, 1935), interest in polycystic ovaries (PCO) and the associated syndrome has evolved from a 'gynaecological curiosity to a multisystem endocrinopathy' (Homburg, 1996). It is probably the most common endocrine disorder in women, accounting for the majority of cases of hirsutism, menstrual disturbance and anovulatory infertility. It is also one of the most poorly defined endocrinological conditions, with a complex pathophysiology that has produced considerable scientific debate. Evidence of the ongoing interest in this disorder is not difficult to find; an electronic search on MEDLINE from 1966 to 1998 using the search term 'polycystic ovary syndrome' produces 3361 citations: of these, 431 are review articles, 1113 relate to diagnosis, 95 relate to aetiology and 130 are randomized controlled trials (Fig. 2.1), and the majority of publications occur after 1980.

Recognition

Although Stein and Leventhal were first in the modern medicine era to describe this condition, an earlier description dating back to 1721 reads:

Young married peasant women, moderately obese and infertile, with two larger than normal ovaries, bumpy, shiny and whitish, just like pigeon eggs. ([translated from Italian] A. Vallisneri, 1721)

There was further recognition in the nineteenth century when sclerocystic changes in the ovary were described (Chereau, 1844), but it was not until Stein and Leventhal first presented their paper at the Central Association of Obstetricians and Gynaecologists in 1935 that the syndrome was more comprehensively described. They reported on seven women who had amenorrhoea, hirsutism, and

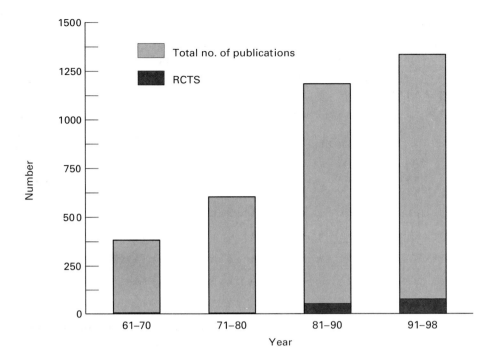

Fig. 2.1   The medical literature on polycystic ovary syndrome.

enlarged ovaries, with multiple small cysts and thickened tunica (Fig 2.2). While there had been reports of menometrorrhagia in women with microcystic disease of the ovary, amenorrhoea had not been recognized or reported in such cases until Stein and Leventhal's report. Stein and Leventhal had also performed ovarian wedge resection which resulted in a return of ovulatory cycles. Of the seven patients who underwent wedge biopsy, all returned to regular menstruation and two conceived. It is not clear whether other cases of the disorder were observed that did not fit this particular pattern. Stein subsequently reported on 75 women who underwent bilateral wedge resection, nearly 90% of whom began to have spontaneous menstrual cycles and 65% of those seeking fertility conceived (Stein, Cohen and Elson, 1948).

The diagnosis of polycystic ovary syndrome

The advances that have taken place in the past century with regard to the diagnosis of this condition have been considerable. Stein and Leventhal's method of diagnosis rested primarily on observing enlarged sclerocystic ovaries at either

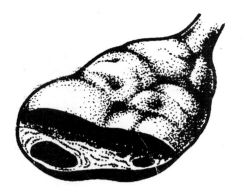

Normal Ovary

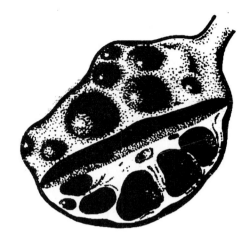

Polycystic Ovary

Fig. 2.2   The polycystic ovary.

pneumoroentgenography or at laparotomy in women who were either anovulatory or hirsute, or both (Stein and Leventhal, 1935). Prior to this, there was little choice but to perform repeated vaginal and rectal examinations which did not always reveal the presence of PCO. At pneumoroentgenography air was admitted into the peritoneum by an abdominal incision and PCO were confirmed when the ovaries were three-quarters as large as the uterine shadow on x-ray. Several examples of this technique are given in Stein and Leventhal's original publication. They often used lipiodal instillations at the same time to outline the fallopian tubes. However, this technique did not really gain popularity, and eventually laparotomy and wedge biopsy became the mainstay of both diagnosis and treatment (Goldzieher and Green, 1962).

With the development of radioimmunoassay techniques in the 1970s and the introduction of clomiphene citrate, laparotomy and biopsy were largely abandoned as a diagnostic method. In 1958, McArthur, Ingersoll and Worcester first described elevated urinary levels of luteinizing hormone (LH) in women with bilateral PCO (McArthur et al., 1958). Throughout the 1970s and 1980s, elevated serum concentrations of LH and testosterone were considered an essential prerequisite for diagnosis (Yen, Vela and Rankin, 1970; Rebar et al., 1976). For example, Yen (1980) stated that 'true PCOS' had typical abnormalities of gonadotrophin and androgen secretion. There have been a number of interesting evolutions in the search for diagnostic criteria. Not only was an elevation in the LH level felt to be necessary, but in time the ratio of LH to follicle stimulating hormone (FSH) was also required to be elevated. Initially the ratio was 2:1, then 3:1 and even 2.5:1 (Yen, 1980; Lobo et al., 1981; Shoupe, Kumar and Lobo, 1983; Chang et al., 1983). Eventually, the concept of a ratio was abandoned and the absolute values were relied on for diagnosis (Fox et al., 1991; Robinson et al., 1992). However, by only defining PCOS in the presence of elevation of LH concentrations, obviously all patients will have the condition (Waldstreicher et al., 1988; Fauser et al., 1991, 1992) and LH becomes a *sine qua non* for the diagnosis (Franks, 1995; Homburg, 1996). Elevations in androgens are similarly unhelpful in defining the syndrome as the levels are modestly and inconsistently elevated (Gadir et al., 1990). Other limitations of the biochemical diagnosis of PCOS included the variable and imprecise nature of the assays and the dynamic nature of hormonal steroidal release from the ovary (Fauser et al., 1991, 1992). LH is secreted in a pulsatile manner and the difference between the peak and nadir of each pulse can be substantial (Santon and Bardin, 1973) and therefore measuring the hormone levels only once may be misleading (Franks, 1989). Furthermore, there were still many women who were noted to have the clinical symptoms but whose LH and testosterone levels did not fall within the diagnostic criteria (Adams et al., 1985). There was a need for a diagnostic test that could observe the ovary without damaging its surface and potentially reducing fertility, but that did not just 'take a snapshot' of the endocrine state of a patient as a single measurement of the serum concentration of ovarian hormones does.

Fortunately, real-time ultrasound was developing into a useful diagnostic tool. Ultrasound examination of the ovary has many advantages over direct observation at laparoscopy or laparotomy: it is non-invasive, simple, allows careful, repeatable measurements and it is possible to see the follicular structures clearly just below the surface of the ovary as well as to demonstrate the dense and frequently increased stroma (Fig. 2.3). Swanson, Sauerbrei and Cooperberg (1981) first reported on the ultrasound description of PCO. The cysts ranged from 2mm to 6 mm and were either peripherally distributed or throughout the parenchyma. Ultrasound descriptions have been shown to correlate with both laparoscopic findings and histological findings (Eden et al., 1989; Saxton et al., 1990). In the study by Eden et al. (1989), direct laparoscopic inspection of the ovaries was considered the reference test for the diagnosis of PCO, and the sensitivity (97%) and specificity (100%) with ultrasound were very good. In the study by Saxton et al. (1990), women who were undergoing open hysterectomy and bilateral oophorectomy had an ultrasound within 24 hours of surgery, when careful measurements and morphological descriptions were made. The measurements were repeated the following day in theatre and again in the histopathology laboratory by independent observers with

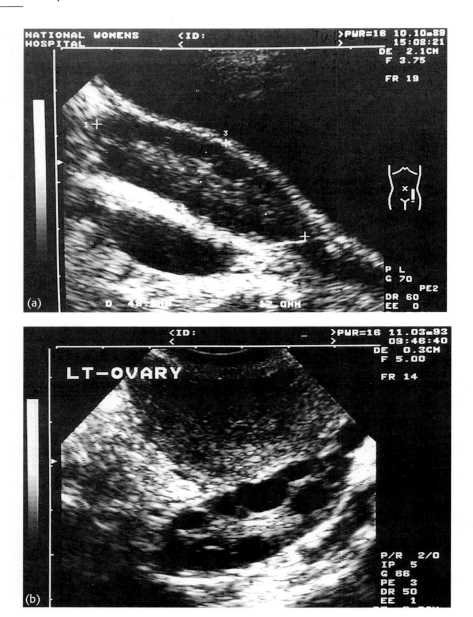

Fig. 2.3   Ultrasound view of polycystic ovary: (a) transabdominal, and (b) transvaginal.

no prior knowledge of the ultrasound findings. There was 100% sensitivity and specificity in the 28 ovaries (of 14 women) that were studied.

Thus, ultrasound has now become the gold standard for the diagnosis of PCO. The diagnostic criteria described by Adams et al. (1985) are frequently cited and although there are ongoing discussions about the number of follicles and the size of the ovary (Fox et al., 1991) there has been little change to these criteria. The ultrasound diagnostic criteria rest on the observation of more than ten discrete follicles of <10mm, usually peripherally arranged around an enlarged, hyperechogenic, central stroma at either transabdominal or transvaginal ultrasound (see Fig. 2.3). The upper limit for ovarian volumes has decreased from >10 cm^3 to as low as >5.5 cm^3 (Orsini, Venturoli and Lorusso, 1985; El Tabbakh et al., 1986; Polson et al., 1988; Ardaens et al., 1991; Farquhar et al., 1994b; Dewailly, 1997). A comparison of transvaginal ultrasound and transabdominal ultrasound by Fox et al. (1991) suggested that the latter failed to detect 30% of PCO compared to an almost 100% detection rate with the former. However, other studies reported similar detection rates for transabdominal and transvaginal ultrasound (Farquhar et al., 1994a) although the latter has many practical advantages. Recent advances in ultrasound include an objective and quantitative method of measuring the ovarian stroma using a computerized ultrasonic technique (Dewailly, 1997) which has demonstrated that women with PCO have a greater stroma than women with normal ovaries. It was concluded that an increased ovarian stroma is the most valuable diagnostic factor for PCOS. However, the absence of stroma does not exclude the diagnosis.

Prevalence studies

When discussing the prevalence in the population, it is important to be clear about the difference between the definitions that are commonly used. Polycystic ovaries should not be confused with the polycystic ovary syndrome. Polycystic ovaries may be diagnosed in the absence of any clinical syndrome (Polson et al., 1988). The polycystic ovary syndrome refers to the presence of PCO in a woman with a particular cluster of symptoms which usually includes amenorrhoea, oligoamenorrhoea, hirsutism, anovulation and other signs of androgen excess such as acne and crown pattern baldness (Franks, 1995; Jacobs, 1996; Homburg, 1996). However, some women with none of these symptoms may be diagnosed with PCO when they have an ultrasound examination for other reasons. Once ultrasound became commonly used in the 1980s it was recognized that PCO were frequently reported in asymptomatic women, and this was one of the reasons that prevalence studies were undertaken. The first prevalence study was reported in a group of patients from a population of volunteers who were predominantly hospital workers and medical students (Polson et al., 1988). The prevalence of PCO in this group was reported to be 23%, but the large majority of these women had clinical manifestations of the syndrome, namely hirsutism or oligoamenorrhoea. Three further prevalence studies have been undertaken (Clayton et al., 1992; Farquhar et al., 1994b; Michelmore et al., 1998), and a prevalence rate of between 16% and 33% was

Table 2.1. Summary of prevalence studies of polycystic ovaries and polycystic ovary syndrome

Reference	Setting	n	PCO (%)	PCOS (%)[a]	Notes
Polson et al. (1988)	Volunteers	258	23	76	Transabdominal ultrasound
Clayton et al. (1992)	GP practice	190	22	30[b]	
Farquhar et al. (1994)	Electoral roll	183	21	59	Transvaginal and transabdominal ultrasound
Michelmore et al. (1988)	GP practice volunteers	224	34	65	Transabdominal ultrasound

Notes:
[a] Defined as either hirsutism or irregular cycles, or both.
[b] Irregular or very irregular cycles (does not include hirsutism).

reported. With the exception of Clayton et al.'s study, the other three prevalence studies found that women with PCO were also more likely to have symptoms suggestive of the PCOS, namely hirsutism or menstrual disturbances. The findings of these prevalence studies are summarized in Table 2.1.

Concept of a spectrum

The prevalence studies have lead to a greater understanding of this condition. It is now widely recognized that there is a continuum or spectrum of clinical presentations (Balen et al., 1995). At one end of the spectrum are the women who ovulate and who have no dermatological manifestations such as acne or hirsutism. These women may have had an ultrasound for some other unrelated reason. At the other end of the spectrum there may be women with menstrual disturbances: oligo-amenorrhoea, increased hair growth, acne, crown pattern baldness, evidence of insulin resistance. The patients described by Stein and Leventhal in 1935 probably represented one extreme of the clinical spectrum. The presence of a woman in this continuum is probably predetermined by genetic factors but her position on the continuum is likely to be related to lifestyle and, in particular, body mass index. Although the exact 'trigger' that 'causes' the expression of the syndrome is unknown, it is likely that body mass index is involved (Balen et al., 1995), and women at the PCO end of the spectrum (without PCOS) may move to the other end of the spectrum if they have an increase in body weight (Homburg, 1996). Weight reduction in a woman with PCOS will often return her to the other end of the spectrum with ovulatory cycles and improved hirsutism (Kiddy et al., 1992; Clark et al., 1995). In clinical practice there is a tendency for only women at the severely affected end of the scale (with PCOS) to be referred to infertility or endo-crine services. An asymptomatic non-obese woman who is diagnosed with PCO on ultrasound should be counselled about the advisability of maintaining a normal body mass index in the future. Should symptoms of amenorrhoea or hyperandro-genism develop, specialist attention should be sought regardless of weight. It is unclear and controversial if all lean women with PCO only should undergo tests for insulin resistance (Franks, 1995; Nestler, 1998).

Clinical manifestations

Polycystic ovary syndrome appears to be a heterogeneous condition with a wide variety of clinical presentations. The more severe the biochemical disturbance, the more likely the woman is to have a clinical presentation (Conway, Honour and Jacobs, 1989; Balen et al., 1995). The majority of women will present with only one or two of the clinical manifestations. It is unclear why some women may present with anovulation with no hyperandrogenic manifestations, while others may present with severe androgenic symptoms but remain ovulatory.

Menstrual disturbances

Oligoamenorrhoea, amenorrhoea and prolonged erratic menstrual bleeding are all aspects of the menstrual disturbances that occur in PCOS. Nearly 90% of women with oligoamenorrhoea have PCO on ultrasound, while PCO are only present in 30% of women with amenorrhoea (Adams, Polson and Franks, 1986; Franks, 1995). The majority of women with anovulatory infertility will have PCOS, although weight-related amenorrhoea and hyperprolactinaemia need to be consid-ered as part of the differential diagnosis.

Hirsutism, acne and alopecia

Increased facial and body hair is one of the most commonly presenting symptoms, and 92% of women with this symptom have PCO on ultrasound (Adams et al., 1986). Acne has also only recently been acknowledged as an endocrine disorder (Bunker et al., 1991) and approximately three-quarters of women who present with acne have PCO on ultrasound (Eden, 1991). Alopecia and crown pattern baldness have been less commonly reported in women with PCOS. All these clinical symp-toms reflect the mild androgenic stimulations of the pilosebaceous unit. Severe signs of virilization such as clitoromegaly, or deepening of the voice, as well as rapid onset of hirsutism are rarely manifestations of PCOS, and an androgen-producing tumour should be excluded (Ehrmann et al., 1994). Similarly, if the testosterone concentration is >4.8 nmol/l, further investigations need to be undertaken (Balen et al., 1995).

Recurrent miscarriage

Polycystic ovaries have been identified as being associated with recurrent miscarriage and early pregnancy loss following in-vitro fertilization (IVF) cycles (Sagle et al., 1988; Homburg et al., 1988; Regan, Owen and Jacobs, 1990; Rai, Clifford and Regan, 1996). Hypersecretion of LH was proposed as the underlying cause of the reproductive loss (Homburg et al., 1988). There have, however, been conflicting reports which have resulted in much debate. For example, Thomas et al. (1989) found no association with LH levels and outcome following IVF, while others have reported no increase in LH in women with recurrent miscarriage and PCO (Tulppala et al., 1993; Liddell, Farquhar and Sowden, 1997). Some authors have advocated lowering elevated LH levels in women trying to conceive by suppression with gonadotrophin releasing hormone (GnRH) analogues (Balen et al., 1995). Although one trial of 106 women with elevated LH levels and PCO who were given GnRH analogues did not show an improvement in pregnancy outcomes (Clifford et al., 1996), further research is needed to evaluate this approach.

Metabolic symptomatology

The metabolic aspects of PCOS are obesity (present in 30–50% of women with PCOS) and insulin resistance, both of which are common. The distribution of fat in women with PCO results in an increased waist:hip ratio (Bringer et al., 1993) and is frequently associated with greater insulin resistance than if fat is distributed predominantly in the lower body segment (Pasquali, Casimirri and Venturoli, 1994). Some women may also present with acanthosis nigricans (a feathering pigmented area of tissue in the neck and axillary regions); this is now recognized as a non-specific marker of moderate to severe insulin resistance (Dunaif, 1992a). Hypersecretion of insulin results in ovarian secretion of androgens, leading to hirsutism and menstrual disturbance (Conway, Clark and Wong, 1993). There is increasing evidence that women with PCOS are at increased risk for the development of Type II diabetes mellitus (Ehrmann et al., 1994) and myocardial infarction (Birdsall, Farquhar and White, 1997; Wild, 1997).

Aetiology

Although uncertainty exists regarding the aetiology of PCOS, genetic factors are strongly implicated. For example, a high percentage of siblings and mothers of women with PCOS have the same morphological appearances at ultrasound (Hague et al., 1988). There is also evidence of an autosomal transmission of the responsible genetic sequences. It is possible that a gene (or series of genes) may render the ovary susceptible to insulin stimulation of androgen secretion while blocking follicular maturation (Nestler, 1997). In men, this genetic predisposition may be expressed as premature balding (Carey et al., 1993). The symptoms frequently begin at puberty, although in many women the syndrome is not fully expressed until later in their reproductive years (Lunde et al., 1989; Dewailly et al., 1994). This topic is expanded in subsequent chapters.

Pathophysiology

It is beyond the scope of this introductory chapter to discuss in detail the pathophysiological processes that lead to the development of PCOS. The topic has certainly resulted in vigorous international debate. Fortunately, there are some areas of agreement. Firstly, establishing the source of the ovarian androgen production is important to the understanding of the aetiology. Secondly, insulin resistance probably contributes to the overall androgen levels. The increased ovarian androgen production seen in PCOS is the result of a series of complex biochemical processes which begins with disordered activity in the enzyme cytochrome P450c 17-alpha, which catalyses 17-hydroxylase and 17/20 lyase activities (Rosenfield et al., 1990), the rate-limiting step in androgen biosynthesis (Barnes et al., 1989). Ovulatory women with PCOS may also demonstrate this disordered activity (Franks and White, 1993). Persistently high levels of LH will produce excessive amounts of androstenedione by causing increased P450 cytochrome activity. Unfortunately, this does not explain increased androgen activity in women who have normal LH levels. Various explanations include failed downgrading of the LH receptor midcycle (Rosenfield et al., 1990), and increased number of LH receptors in women with PCOS . Insulin-like growth factor (IGF-1) potentiates the expression of LH receptors (Adashi et al., 1985) and stimulates LH-induced androgen production and the accumulation of androgens in the ovary (Barbieri et al., 1986; Cara and Rosenfield, 1988). Although there is no increase in the levels of IGF-1 in women with PCOS (Homburg et al., 1992), there is evidence of increased biological activity. IGF-1 actively induces insulin resistance and also increases androgen secretion. It is likely that IGF-1 stimulates 17β-oestradiol production by a combination of granulosa cell proliferation and stimulation of the aromatase complex (Adashi et al., 1985). It may also act as an amplifier of the action of FSH by interacting with FSH transduction signal at multiple sites (Adashi, Resnick and Hernandez, 1988).

Evidence of insulin resistance and consequent hyperinsulinaemia in women with PCOS is plentiful (Khan et al., 1976; Burghen, Givens and Kitabehi, 1980; Dunaif, 1997). Insulin resistance is most evident in women with a high body mass index (Pasquali et al., 1994; Dunaif, 1997). It occurs in 30–60% of women with PCOS (Dunaif, 1992a). In spite of insulin resistance at peripheral sites, e.g. adipose tissue, the ovary remains sensitive to insulin and other stimulatory peptides, e.g.

IGF (Bergh et al., 1993; Willis and Franks, 1995). This phenomenon has been described in women with PCOS with both normal and high body mass indices (Plymate et al., 1981; Dunaif, 1992b). The action of insulin on the liver leads to a decrease in the production of sex hormone-binding globulin and IGF-1-binding protein, which results in an increase in unbound testosterone. Thus, although the ovary is the major site of increased androgen production in PCOS, insulin resistance may contribute to the overall androgen levels.

Advances in management

The initial management of diagnosed PCOS will depend upon the clinical problem – anovulation or hirsutism. Other issues that need to be considered subsequently include the avoidance of long-term sequelae of the syndrome.

Hirsutism

The mainstay of management in the first half of the twentieth century depended on hair removal techniques. In moderate cases this may still be the choice of treatment, especially if fertility is sought. Anti-androgen therapy was introduced in the 1960s. Spironolactone, cyproterone acetate and, more recently, flutamide are successful treatments for symptoms of hyperandrogenism, including acne. Antibiotic therapy is also useful for the management of acne. Androgen-dependent alopecia is generally irreversible. Anti-androgens are usually prescribed with a low-dose oral contraceptive in order to induce regular withdrawal bleeding and provide contraceptive cover.

Anovulation

The first human pituitary FSH was used successfully to induce ovulation in anovulatory women in 1958 (Gemzell, Diczfalusy and Tillinger, 1958). However, the initial enthusiasm was somewhat dampened by the high fetal and maternal complication rates, mostly resulting from multiple ovulations and pregnancies. In 1961, Greenblatt and associates reported successful induction of ovulation using the compound clomiphene citrate (Greenblatt, 1961). Clomiphene citrate is chemically related to the non-steroidal oestrogen chlorotrianisence. The advantages of clomiphene citrate were obvious: it is inexpensive, has low toxicity and few side-effects. Ovulation occurred in 70–80% of cases and pregnancy resulted in 30–40% (Kistner, 1966; Cudmore and Tupper, 1966; MacLeod et al., 1970). Clomiphene is thought to act essentially through competition with oestrogen at hypothalamic receptor sites, stimulating the release of GnRH and thus gonadotrophins by negative feedback (Ginsburg et al., 1975). Following the favourable outcomes with clomiphene, the indications for gonadotrophins (with the exception of assisted reproductive technology) in anovulatory woman with PCOS became limited to those who did not respond to clomiphene citrate (usually at 150 mg/day).

Pituitary gonadotrophins were replaced with urinary derived human menopausal gonadotrophins in the early 1960s (Thompson and Hansen, 1970). The initial regimens resulted in pregnancy and miscarriage rates of less than 30%, high multiple pregnancy rates (30%) and ovarian hyperstimulation syndrome rates <5% (Wang and Gemzell, 1980). The development of a low-dose schedule of gonadotrophins has now reduced the sequelae of multiple follicles (Polson et al., 1987; Sagle et al., 1991; Hamilton-Fairley et al., 1991, 1992; Shoham, Patel and Jacobs, 1991). By aiming for a single preovulatory follicle, multiple pregnancy rates of 5–7% with few multiples greater than two have resulted. In the 1980s, the urinary product was purified successfully to produce a 'pure' FSH (Seibel et al., 1984). As there was concern that LH was detrimental to a successful outcome, there were high hopes for better ovulation and pregnancy rates with a pure FSH product. However, this hope of improved pregnancy outcomes was not borne out by the clinical trials although the incidence of ovarian hyperstimulation syndrome was reduced (Hughes, Collins and Vandekerckhove, 1999a). Further developments in the 1990s include the production of a recombinantly derived FSH (Recombinant Human FSH Study Group, 1995; Shoham and Insler, 1996) which in the future may eliminate the need for urinary products which are time consuming and inconvenient to collect and prepare.

The introduction of GnRH analogues also seemed to offer hope for better treatment regimens and outcomes when used in combination with gonadotrophins (Yen, 1983; Insler et al., 1988). Once again, this initial enthusiasm has not been borne out by evidence from clinical trials as neither the pregnancy rates nor the ovarian hyperstimulation syndrome rates are improved (Hughes, Collins and Vandekerckhove, 1999b).

With the advent of laparoscopic surgery in the 1980s, surgical management of PCOS once again regained some favour (Gjonnaess, 1984). Diathermy or 'drilling' of the ovarian stroma at laparoscopy has been shown to restore ovulatory cycles in women with clomiphene-resistant PCOS. Cohort studies report ovulatory rates of 70–90% and pregnancy rates of 40–70% (Li et al., 1989; Donesky and Adashi, 1995). Only one randomized controlled trial comparing ovarian diathermy with gonadotrophins has been published (Gadir et al., 1990) and further studies are underway (Vegetti et al., 1998). No large, long-term studies have been reported, but the incidence of adhesions is of concern. However, as the pregnancy rates are reported to be >40%, the impact of adhesions is not likely to be great. Furthermore, Greenblatt and Casper (1993) conducted repeat laparoscopy six months after ovarian diathermy and showed that the adhesions were often minimal. The duration of effect is also poorly studied, but appears to be 12–18 months. There is also some evidence that ovulation induction with gonadotrophins following laparoscopic ovarian drilling may be improved (Fahri, Soule and Jacobs, 1995). However, the long-term consequences of ovarian drilling are as yet unclear and there is concern about the future occurrence of premature menopause.

Summary

Polycystic ovary syndrome is a subject that continues to lead to an enormous amount of debate amongst the medical and scientific communities. Over the past 60 years, tremendous advances have been made in diagnosis and management. It is one of the most common endocrine disorders and in the future the focus of management is likely to be the prevention of the long-term sequelae associated with insulin resistance.

REFERENCES

Adams, J., Franks, S., Polson, D.W. et al. (1985). Multifollicular ovaries: clinical and endocrine features and response to pulsatile gonadotropin releasing hormone. *Lancet* **2**, 1375–9.

Adams, J., Polson, D.W. and Franks, S. (1986). Prevalence of polycystic ovaries in women with anovulation and idiopathic hirsutism. *British Medical Journal* **293**, 355–9.

Adashi, E.Y., Resnick, C.E., D'Ercole, J., Svoboda, M.E. and Van Wyk, J.J. (1985). Insulin-like growth factors as intraovarian regulators of granulosa cell growth and function. *Endocrinology Review* **6**, 400–20.

Adashi, E.Y., Resnick, C.E. and Hernandez, E.R. (1988). Insulin-like growth factor 1 as an amplifier of FSH: studies on mechanism(s) and site(s) of action in cultured rat granulosa cells. *Endocrinology* **122**, 1583–91.

Ardaens, Y., Robert, Y., Lemaitre, L. et al. (1991). Polycystic ovarian disease: contribution of vaginal endosonography and reassessment of ultrasonic diagnosis. *Fertility and Sterility* **55**, 1062–8.

Balen, A.H., Conway, G.S., Kaltsas, G. et al. (1995). Polycystic ovary syndrome: the spectrum of the disorder in 1741 patients. *Human Reproduction* **10**, 2107–11.

Barbieri, R.L., Makris, A., Randall, R.W. et al. (1986). Insulin stimulates androgen accumulation in incubations of ovarian stroma obtained from women with hyperandrogenism. *Journal of Clinical Endocrinology and Metabolism* **62**, 904–10.

Barnes, R.B., Rosenfield, R.L., Burstein, S. and Ehrmann, D.A. (1989). Pituitary–ovarian responses to nafarelin testing in the polycystic ovary syndrome. *New England Journal of Medicine* **320**, 559–65.

Bergh, C., Carlsson, B., Olsson, J.H., Selleskog, U. and Hiullensjo, T. (1993). Regulation of androgen production in activated human thecal cells by IGF-1 + insulin. *Fertility and Sterility* **59**, 323–31.

Birdsall, M., Farquhar, C.M. and White, H. (1997). Association between polycystic ovaries and extent of coronary artery disease in women having cardiac catheterization. *Annals of International Medicine* **126**, 32–5.

Bringer, J., Lefebvre, P., Boulet, F. et al. (1993). Body composition and regional fat distribution in polycystic ovarian syndrome. Relationship to hormonal and metabolic profiles. *Annals of the New York Academy of Sciences* **687**, 115–23.

Bunker, C.B., Newton, J.A., Conway, G.S. et al. (1991). The hormonal profile of women with acne and polycystic ovaries. *Clinical and Experimental Dermatology* **16**, 420–3.

Burghen, G.A., Givens, J.R. and Kitabehi, A.E. (1980). Correlation of hyperandrogenism with hyperinsulinism in polycystic ovarian disease. *Journal of Clinical Endocrinology and Metabolism* **50**, 113–16.

Cara, J.F. and Rosenfield, R. (1988). Insulin-like growth factor-1 and insulin potentiate luteinizing hormone-induced androgen synthesis by rat ovarian thecal-interstitial cells. *Endocrinology* **123**, 733–9.

Carey, A.H., Chank, L., Short, F. et al. (1993). Evidence for a single gene effect causing polycystic ovaries and male pattern baldness. *Clinical Endocrinology* **38**, 653–8.

Chang, R.J., Nakamura, R.M., Judd, H.L. and Kaplan, S.A. (1983). Insulin resistance in non-obese patients with polycystic ovarian disease. *Journal of Clinical Endocrinology and Metabolism* **57**, 356–9.

Chereau, A. (1844) *Memoire pour Servir a l'Etude des Maladies des Ovaries.* Paris: Fortin, Masson and Cie.

Clark, A.M., Ledger, W., Galletly, C. et al. (1995). Weight loss results in significant improvement in pregnancy and ovulation rates in anovulatory obese women. *Human Reproduction* **10**, 2705–12.

Clayton, R.N., Ogden, V., Hodgkinson, J. et al. (1992). How common are polycystic ovaries in normal women and what is their significance for the fertility of the population. *Clinical Endocrinology* **37**, 127–34.

Clifford, K., Rai, R., Watson, H., Franks, S. and Regan, L. (1996). Randomized controlled trial of pituitary suppression of high LH concentrations in women with recurrent miscarriage. Abstracts of the 12th Annual Meeting ESHRE, Maastricht, 25–6 (A054).

Conway, G.S., Clark, P.M. and Wong, D. (1993). Hyperinsulinaemia in the polycystic ovary syndrome confirmed with a specific immunoradiometric assay for insulin. *Clinical Endocrinology (Oxford)* **38**, 219–22.

Conway, G.S., Honour, J.W. and Jacobs, H.S. (1989). Heterogeneity of the polycystic ovary syndrome: clinical, endocrine and ultrasound features in 556 patients. *Clinical Endocrinology* **30**, 459–70.

Cudmore, D.W. and Tupper, W.R.C. (1966). Induction of ovulation with clomiphene citrate. A double-blind study. *Fertility and Sterility* **17**, 363–73.

Dewailly, D. (1997). Definition and significance of polycystic ovaries. *Baillière's Clinical Obstetrics and Gynaecology* **11**, 349–68.

Dewailly, D., Robert, Y., Helin, I. et al. (1994). Ovarian stromal hypertrophy in hyperandrogenic women. *Clinical Endocrinology* **41**, 557–62.

Donesky, B.W. and Adashi, E.Y. (1995). Surgically induced ovulation in the polycystic ovary syndrome: wedge resection revisited in the age of laparoscopy. *Fertility and Sterility* **63**, 439–63.

Dunaif, A. (1992a). Insulin resistance and ovarian hyperandrogenism. *Endocrinologist* **2**, 248–60.

Dunaif, A. (1992b). *The Polycystic Ovary Syndrome.* Cambridge, MA: Blackwell Scientific.

Dunaif, A. (1997). Insulin resistance and the polycystic ovarian syndrome: mechanisms and implications for pathogenesis. *Endocrine Review* **18**, 774–800.

Eden, J.A. (1991). The polycystic ovary syndrome presenting as resistant acne successfully treated with cyproterone acetate. *Medical Journal of Australia* **155**, 677–80.

Eden, J.A., Place, J., Carter, G.D. et al. (1989). The diagnosis of polycystic ovaries in subfertile women. *British Journal of Obstetrics and Gynaecology* **96**, 809–15.

Ehrmann, D.A., Barnes, R.B. and Rosenfield, R.L. (1994). Hyperandrogenism, hirsutism and the polycystic ovary syndrome. In *Endocrinology*, 3rd edn, Vol. 3, ed. L.J. De Groot, M. Berse, H.G. Burger et al. pp. 2093–112. Philadelphia: W.B. Saunders.

El Tabbakh, G.H., Lotfy, I., Azab, I. et al. (1986). Correlation of the ultrasonic appearance of the ovaries in polycystic ovarian disease and the clinical, hormonal, and laparoscopic findings. *American Journal of Obstetrics and Gynecology* **154**, 892–5.

Fahri, J., Soule, S. and Jacobs, H.S. (1995). Effect of laparoscopic ovarian electrocautery on ovarian response and outcome of treatment with gonadotropins in clomiphene citrate-resistant patients with polycystic ovary syndrome. *Fertility and Sterility* **64**, 930–5.

Farquhar, C.M., Birdsall, M., Manning, P. and Mitchell, J.M. (1994a). Transabdominal versus transvaginal ultrasound in the diagnosis of polycystic ovaries on ultrasound scanning in a population of randomly selected women. *Ultrasound Obstetrics and Gynecology* **4**, 54–9.

Farquhar, C.M., Birdsall, M., Manning, P., Mitchell, J.M. and France, J.T. (1994b). The prevalence of polycystic ovaries on ultrasound scanning in a population of randomly selected women. *Australian and New Zealand Journal of Obstetrics and Gynaecology* **34**, 67–72.

Fauser, B.C., Pache, T.D., Hop, W.C., de Jong, F.H. and Dahl, K.D. (1992). The significance of a single serum LH measurement in women with cycle disturbance: discrepancies between immunoreactive and bioactive hormone estimates. *Clinical Endocrinology (Oxford)* **37**, 445–52.

Fauser, B.C., Pache, T.D., Lamberts, S.W. et al. (1991). Serum bioactive and immunoreactive luteinizing hormone and follicle-stimulating hormone levels in women with cycle abnormalities, with or without polycystic ovarian disease. *Journal of Clinical Endocrinology and Metabolism* **73**, 811–17.

Fox, R., Corrigan, E., Thomas, P.A. and Hull, M.G. (1991). The diagnosis of polycystic ovaries in women with oligo-amenorrhoea: predictive power of endocrine tests. *Clinical Endocrinology* **34**, 127–31.

Franks, S. (1989). Polycystic ovary syndrome: a changing perspective. *Clinical Endocrinology* **31**, 87–120.

Franks, S. (1995). Polycystic ovary syndrome. *New England Journal of Medicine* **333**, 853–61.

Franks, S. and White, D.M. (1993). Prevalence of and aetiological factors in polycystic ovary syndrome. In *Polycystic Ovary Syndrome. A New Approach to Treatment*, ed. S. Franks and F. Neuman, pp. 19–21. Chester, UK.

Gadir, A.A., Mowafi, R.S., Alnaser, H.M. et al. (1990). Ovarian electrocautery versus human menopausal gonadotrophins and pure follicle stimulating hormone therapy in the treatment of patients with polycystic ovarian disease. *Clinical Endocrinology (Oxford)* **33**, 585–92.

Gemzell, C.A., Diczfalusy, E. and Tillinger, K.G. (1958). Clinical effect of human pituitary follicle-stimulating hormone (FSH). *Journal of Clinical Endocrinology and Metabolism* **18,** 1333.

Ginsburg, J., Isaacs, A.J., Gore, M.B.R. and Havard, C.W.H. (1975). Use of clomiphene and luteinizing hormone/follicle stimulating hormone-releasing hormone in investigation of ovulatory failure. *British Medical Journal* 3,130–3.

Gjonnaess, H. (1984). Polycystic ovarian syndrome treated by ovarian electrocautery through the laparoscope. *Fertility and Sterility* **41,** 20–5.

Goldzieher, J.W. and Green, J.A. (1962). The polycystic ovary I. Clinical and histological features. *Journal of Clinical Endocrinology and Metabolism* **22,** 325–8.

Greenblatt, E. and Casper, R. (1993). Adhesion formation after laparoscopic ovarian cautery for polycystic ovarian syndrome: lack of correlation with pregnancy rate. *Fertility and Sterility* **60,** 766–70.

Greenblatt, R.B. (1961). Chemical induction of ovulation. *Fertility and Sterility* **12,** 402.

Hague, W.M., Adams, J., Reeders, S.T., Peto, T.E. and Jacobs, H.S. (1988). Familial polycystic ovaries: a genetic disease: *Clinical Endocrinology (Oxford)* **29,** 593–605.

Hamilton-Fairley, D., Kiddy, D., Watson, H., Paterson, C. and Franks, S. (1992). Association of moderate obesity with a poor pregnancy outcome in women with polycystic ovary syndrome treated with low dose gonadotrophin. *British Journal of Obstetrics and Gynaecology* **99,** 128–31.

Hamilton-Fairley, D., Kiddy, D., Watson, H., Sagle, M. and Franks, S. (1991). Low dose gonadotrophin therapy for induction of ovulation in 100 women with polycystic ovary syndrome. *Human Reproduction* **6,** 1095–9.

Homburg, R. (1996). Polycystic ovary syndrome – from gynaecological curiosity to multisystem endocrinopathy. *Human Reproduction* **11,** 29–39.

Homburg, R., Armar, N.A., Eshel, A., Adams, J. and Jacobs, H.S. (1988). Influence of serum luteinizing hormone concentrations on ovulation, conception and early pregnancy loss in polycystic ovary syndrome. *British Medical Journal* **297,** 1024–6.

Homburg, R., Pariente, C., Lunenfeld, B. and Jacobs, H.S. (1992). The role of insulin-like growth factor-1 (IGF-1) and IGF binding protein-1 (IGF-BP-1) in the pathogenesis of polycystic ovary syndrome. *Human Reproduction* **7,** 1379–83.

Hughes, E., Collins, J. and Vandekerckhove, P. (1999a). Ovulation induction with urinary follicle stimulating hormone versus human menopausal gonadotrophin for clomiphene-resistant polycystic ovary syndrome (Cochrane Review). In The Cochrane Library, Issue 1. Oxford: Update Software.

Hughes, E., Collins, J. and Vandekerckhove, P. (1999b). Gonadotrophin-releasing hormone analogue as an adjunct to gonadotropin therapy for clomiphene resistant polycystic ovarian syndrome (Cochrane Review). In The Cochrane Library, Issue 1. Oxford: Update Software.

Insler,V., Potashnik, G., Lunenfeld, E., Meizner, I. and Levy, J. (1988). Ovulation induction with hMG following down regulation of the pituitary–ovarian axis by LH–RH analogues. *Gynecological Endocrinology* **2,** 67.

Jacobs, H.S. (1996). Polycystic ovary syndrome: the present position. *Gynecological Endocrinology* **10,** 427–33.

Khan, C.R., Flier, J.S., Bar, R.S., Archal, J.A. and Gorden, P. (1976). The syndromes of insulin resistance and acanthosis nigricans: insulin receptor disorders in man. *New England Journal of Medicine* **294**, 739–45.

Kiddy, D.S., Hamilton-Fairley, D., Bush, A. et al. (1992). Improvement in endocrine and ovarian function during dietary treatment of obese women with polycystic ovary syndrome. *Clinical Endocrinology (Oxford)* **36**, 105–11.

Kistner, R.W. (1966). Use of clomiphene citrate, human chorionic gonadotrophin, and human menopausal gonadotrophin for induction of ovulation in the human female. *Fertility & Sterility* **17**, 569.

Li, T.C., Saravelos, H., Chow, M.S., Chisabingo, R. and Cooke, I.D. (1989). Factors affecting the outcome of laparoscopic ovarian drilling for polycystic ovarian syndrome in women with anovulatory infertility. *British Journal of Obstetrics and Gynaecology* **105**, 338–44.

Liddell, H., Farquhar, C.M. and Sowden, C. (1997). The association of polycystic ovaries and recurrent miscarriage. *New Zealand Medical Journal* **37**, 402–6.

Lobo, R.A., Granger, L., Goebelsmann, U. and Mishell, J.R. (1981). Elevations in unbound serum estradiol as a possible mechanism for inappropriate gonadotrophin secretion in women with PCO. *Journal of Clinical Endocrinology and Metabolism* **52**, 156–8.

Lunde, O., Magnus, P., Sandvik, L. and Hoglo, S. (1989). Familial clustering in the polycystic ovarian syndrome. *Gynecologic and Obstetric Investigation* **28**, 23–30.

MacLeod, S.C., Mitton, D.M., Parker, A.S. and Tupper, W.R.C. (1970). Experience with induction of ovulation. *American Journal of Obstetrics and Gynecology* **1**, 814–24.

McArthur, J.W., Ingersoll, F.W. and Worcester, J. (1958). The urinary excretion of interstitial-cell and follicle-stimulating hormone activity by women with diseases of the reproductive system. *Journal of Clinical Endocrinology and Metabolism* **18**, 1202–15.

Michelmore, K., Balen, A., Dunger, D. et al. (1998). Prevalence and clinical features of polycystic ovary syndrome in 224 young female volunteers. *Human Reproduction* Abstract 0024, **13**.

Nestler, J.E. (1997). Insulin regulation of human ovarian androgens. *Human Reproduction* **12** (Suppl.), 52–62.

Nestler, J.E. (1998). Polycystic ovary syndrome: a disorder for the generalist. *Fertility and Sterility* **70**, 811–12.

Orsini, L.F., Venturoli, S. and Lorusso, R. (1985). Ultrasonic findings in polycystic ovarian disease. *Fertility and Sterility* **43**, 709–14.

Pasquali, R., Casimirri, F. and Venturoli, D. (1994). Body fat distribution has weight-independent effects on clinical, hormonal and metabolic features of women with polycystic ovary syndrome. *Metabolism* **6**, 706–13.

Plymate, S.R., Fariss, B.L., Basset, M.L. and Matej, L. (1981). Obesity and its role in polycystic ovary syndrome. *Journal of Clinical Endocrinology and Metabolism* **66**, 1246–8.

Polson, D.W., Adams, J., Wadsworth, J. and Franks, S. (1988). Polycystic ovaries – a common finding in normal women. *Lancet* **1**, 870–2.

Polson, D.W., Mason, H.D., Saldanha, M.B. and Franks, S. (1987). Ovulation of a single dominant follicle during treatment with low dose pulsatile follicle stimulating hormone in women with polycystic ovary syndrome. *Clinical Endocrinology* **26**, 205–12.

Rai, R., Clifford, K. and Regan, L. (1996). The modern preventative treatment of recurrent miscarriage. *British Journal of Obstetrics and Gynaecology* **103**, 106–10.

Rebar, R., Judd, H.L., Yen, S.C.C. et al. (1976). Characterization of the inappropriate gonado-tropin secretion in polycystic ovary syndrome. *Journal of Clinical Investigation* 57, 1320–9.

Recombinant Human FSH Study Group (1995). Clinical assessment of recombinant human fol-licle-stimulating ovarian follicle development before in vitro fertilization. *Fertility and Sterility* 63, 77–86.

Regan, L., Owen, E.J. and Jacobs, H.S. (1990). Hypersecretion of luteinising hormone, infertility and miscarriage. *Lancet* 336, 1141–4.

Robinson, S., Rodin, D.A., Deacon, A., Wheeler, M.J. and Clayton, R.N. (1992). Which hormone tests for the diagnosis of polycystic ovary syndrome? *British Journal of Obstetrics and Gynaecology* 99, 232–8.

Rosenfield, R.L., Barnes, R.B., Cara, J.F. and Lucky, A.W. (1990). Dysregulation of cytochrome P450c 17 alpha as the cause of polycystic ovarian syndrome. *Fertility and Sterility* 53, 785–91.

Sagle, M., Bishop, K., Ridley, N. et al. (1988). Recurrent early miscarriage and polycystic ovaries. *British Medical Journal* 297, 1027–8.

Sagle, M.A., Hamilton-Fairley, D., Kiddy, D.S. and Franks, S. (1991). A comparative randomized study of low dose human menopausal gonadotropin and follicle stimulating hormone in women with polycystic ovarian syndrome. *Fertility and Sterility* 55, 56–60.

Santon, R.J. and Bardin, C.W. (1973). Episodic LH secretion in man. Pulse analysis, clinical inter-pretation, physiologic mechanisms. *Journal of Clinical Investigation* 52, 2617–28.

Saxton, D.W., Farquhar, C.M., Rae, T. et al. (1990). Accuracy of ultrasound measurements of female pelvic organs. *British Journal of Obstetrics and Gynaecology* 97, 695–9.

Seibel, M.M., Kamrava, M.M., McArdle, C. and Taymor, M.L. (1984). Treatment of polycystic ovarian disease with chronic low dose follicle stimulating hormone: biochemical changes and ultrasound correlation. *International Journal of Fertility* 29, 39–43.

Shoham, Z. and Insler, V. (1996). Recombinant technique and gonadotropins production: new era in reproductive medicine. *Fertility and Sterility* 66, 187–201.

Shoham, Z., Patel, A. and Jacobs, H.S. (1991). Polycystic ovary syndrome: safety and effective-ness of stepwise and low dose administration of purified follicle stimulating hormone. *Fertility and Sterility* 55, 1051–6.

Shoupe, D., Kumar, D.D. and Lobo, R.A. (1983). Insulin resistance in polycystic ovary syndrome. *American Journal of Obstetrics and Gynecology* 147, 588–92.

Stein, I.F., Cohen, M.R. and Elson, R.E. (1948). Results of bilateral ovarian wedge resection in 47 cases of sterility. *American Journal of Obstetrics and Gynecology* 58, 267–73.

Stein, I.F. and Leventhal, M.L. (1935). Amenorrhoea associated with bilateral polycystic ovaries. *American Journal of Obstetrics and Gynecology* 29, 181–91.

Swanson, M., Sauerbrei, E.E. and Cooperberg, P.L. (1981). Medical implications of ultrasonically detected polycystic ovaries. *Journal of Clinical Ultrasound* 9, 219–22.

Thomas, A., Okamoto, S., O'Shea, F. et al. (1989). Do raised serum luteinizing hormone levels during stimulation for in-vitro fertilization predict outcome? *British Journal of Obstetrics and Gynaecology* 96, 1328–32.

Thompson, C.R. and Hansen, L.M. (1970). Pergonal (menotropins): a summary of clinical expe-rience in the induction of ovulation and pregnancy. *Fertility and Sterility* 21, 844–53.

Tulppala, M., Stenman, U-H., Cacciatore, B. and Ylikorkala, O. (1993). Polycystic ovaries and levels of gonadotrophins and androgens in recurrent miscarriage: prospective study in 50 women. *British Journal of Obstetrics and Gynaecology* **100**, 348–52.

Vallisneri, A. (1721). Cited in Insler, V. and Lunenfeld, B. (1990). Polycystic ovarian disease: a challenge and controversy. *Gynecological Endocrinology* **4**, 51–70.

Vegetti, W., Ragni, G., Baroni, E. et al. (1998). Laparoscopic ovarian drilling versus low-dose pure FSH in anovulatory clomiphene-resistant patients with polycystic ovarian syndrome: randomized prospective study. Human Reproduction Abstracts of the 14th Annual Meeting of ESHRE, Goteborg, p. 120.

Waldstreicher, J., Santoro, N.F., Hall, J.E., Filicori, M. and Crowley Jr, W.F. (1988). Hyperfunction of the hypothalamic–pituitary axis in women with polycystic ovarian disease: indirect evidence for partial gonadotroph desensitization. *Journal of Clinical Endocrinology and Metabolism* **66**, 165–72.

Wang, C.F. and Gemzell, C. (1980). The use of human gonadotropins for induction of ovulation in women with polycystic ovarian disease. *Fertility and Sterility* **33**, 479–86.

Wild, R.A. (1997). Cardiovascular and lipoprotein abnormalities in androgen excess. In *Androgen Excess Disorders in Women*, ed. R. Azziz, J.E. Nestler, D. Dewailly, pp. 681–8. Philadelphia: Lippincott-Raven.

Willis, D. and Franks, S. (1995). Insulin action in human granulosa cells from normal and polycystic ovaries is mediated by the insulin receptor and not the type-I insulin-like growth factor receptor. *Journal of Clinical Endocrinology and Metabolism* **80**, 3788–90.

Yen, S.S.C. (1980). The polycystic ovary syndrome. *Clinical Endocrinology* **12**, 177–207.

Yen, S.S.C. (1983). Clinical application of gonadotropin releasing hormone analogues. *Fertility and Sterility* **39**, 257.

Yen, S.S.C., Vela, P. and Rankin, J. (1970). Inappropriate secretion of follicle-stimulating hormone and luteinizing hormone in polycystic ovarian disease. *Journal of Clinical Endocrinology and Metabolism* **30**, 435–42.

3

The inheritance of polycystic ovary syndrome

Stephen Franks, Ester Cela, Neda Gharani, Dawn Waterworth and Mark McCarthy

Introduction

Polycystic ovary syndrome (PCOS) shows a strong familial aggregation, suggesting a major genetic component to its aetiology. It is unlikely that there is a single cause for the syndrome, but it is likely that much of the clinical and biochemical variability of PCOS can be explained by an oligogenic pattern of inheritance, with the interaction of environmental factors (notably weight) with a small number of major causative genes.

There are several problems faced by those who wish to study the genetics of PCOS (Franks et al., 1997). Firstly, this is a disorder that affects women of reproductive age, and it is therefore very difficult for segregation studies to span more than one generation. In addition, there is no commonly accepted male phenotype. Lastly, the high prevalence of PCOS in the population means that large pedigrees may include subjects with PCOS arising from different genotypes. All this is compounded by the lack of universally acceptable clinical or biochemical diagnostic criteria, which make comparisons of studies from different groups difficult.

Our studies have taken a candidate gene approach, focusing primarily on genes involved in androgen production and in insulin secretion or action. The evidence for a genetic basis for PCOS and the work done on several candidate genes are reviewed here.

Familial studies in polycystic ovary syndrome

Studies of familial clustering

Over the last 30 years, several small clinical studies and some very good reviews have been published which draw attention to the phenomenon of familial clustering in PCOS. The criteria used to identify probands and affected family members have varied considerably between studies, and it is therefore not surprising that there has been no general agreement about the mode of inheritance of PCOS. This

Table 3.1. Summary of family studies in polycystic ovary syndrome

Reference	Number of women/families	Proposed mode of inheritance
Cooper et al. (1968)	18 women	Autosomal dominant
Givens (1988)	3 multiply affected families	? X-linked dominant
Ferriman and Purdie (1979)	381 women	Autosomal dominant
Hague et al. (1988)	132 women	Unclear
Lunde et al. (1989)	50 women	Exceeded autosomal dominant
Norman et al. (1996)	5 multiply affected families	Not stated
Legro et al. (1998a)	80 sib-pairs	Autosomal dominant
Govind et al. (1999)	29 multiply affected families	Autosomal dominant
St Mary's family database	17 multiply affected families	Oligogeic

problem was further complicated by the fact that most of the studies suffered from ascertainment bias, in that families with multiple affected females were preferentially studied (see Table 3.1).

The first large study of familial PCOS was carried out in 1968 by Cooper and colleagues in which first-degree female relatives of women with PCOS (diagnosed on wedge resection or culdoscopy) were found to have a higher prevalence of oligomenorrhoea than a control population. This study suggested an autosomal dominant mode of inheritance with reduced penetrance. Givens (1988) conducted several family-based studies between 1971 and 1988, and was the first to identify some of the metabolic abnormalities that may accompany the syndrome. They initially suggested an X-linked mode of inheritance, but subsequently a probable dominant mode of inheritance was emphasized. They also reported that males from some families were found to have elevated luteinizing hormone (LH) levels and oligospermia.

Ferriman and Purdie in 1979 studied 700 women (selected on the basis of hirsutism with or without enlarged ovaries on gynaecography) and their relatives by postal questionnaire. They found a high prevalence of symptoms amongst first-degree female relatives (hirsutism, oligomenorrhoea), and amongst first-degree male relatives (premature balding). They concluded that the mode of inheritance was 'modified dominant'.

Hague et al. in 1988 studied women ascertained on the basis of polycystic ovarian morphology on ultrasound scan with associated symptoms. Affected status was assigned to first-degree female relatives on the basis of ovarian morphology on ultrasound scan. The segregation ratios for the inheritance of PCOS were in excess of those expected in an autosomal dominant pattern of inheritance. Lunde et al. in 1989 studied women identified as having 'multicystic ovaries' on wedge resection, plus a symptom of PCOS. Relatives were studied in part by direct contact and in part by postal questionnaire. Their results were similar to those described by Ferriman and Purdie, in that they found a higher prevalence of hirsutism and oligomenorrhoea amongst first-degree female relatives and of premature balding in first-degree male relatives. No clear mode of inheritance was determined.

Norman, Masters and Hague in 1996 studied five families of women selected on the basis of polycystic ovarian morphology on ultrasound, plus hyperandrogenaemia. They again found higher rates of symptoms in both female and male relatives, and were the first to describe biochemical abnormalities (hyperinsulinaemia and hypertriglyceridaemia) in relatives of women with PCOS.

Legro et al. (1998a, 1998b)in 1998 examined 155 sisters of 80 women with PCOS. As their hypothesis was that hyperandrogenaemia may be a genetic trait per se, they assigned affected status to probands on the basis of oligomenorrhoea and a raised serum androgen concentration, with no mention of ovarian morphology on ultrasound scan. They found that 22% of sisters had oligomenorrhoea and hyperandrogenaemia, and that 24% of sisters had hyperandrogenaemia and regular menses. They concluded that there is familial aggregation of hyperandrogenaemia in PCOS kindred, and they suggest an autosomal dominant mode of inheritance.

Govind, Obhrai and Clayton in 1999 studied 29 families in which the probands had polycystic ovarian morphology and symptoms of PCOS. They found that 66% of first-degree female relatives were affected (polycystic ovarian morphology), as were 22% of first-degree male relatives (premature balding). Of a total of 71 siblings of PCOS probands, 39 were affected, giving a segregation ratio of 55%, which is consistent with an autosomal dominant mode of inheritance.

Our own group (Carey et al. 1993) has studied 23 multiply affected families of women with polycystic ovarian morphology on ultrasound, who presented with at least one symptom of PCOS (see Fig. 3.1). Assignment of affected status was made on the basis of ultrasound evidence of polycystic ovaries in the female relatives and premature onset of balding in the male relatives. The segregation analysis of the first ten families pointed to an autosomal dominant mode of inheritance, but as existing pedigrees were expanded and new ones added, it became obvious that the picture is somewhat more complex than it appeared initially. Although the final results are not incompatible with an autosomal dominant model, it would appear more likely that PCOS can be best explained by the interaction of a small number of causative genes, the so-called oligogenic mode of inheritance.

Twin studies

There have been a few case reports of twins with PCOS (Hutton and Clark, 1984); however, there has only been one substantial study involving twins. Jahanfar in 1995 studied 34 (19 monozygotic and 15 dizygotic) pairs of twins (Jahanfar et al.,

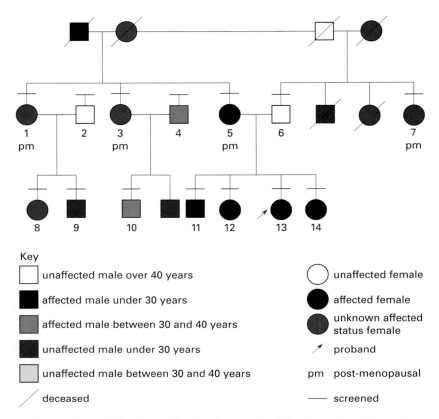

Fig. 3.1   Pedigree of a multiply affected family, showing the following points: (a) problems associated with assigning definite affected status to post-menopausal women; (b) difficulty in assigning definite affected status to men; (c) multiply affected siblings.

1995). Of these, five monozygotic and six dizygotic pairs were scan discordant. This study suggested that PCOS is not the result of a single autosomal dominant genetic defect, but rather that it may be X-linked or autosomal recessive, with the influence of environmental factors. However, this analysis highlighted the importance of genetic factors in determining insulin levels and body mass index.

Pathophysiological basis for candidate gene approach

Ovarian hyperandrogenism

Hyperandrogenism (together with raised serum LH concentrations) is the most frequent finding in women with PCOS, but its prevalence in various studies obviously depends on the criteria used to define PCOS and hence to recruit patients.

In women, the predominant androgens are androstenedione and dihydroepiandrosterone, and both can be metabolized to testosterone. Testosterone and di-hydrotesosterone are the most biologically active androgens, with 50% of testosterone being secreted from the ovary and adrenals, and 50% deriving from peripheral conversion of androstenedione. Serum testosterone and androstenedione are elevated in women with PCOS (50–100% higher than in controls), and there is a huge variation between patients. Women with anovulation but no symptoms of hyperandrogenaemia may have elevated serum androgen levels, and women with hirsutism may have normal serum androgen levels. This probably reflects variable sensitivities of the hair follicle to androgens, and variable rates of clearance of androgens by peripheral tissues. The clearance and bioavailability of testosterone are affected by the serum concentration of sex-hormone-binding globulin, which in turn is mediated by nutritional factors.

The main source of excess androgens in women with PCOS appears to be the ovary (Franks, 1995), and if the pituitary–ovarian axis is suppressed in these patients, circulating levels of androstenedione and testosterone fall to within the normal range (Steingold, De Ziegler and Cedars, 1987).

A few studies have looked at the role of 17α-hydroxylase/17,20 lyase (P450c17α) in the genesis of ovarian androgen production. Rosenfield and colleagues (Rosenfield et al., 1989; Barnes et al., 1989) have assessed the response of the pituitary and ovary to gonadotrophin releasing hormone (GnRH) in women with hyperandrogenaemic PCOS whose adrenal androgen production had been suppressed. They found that serum concentrations of both androstenedione and 17-hydroxyprogesterone were significantly higher both before and after administration of GnRH agonist. These findings were later confirmed in other studies (White et al., 1995). These data support the hypothesis that in PCOS there may be an abnormal regulation of 17α-hydroxylase/17,20 lyase activity in the ovary. This fact, taken together with the finding that hyperandrogenaemia in ovulatory and anovulatory women with polycystic ovaries is similar, even though LH levels are much higher in the latter (White et al., 1995), gives some evidence that hyperandrogenism in PCOS may therefore represent an intrinsic abnormality of ovarian theca–interstitial cell function.

Our group therefore studied androgen production by human ovarian theca cells *in vitro* (Gilling-Smith et al., 1994), both in women with polycystic ovaries (PCO) and in normal controls. Production of androstenedione, 17-hydroxyprogesterone and progesterone was significantly higher in PCO theca cells than in normal theca cells. This suggests increased activity of 17-hydroxylase/17,20 lyase as an intrinsic property of PCO theca cells. However, the raised concentration of progesterone as well as 17-hydroxyprogesterone raises the possibility that abnormal steroidogenesis by PCO theca cells includes upregulation of the activity of P450 cholesterol side-chain cleavage.

Abnormalities of insulin secretion and action

Since an initial report in 1980 of the association between PCOS and hyperinsulinaemia (Burghen, Givens and Kitabchi, 1980), it has become apparent that women with PCOS are both hyperinsulinaemic and insulin resistant in relation to weight-matched controls (Dunaif, 1995; Holte, 1996). The insulin resistance of women with PCOS must be regarded as a distinct clinical entity (Dunaif et al., 1989) and can be distinguished from the rare genetic syndromes of severe insulin resistance.

Insulin resistance is defined as 'a state in which greater than normal amounts of insulin are required to elicit a quantitatively normal response'. Euglycaemic glucose clamp studies have demonstrated a significant and substantial decrease in insulin-mediated glucose disposal in women with PCOS, a measure of peripheral sensitivity to insulin. In the presence of this peripheral insulin resistance, pancreatic insulin secretion increases in a compensatory fashion. Hyperinsulinaemia may be further compounded by decreased hepatic insulin clearance of insulin, even though the evidence for this is not conclusive. Diabetes develops when the compensatory increase in insulin in response to insulin resistance is no longer sufficient to maintain euglycaemia.

Controversy remains as to the pathogenesis of the insulin resistance. As with all studies of PCOS, conflicting results between different groups can often be explained by differing diagnostic criteria for PCOS. Studies relating insulin dynamics to menstrual history suggest that insulin resistance is present mainly in anovulatory hyperandrogenaemic women, whereas women with regular ovulatory menses and hyperandrogenaemia are not insulin resistant (Dunaif et al., 1987). Insulin resistance is present in both lean and obese women, and has been found in all major ethnic groups. There is a complex relationship between insulin resistance, central adiposity and hyperandrogenaemia.

There is evidence that, in a proportion of women with PCOS, there is a post-receptor defect characterized by an abnormality of serine–threonine phosphorylation of the insulin receptor in response to insulin (Dunaif et al., 1995). There is also evidence that women with PCOS, in addition to insulin resistance, also have a primary pancreatic β-cell dysfunction.

Hyperinsulinaemia and insulin resistance may contribute to anovulation in obese women with PCOS. During calorie-restricted diets, changes in insulin concentrations precede resumption of ovulatory cycles (Kiddy et al., 1992). It seems unlikely, however, that hyperinsulinaemia and insulin resistance play an obligatory role in the development of ovarian hyperandrogenism (Franks, Robinson and Willis, 1996).

The prevalence of impaired glucose tolerance in obese women with PCOS is significantly increased compared to weight-matched controls (30% vs 10%) (Dunaif et al., 1989). This is particularly evident in women in their thirties and forties, but

impaired glucose tolerance can occur in pubescent girls. A study of postmenopausal women with PCOS found a prevalence of type II diabetes mellitus
(NIDDM) of 15% (vs 5% in a control population), suggesting that PCOS is a major
risk factor for the development of type II diabetes mellitus (Dahlgren et al., 1992).

The relationship between insulin resistance and hyperandrogenaemia in women
with PCOS is complicated, and it has proved difficult to establish whether these two
conditions coexist simply because they are two common endocrine abnormalities
in women with PCOS, or because one causes the other.

The earliest reports linking hyperandrogenaemia and insulin resistance were in
women with acanthosis nigricans who also had features of PCOS. In 1980, Burghen
et al. first demonstrated a positive correlation between plasma androgen and
fasting insulin levels in obese women with PCOS, and since then several studies
have confirmed the association in lean women with PCOS.

Studies on women exposed to androgens (women with congenital adrenal
hyperplasia, women on 'androgenic' combined oral contraceptives, female-to-male
transexuals) have given evidence that even the modest hyperandrogenaemia characteristic of PCOS may contribute to insulin resistance. However, suppressing
androgen levels does not restore normal insulin sensitivity (Dunaif et al., 1990),
and androgen administration does not produce insulin resistance, and therefore
additional factors are necessary to explain insulin resistance in PCOS.

Conversely, the syndromes of extreme insulin resistance are often associated with
hyperandrogenaemia, and in women with PCOS, lowering insulin levels ameliorates but does not abolish hyperandrogenaemia (Nestler, Barlascini and Matt,
1990).

Candidate genes for polycystic ovary syndrome

These are discussed in detail in Chapter 4, so only a brief summary is given here.

Genes coding for steroidogenic enzymes

Because of the evidence that an underlying disorder of androgen metabolism is
involved in the aetiology of PCOS, several genes coding for steroidogenic enzymes
have been studied.

CYP11a (cholesterol side-chain cleavage gene)

In steroidogenic tissues, including the ovary, the initial and rate-limiting step in the
pathway leading from cholesterol to steroid hormones is the cleavage of the side-
chain of cholesterol to yield pregnenolone. This reaction is known as cholesterol
side-chain cleavage, and is catalysed by a specific form of cytochrome P450 known
as P450 side-chain cleavage (P 450 scc). CYP11a encodes P450 scc.

Gharani et al. (1997) analysed the segregation of *CYP11a* with PCO phenotype in 20 multiply affected families using a number of polymorphic markers in the region of *CYP11a*. Non-parametric linkage analysis showed evidence of excessive allele sharing (i.e. linkage) at the *CYP11a* locus, giving a maximum non-parametric linkage score of 3.03 ($p = 0.003$), thus suggesting that *CYP11a* is a major genetic susceptibility locus for PCOS. In a case-control study of 148 consecutively recruited women with PCOS and 59 matched normal control women, they also showed an association between the most common polymorphism of *CYP11a* and both PCOS and serum testosterone concentrations. The distribution of genotype was found to vary significantly if subjects were further divided according to the presence of hirsutism/ raised serum androgens.

CYP19 (gene encoding P450 aromatase)

Several studies have been published which point to abnormal regulation of aromatase in women with PCOS. Gharani et al. (1997), however, showed no association of alleles of *CYP19* with PCO, and no evidence for excessive allele sharing.

CYP17 (17-hydroxylase/17,20-lyase gene)

17-hydroxylase/17,20-lyase is a known rate-limiting enzyme in androgen biosynthesis, and clinical studies point to abnormal regulation in women with PCOS. Initial studies on *CYP17* were encouraging (Carey et al., 1994), and suggested an association between a variant allele of *CYP17* and women with PCOS. However, further studies were able to exclude *CYP17* as a major causative gene for PCOS (Gharani et al., 1996; Franks, 1997; Techatraisak, Conway and Rumsby, 1997).

Genes involved in the secretion and action of insulin

Numerous metabolic studies have shown that women with PCOS have abnormalities of both insulin secretion and action, and therefore this raises the possibility that genes coding for insulin may have a role in the aetiology of PCOS.

Insulin gene

Abnormalities of insulin secretion, and in particular in first phase insulin secretion, have been demonstrated in women with PCOS (Holte et al., 1996). This suggests an underlying defect in pancreatic β-cell function, and therefore the role of the insulin gene in the aetiology of PCOS has been studied.

The VNTR (variable number tandem repeats) locus upstream of the insulin gene regulates insulin expression (Bennett, Lucassen and Gough, 1995). Waterworth et al. (1997) examined the VNTR minisatellite 5′ to the insulin gene, a locus that has been implicated in susceptibility to type II diabetes mellitus and to hyperinsulinaemia related to central obesity. They found that class III alleles were associated with PCOS, particularly with anovulatory PCOS. This is in keeping with the observation that hyperinsulinaemia is more prominent in anovulatory women. Non-parametric linkage analysis showed evidence for excessive allele sharing at the insulin VNTR locus. These findings suggest that the VNTR of the insulin gene is a major susceptibility locus for PCOS, particularly in anovulatory women, and may contribute to the mechanism of hyperinsulinaemia.

Insulin receptor gene

The demonstration of impaired sensitivity to insulin action led to the hypothesis that a genetic abnormality of the insulin receptor/post-receptor signalling was involved in the aetiology of PCOS. Talbot et al. (1996) investigated whether mutations in the insulin receptor gene could explain the insulin resistance in women with PCOS, and concluded that mutations in the insulin receptor gene were rare in women with PCOS. Conway, Avey and Rumsby (1996) found no abnormalities in the tyrosine kinase domain of the insulin receptor gene in hyperinsulinaemic women with PCOS.

A genetic basis for the reported abnormality of serine–threonine phosphorylation in insulin signalling is possible. As this has recently been shown to be involved in androgen secretion in steroidogenic tissues, a plausible hypothesis is that there is a common aetiology for both insulin resistance and hyperandrogenism in PCOS (Legro et al., 1998b).

Glycogen synthetase gene

Rajkhowa et al. (1996) concluded that variation in this gene was not a feature of PCOS, and that it did not relate to indices of insulin sensitivity or glucose intolerance.

Future avenues

The strategy of assessing candidate genes remains a reasonable approach in a disorder in which biochemical sub-phenotypes can be characterized. An 'anonymous' genome-wide scan to identify other susceptibility loci is also useful but requires many subjects. The use of affected sibling sister pairs with PCOS bypasses the problems that arise from attempting to characterize a male phenotype, as does the application of the transmission–disequilibrium test to the analysis of DNA from patient–parent 'trios'.

Conclusion

Polycystic ovary syndrome is a disorder of unknown aetiology, but which appears to have a major genetic component. The exact mode of inheritance remains unknown, but clinical genetic studies have pointed to an autosomal dominant mode of inheritance or an oligogenic mode of inheritance. Our group has found evidence for two key genes in the aetiology of PCOS. Differences in *CYP11a* could account for variation in androgen production, and subjects who are homozygous or heterozygous for class III alleles at the insulin gene VNTR locus are more likely to have disturbances of insulin secretion and action. This genotype would predispose to menstrual irregularities and type II diabetes mellitus.

REFERENCES

Barnes, R.B., Rosenfield, R.L., Burstein, S. and Ehrmann, D.A. (1989). Pituitary–ovarian responses to nafarelin testing in the polycystic ovary syndrome. *New England Journal of Medicine* 320, 559–65

Bennett, S.T., Lucassen, A.M. and Gough, S.C.L. et al. (1995). Susceptibility to human type 1 diabetes at *IDDM2* is determined by tandem repeat variation at the insulin gene minisatellite locus. *Nature Genetics* 9, 284–92

Burghen, G.A, Givens, G.R. and Kitabchi, A.E. (1980). Correlation of hyperandrogenism with hyperinsulinism in polycystic ovarian disease. *Journal of Clinical Endocrinology and Metabolism* 50, 113–16.

Carey, A.H., Chan, K.L., Short, F. et al. (1993). Evidence for a single gene effect in polycystic ovaries and male pattern baldness. *Clinical Endocrinology* 38, 653–8

Carey, A.H., Waterworth, D., Patel, K. et al. (1994). Polycystic ovaries and premature male pattern baldness are associated with one allele of the steroid metabolism gene CYP 17. *Human and Molecular Genetic*s 3, 1873–6

Conway, G.S., Avey, C. and Rumsby, G. (1996). The tyrosine kinase domain of the insulin receptor gene in women with polycystic ovary syndrome. *Journal of Clinical Endocrinology and Metabolism* 81, 1979–83.

Cooper, H.E., Spellacy, W.N., Prom, K.A. and Cohon, W.D. (1968). Hereditary factors in the Stein–Leventhal syndrome. *American Journal of Obstetrics and Gynecology* 100, 371–87.

Dahlgren, E., Johansson, S., Lindstedt, G. et al. (1992). Women with polycystic ovary syndrome wedge resected in 1956 to 1965: a long term follow-up focussing on natural history and circulating hormones. *Fertility and Sterility* 57, 505–13

Dunaif, A. (1995). Hyperandrogenic anovulation (PCOS): a unique disorder of insulin action associated with an increased risk of non-insulin dependent diabetes mellitus. *American Journal of Medicine* 98(1A), 33S–39S.

Dunaif, A., Graf, M., Mandeli, J., Laumas, V. and Dobrjansky, A. (1987). Characterization of groups of hyperandrogenic women with acanthosis nigricans, impaired glucose tolerance and/or hyperinsulinemia. *Journal of Clinical Endocrinology and Metabolism* 65,499–507

Dunaif, A., Green, G., Futterweit, W. and Dobrjansky, A. (1990). Suppression of ovarian hyperandrogenism does not improve peripheral or hepatic insulin resistance in the polycystic ovary syndrome. *Journal of Clinical Endocrinology and Metabolism* 70, 699–704.

Dunaif, A., Segal, K.R. and Shelley, D.R. (1989). Evidence for distinctive and intrinsic defects in insulin action in the polycystic ovary syndrome. *Diabetes* 38, 1165–74.

Dunaif, A., Xia, J., Book, C-B., Schenker, E. and Tang, Z. (1995). Excessive insulin receptor phosphorylation in cultered fibroblasts and in skeletal muscles. *Journal of Clinical Investigation* **96**, 801–10.

Ferriman, D. and Purdie, A.W. (1979). The inheritance of polycystic ovarian disease and a possible relationship to premature balding. *Clinical Endocrinology* **11**, 291–300.

Franks, S. (1995). Medical progress article: polycystic ovary syndrome. *New England Journal of Medicine* **333**, 853–61.

Franks S. (1997) The 17α-hydroxylase-17,20-lyase gene (CYP 17) and polycystic ovary syndrome (commentary). *Clinical Endocrinology* **46**, 135–6

Franks, S., Gharani, N., Waterworth, D. et al. (1997). The genetic basis of polycystic ovary syndrome. *Human Reproduction* **12**, 2641–8.

Franks, S., Robinson, S. and Willis, D. (1996). Nutrition, insulin and polycystic ovary syndrome. *Review of Reproduction* **1**, 47–53.

Gilling-Smith, C., Willis, D.S., Beard, R.W. and Franks, S. (1994). Hypersecretion of androstenedione by isolated theca cells from polycystic ovaries. *Journal of Clinical Endocrinology and Metabolism* **79**, 1158–65

Givens, J.R. (1988). Familial polycystic ovarian disease. *Endocrinology and Metabolism Clinics of North America* **17**, 771–83.

Gharani, N., Waterworth, D.M., Batty, S. et al. (1997). Association of the steroid synthesis gene CYP11a with polycystic ovary syndrome and hyperandrogenism. *Human Molecular Genetics.* **6**, 397–402.

Gharani, N., Waterworth, D.M., Williamson, R. and Franks, S. (1996). 5′ polymorphism of the CYP17 gene is not associated with serum testosterone levels in women with polycystic ovary syndrome. (Letter.) *Journal of Clinical Endocrinology and Metabolism* **81**, 4174.

Govind, A., Obhrai, M.S. and Clayton, R.N. (1999). Polycystic ovaries are inherited as an autosomal dominant trait: analysis of 29 polycystic ovary syndrome and 10 control families. *Journal of Clinical Endocrinology and Metabolism* (1999) **84** (**1**), 38–43.

Hague, W.M., Adams, J., Algar, V. et al. (1988). Familial polycystic ovaries: a genetic disease? *Clinical Endocrinology* **32**, 407–15.

Holte, J. (1996). Disturbances in insulin secretion and sensitivity in women with the polycystic ovary syndrome. *Ballière's Clinical Endocrinology and Metabolism* **10**, 221–47.

Hutton, C. and Clark, F. (1984). Polycystic ovarian syndrome in identical twins. *Postgraduate Medical Journal* **60**, 64–5.

Jahanfar. S, Eden. J.A., Warren, P.W, Seppala, M. and Nguyen, T.V. (1995). A twin study of polycystic ovary syndrome. *Fertility and Sterility* **63** (**3**), 478–86

Kiddy, D.S., Hamilton-Fairley D., Bush, A. et al. (1992). Improvement in endocrine and ovarian function during dietary treatment of obese women with polycystic ovary syndrome. *Clinical Endocrinology* **36**, 105–11.

Legro, R,S., Driscoll, D., Strauss, J.F., Fox, J. and Dunaif, A. (1998). Evidence for a genetic basis for hyperandrogenemia in polycystic ovary syndrome. *Proceedings of the National Academy of Sciences USA* **95**, 14956–60

Legro, S.L., Spielman, R., Urbanek, M. et al. (1998) Phenotype and genotype in polycystic ovary syndrome. *Recent Progress in Hormone Research* **53**, 217–56.

Lunde, O., Magnus, P., Sandvik, L. and Hoglo, S. (1989). Familial clustering in the polycystic ovarian syndrome. *Gynecology and Obstetric Investigation* 28, 23–30.

Nestler, J.E., Barlascini, C.O. and Matt, D.W. (1990). Suppression of serum insulin by diazoxide reduced serum testosterone levels in obese women with polycystic ovary syndrome. *Journal of Clinical Endocrinology and Metabolism* 68,1027.

Norman, R.J., Masters, S. and Hague, W. (1996). Hyperinsulinemia is common in family members of women with polycystic ovary syndrome. *Fertility and Sterility* 66, 942–7.

Rajkhowa, M., Talbot, J.A., Jones, P.W. and Clayton, R.N. (1996). Polymorphism of glycogen synthetase gene in polycystic ovary syndrome. *Clinical Endocrinology* 44 (1), 85–90.

Rosenfield, R.L., Barnes, R.B., Cara, J.F. and Lucky, A.W. (1990). Dysregulation of cytochrome P450c 17 alpha as the cause of polycystic ovary syndrome. *Fertility and Sterility* 53, 785–91.

Steingold, K., De Ziegler, D. and Cedars, M. (1987). Clinical and hormonal effects of chronic gonadotrophin-releasing hormone agonist treatment in polycystic ovarian disease. *Journal of Clinical Endocrinology and Metabolism* 65, 773–8.

Talbot, J.A., Bicknell, E.J., Rajkhowa, M. et al. (1996). Molecular scanning of the insulin receptor gene in women with polycystic ovary syndrome. *Journal of Clinical Endocrinology and Metabolism* 81(5), 1979–83.

Techatraisak, K., Conway, G.S. and Rumsby, G. (1997). Frequency of a polymorphism in the regulatory region of the 17 (α-hydroxylase-17,20 lyase (CYP17) gene in the hyperandrogenic states. *Clinical Endocrinology* 46, 131–4.

Waterworth, D.M., Bennet, S.T., Gharani, N. et al. (1997). Linkage and association of the insulin gene VNTR regulatory polymorphism with polycystic ovary syndrome. *Lancet* 349, 986–9.

White, D.W., Leigh, A., Wilson, C., Donaldson, A. and Franks, S. (1995). Gonadotrophin and gonadal steroid response to a single dose of a long acting agonist of gonadotrophin releasing hormone in ovulatory and anovulatory women with polycystic ovary syndrome. *Clinical Endocrinology* 42, 475–81.

4

The genetic basis of polycystic ovary syndrome

Lee-Chuan Kao, Margrit Urbanek, Deborah Driscoll, Richard S. Legro, Andrea Dunaif, Richard S. Spielman and Jerome F. Strauss III

Introduction

Genetic factors determine disease susceptibility and response to therapeutic interventions. A number of mutations and genetic variants (polymorphisms) have been found to predispose individuals to specific conditions, including cardiovascular disease, diabetes, and Alzheimer's disease. The reductionist view of human biology, that genes are the determinants of disease risk, is more difficult to argue in the case of complex disorders in which the underlying pathophysiology is obscure, as is the case for polycystic ovary syndrome (PCOS). Unfortunately, the exploration of the genetics of PCOS has been plagued by debate about disease phenotypes and the lack of appropriate animal models which could be informative regarding the genetics of the disorder. The phenotype issue is not trivial, since any rigorous genetic analysis demands that individuals be accurately assigned to affected status. The larger the number of distinct phenotypes within the affected category that need to be considered, the more complex the analysis and the greater the likelihood that investigators using different diagnostic criteria will arrive at different conclusions. In addition, the lack of a secure male phenotype makes formal segregation analysis as well as genetic linkage studies more difficult. It is no wonder that many scholars have privately concluded that PCOS is a multigenic disorder that is beyond the comprehension of contemporary genetic analysis. The authors' personal bias is that this resignation is unwarranted, even at a time when relatively limited information is available, and that careful investigation will ultimately disclose dominant genetic factors that contribute to PCOS susceptibility. This chapter reviews evidence for a genetic basis for PCOS and summarizes current research focusing on association and genetic linkage studies.

Family studies

The foundation of genetic studies is the evidence that some diseases cluster in families. Therefore, it is important to review the major published work suggesting that PCOS is a familial condition. As a preamble to this review it should be noted that none of the existing family studies convincingly establishes a mode of inheritance, because the number of families studied was too small, or the parental phenotypes could not be firmly established, or the male phenotype was uncertain. Moreover, the diagnostic criteria used to assign affected status differed among the studies, as did the methods with which the status of first-degree and second-degree relatives were ascertained. By and large, ovarian morphology determined from tissue biopsy, direct visualization or diagnostic imaging, in association with menstrual disturbances and evidence for hyperandrogenism have been used in most studies as the criteria for diagnosing PCOS in probands. When considered, the male phenotype has primarily been balding before the age of 30 or increased pilosity. However, as mentioned above, the rigor with which these phenotypes were identified, particularly in relatives of the probands, ranged from the use of questionnaires to variable levels of clinical and biochemical evaluation. Despite the heterogeneity in study design and the inability to obtain comprehensive phenotype information to permit a formal segregation analysis, collectively the existing literature strongly suggests the clustering of PCOS in families, with a mode of inheritance that is consistent with an autosomal dominant pattern (Legro et al., 1998b). These family studies are described in detail in Chapter 3, so that only a few comments will be added here.

Our group (Legro et al., 1998a) conducted a prospective study of 80 PCOS women and 115 of their sisters. The probands were identified on the basis of oligomenorrhoea (fewer than six menses/year) and hyperandrogenaemia defined as a total or biologically available testosterone level that was greater than 2 standard deviations above the mean values of an age-matched and body mass index-matched control group of women. This study concluded that there is familial clustering of hyperandrogenaemia with or without oligomenorrhoea, indicating that hyperandrogenaemia is a dominant trait. A recent report of Carmina and Lobo (1999) also noted that hyperandrogenic women display evidence for PCOS on diagnostic testing, including a polycystic ovarian morphology on ultrasound and an increased 17-hydroxyprogesterone response to a leuprolide acetate challenge despite normal menses. The Legro et al. (1998a) study, although conducted on a relatively small population, suggested that testosterone levels in sisters of PCOS women had a bimodal distribution, which could be consistent with a monogenic trait controlled by two alleles at an autosomal locus.

Karyotype studies

The study of chromosome number and morphology has disclosed the genetic basis of a number of diseases and syndromes. Although there are reports of X chromosome aneuploidies (Netter et al., 1961; Bishun and Morton, 1964), an increased frequency of tetraploidy in cultured lymphocytes (Rojanasakul et al., 1985), as well as other cytogenetic abnormalities (Nur et al., 1987) associated with PCOS in a limited number of subjects, larger cytogenetic analyses have failed to identify karyotypic abnormalities (Knorr, Knorr-Gartner and Webele-Kallhardt, 1969; Stenchever et al., 1968). Thus, it appears that gross alterations in chromosome number or structure are not associated with PCOS.

Association and linkage studies

The identification of genes linked to complex diseases has been pursued using a number of strategies, including association studies and linkage analysis for candidate genes, and genome-wide scanning using non-parametric methods. The latter approach is ideal because it makes no assumptions regarding the gene(s) involved, the mode of inheritance, disease penetrance, or prevalence. The screen is based on the analysis of genomic DNA collected from a large number of families with one or more affected sibs for informative markers spaced at 10–20 cM across the genome where parental DNA samples are also available so that identity by descent of alleles can be established. Unfortunately, no investigative team has yet assembled a sufficient number of families with affected sib-pairs (in the order of several hundred) to perform a genome-wide screen. Consequently, the existing literature is based exclusively on association and linkage studies for selected candidate genes (Franks et al., 1997; Urbanek et al., 1999). This does not reflect a cavalier attitude towards the genetic methodology, but rather the difficulty in accruing families with multiple affected sisters and available parents, despite the fact that PCOS is a common disorder.

Association studies test for over-representation of a specific allele of a candidate gene in a population of unrelated affected individuals compared to a cohort of unrelated unaffected individuals. This type of case control study can be used to explore diseases in which the modes of inheritance and penetrance are not understood. These studies do not establish linkage of a disease phenotype with the allele and they are subject to error because the test assumes that the frequencies of the alleles examined are similar in the populations studied. Consequently, studies incorporating mixed populations of ethnic groups where allele frequencies may vary can yield spurious results. Bias may also enter into these studies through the manner in which the control populations are selected. In addition, some investigators have studied the same populations for association with several different markers and have failed to make appropriate compensation in their statistical analyses for multiple tests. It is, therefore, of no surprise that the PCOS literature contains a number of conflicting reports.

Testing available family DNA sets for candidate genes is not an unreasonable exercise in the absence of sufficient populations to conduct a genome-wide scan. Indeed, the candidate approach has been highly successful in identifying genes involved in a number of reproductive endocrine disorders, including congenital lipoid adrenal hyperplasia, ovarian dysgenesis due to follicle-stimulating hormone (FSH) receptor gene mutations and hypogonadotrophic hypogonadism due to gonadotrophin releasing hormone (GnRH) receptor gene mutations. However, in the latter cases the universe of possible candidates to choose from was better defined than in the case of PCOS, for which multiple endocrine and metabolic abnormalities must be accounted. Hence, one might predict that the number of wrong guesses for PCOS candidate genes would be high, and perhaps may continue to be close to a turn at the roulette wheel, until the pathophysiology is crystallized and a gene or genes become 'obvious' candidates. Wrong guesses are not necessarily without value, since the exclusion of loci when sample size is sufficient to do so, or their relegation to low priority, helps to narrow the field of possibilities and may adjust the level to which the gene products are emphasized in models of PCOS pathophysiology.

To date, the candidate genes that have been investigated include those involved in steroid hormone synthesis and action, genes involved in carbohydrate metabolism and fuel homeostasis, genes involved in gonadotrophin action and regulation, and genes in the major histocompatibility region.

Genes involved in steroid hormone synthesis and action

Rationale

Abnormalities in ovarian steroidogenesis, particularly androgen production, are a prominent feature of PCOS. Although there has been intensive interest in the regulation of the gene encoding the gateway to androgen synthesis, 17α-hydroxylase/17,20-lyase (*CYP17*) (Rosenfield, Barnes and Ehrmann, 1994; Gilling-Smith et al., 1997), studies on isolated thecal cells from ovaries of women with PCOS reveal alterations in steroidogenesis that extend beyond *CYP17* activity and include increased progesterone production and reduction of the 17 keto group of C19 steroids (Gilling-Smith et al., 1994; Nelson et al., 1999). Because symptoms of hirsutism and acne are common in PCOS women, androgen action as well as androgen production has been explored.

CYP17

A single nucleotide polymorphism (T→C) at base pair −34 in the *CYP17* promoter initially attracted attention because of the critical role *CYP17* plays in governing androgen biosynthesis. This substitution of a C at this site creates a new potential Sp1 binding site in the rarer allele that could enhance promoter function. Carey et al. (1994) studied 14 caucasian families with 81 affected individuals and found that carriers of the rarer allele (allele 2) had increased susceptibility for PCOS compared to controls. However, in analysing a larger population, these authors failed to confirm a significantly different allele frequency in PCOS women compared to their control group of women (Franks, 1997). Others have also failed to identify mutations in the *CYP17* gene or association of the −34 polymorphism with PCOS (Techatraisak, Conway and Rumsby, 1997; Liovic et al., 1997), or premature pubarche, hirsutism and oligomenorrhoea in adolescence (Witchel et al., 1998).

CYP11A

Gharani et al. (1997) examined 20 families with multiple affected women and found evidence for linkage to the *CYP11A* locus on chromosome 15. Allowing for genetic heterogeneity, these authors estimated that 60% of the 20 families studied had the linked form. An association study conducted on 97 PCOS women and matched controls revealed significant association with D15S520, a pentanucleotide repeat (tttta)n polymorphism at position −528 from the ATG initiation codon in the 5′-region of the *CYP11A* gene, and total serum testosterone levels. Allele 5 of D15S520 was found less frequently in women with hyperandrogenaemia. Although no regulatory role has been assigned to this polymorphism in terms of *CYP11A* gene transcription, the investigators suggested that allelic variants in the *CYP11A* gene have a role in the hyperandrogenaemia of PCOS. Urbanek et al. (1999) analysed two markers (D15S519 and D15S520) included in the study of Gharani et al. (1997) and found only modest evidence for linkage. Using the transmission disequilibrium test in 150 families, Urbanek and colleagues found no significant association between hyperandrogenaemia and any allele at D15S520 or the closely linked marker D15S519. Allele 5 of D15S520 was transmitted at a slightly reduced frequency to affected females, but the difference was not statistically significant.

CYP19

Linkage and association of the *CYP19* gene, also located on chromosome 15, were excluded as a major PCOS locus in the study of Gharani et al. (1997), who used a parametric linkage analysis. Urbanek et al. (1999) also found no evidence for linkage of *CYP19* with PCOS.

HSD17B3

The 17β-hydroxysteroid dehydrogenase responsible for the synthesis of testosterone is encoded by the type 3 gene *HSD17B3*. This gene is not normally expressed in the human ovary (Zhang et al., 1996). An apparently silent polymorphism in exon 11 of the type 3 17β-hydroxysteroid dehydrogenase gene which results in the substitution of a serine residue for a glycine at codon 289 has been studied in normal and PCOS women. This amino acid substitution does not change the enzyme's substrate specificities or its kinetic constants. The frequencies of the two alleles were similar in normal and PCOS women (Moghrabi et al., 1998).

Androgen receptor

Jakubiczka et al. (1997) found no association between the number of repeats in the polymorphic CAG repeat of the first exon of the androgen receptor and PCOS. Using the transmission disequilibrium test, which tests for excess transmissions of alleles to affected individuals, Urbanek et al. (1999) studied 150 families for the trinucleotide repeat polymorphism and failed to find evidence for association with PCOS.

Genes involved in carbohydrate metabolism and fuel homeostasis
Rationale

The common occurrence of insulin resistance and pancreatic beta cell dysfunction in association with PCOS and the increased risk for development of type 2 diabetes mellitus are now well recognized. Moreover, insulin acting through its own receptor, and at high concentrations through the IGF-I receptor, stimulates steroidogenesis (Barbieri et al., 1986; Willis and Franks, 1995; Willis et al., 1996). This has led investigators to focus on insulin resistance as a potential central abnormality in PCOS (Dunaif, 1997). The ability of insulin to act through different signalling pathways to control glucose uptake as well as cell growth and differentiation (Virkamaki, Ueki and Kahn, 1999), could account for insulin resistance in certain tisues with maintenance of insulin sensitivity in others.

Insulin receptor

Mutations in the insulin receptor gene cause severe insulin resistance (the type A syndrome) associated with acanthosis nigricans and PCOS (Moller and Flier, 1988; Taylor et al., 1992; Moller et al., 1994). A number of studies have examined the insulin receptor gene structure in PCOS women with and without insulin resistance (Conway, Avey and Rumsby, 1994; Sorbara et al., 1994; Talbot et al., 1996). However, none of these studies has found common mutations or polymorphisms that are linked to PCOS. In a screen of 37 candidate genes, Urbanek et al. (1999) found the strongest association with PCOS at a marker in the insulin receptor region (marker D19S884). This finding was no longer significant, however, after taking into account the large number of markers and alleles that were tested.

Glycogen synthetase

Glycogen synthetase is positioned in the metabolic pathways for fuel homeostasis to regulate glucose availability. Rajkhowa et al. (1996) looked for association of a Xba1 polymorphism in this gene with insulin sensitivity assessed by fasting insulin levels, oral glucose tolerance and intravenous insulin tolerance tests in women with PCOS. The Xba1 polymorphism was not over-represented in the PCOS women or with measures of insulin resistance in these subjects.

Insulin gene

Waterworth et al. (1997) examined the role of a variable number tandem repeat (VNTR) in the 5′ region of the insulin gene in PCOS. This locus has a bimodal distribution of repeats which have been divided into class I alleles (averaging 40 repeats) and class III alleles with a larger number of repeats (average 157). Linkage of PCOS to this locus was examined in 17 families in which there were multiple individuals affected with polycystic ovaries on ultrasound scan or pre-mature male balding (before the age of 30) and the association of these alleles with polycystic ovaries in two additional populations. The authors found that the class III allele was preferentially transmitted from heterozygous fathers but not from mothers to affected individuals. Linkage analysis suggested increased sharing of the locus in affected sibs. The authors concluded that they had discovered strong linkage and association between alleles at the variable nucleotide tandem repeat (VNTR) in the 5′-region of the insulin gene and PCOS. However, others reviewing the study, data analysis and use of the Genehunter program to identify linkage pointed out concerns (McKeigue and Wild, 1997). Moreover, Urbanek et al. (1999) did not find any evidence for linkage of the insulin gene in their analysis or of association between the class III alleles of the insulin VNTR and hyperandrogenaemia.

Tumour necrosis factor α

Tumour necrosis factor α (TNF-α) is produced by inflammatory cells and adipose tissue. It causes insulin resistance and inhibits steroidogenesis (Almahbobi and Trounson, 1996). Polymorphisms have been identified in the TNF-α promoter, and the association between allelic variants at base pair −308 has been examined in PCOS and normal women (Milner et al., 1999). The rarer allele has been associated with a variety of inflammatory conditions. In the study of Milner et al. no associations were found between either of the two −308 (G→A) alleles with polycystic ovaries, identified by ultrasound in women with normal menstrual cycles, or with PCOS, diagnosed by the ultrasound morphology of the ovary in association with menstrual abnormalities. However, the rarer allele (TNF2) was significantly associated with lower glucose levels in glucose tolerance tests.

Genes involved in gonadotrophin action and regulation

Rationale

Abnormalities in gonadotrophin secretion, particularly luteinizing hormone (LH), are characteristic of PCOS. Since LH plays a permissive role in driving thecal androgen production, there has been interest in exploring genes related to the regulation of LH secretion, LH bioactivity and LH action.

Luteinizing hormone β-subunit gene

Polymorphisms have been identified in the human LH β-subunit (W8R and I15T) which result in an immunologically distinctive form of the gonadotrophin. The association of this LH variant with PCOS has been examined in several studies (Rajkhowa et al., 1995; Elter et al., 1999). The consensus is that the LH variants are present with similar frequencies in PCOS and normal women. However, both over-representation and under-representation of these alleles in obese women with PCOS have been reported.

Dopamine receptor genes

Dopamine inhibits GnRH and prolactin secretion. Polymorphisms have been identified in the dopamine D2 and D3 receptor genes. Homozygosity for the rare allele (allele 2) of the D3 receptor has been associated with PCOS and clomiphene resistance in Hispanic women (Legro et al., 1995). However, a subsequent case-control study carried out in non-Hispanic white women failed to show a significant association with alleles of the dopamine D3 receptor and PCOS (Kahsar-Miller et al., 1999). D2 receptor gene polymorphisms in intron 5 and exon 6 have also been associated with fecundity but not with PCOS (Legro et al., 1994).

Follistatin

In the study of Urbanek et al. (1999) the follistatin locus emerged as a promising candidate from the study of 39 affected sib-pairs. Follistatin, an activin binding protein, is widely expressed, as is activin, and could play an important role in regulating ovarian, pituitary and beta cell function consistent with abnormalities associated with PCOS. Activin stimulates pituitary FSH secretion and acts directly on the ovary to promote follicular maturation (Mather, Moore and Li, 1997). Neutralization of activin would be expected to cause reductions in FSH levels and arrested follicular maturation, as occurs in transgenic mice overexpressing follistatin (Guo et al., 1998). In addition, activin inhibits thecal androgen biosynthesis, and its removal by binding to follistatin might lead to unrestrained theca androgen synthesis driven by LH. Finally, activin has been shown to stimulate insulin secretion, and loss of local activin action might impair beta cell function. Although this collection of facts would seem to constitute an attractive argument for follistatin as a candidate gene, particularly for a mutation or variant leading to increased follistatin expression or activity, such a mutation or allelic variant in the human follistatin gene has yet to be identified.

The major histocompatibility region
Rationale

Linkage of disorders to the major histocompatibility locus encoding human leukocyte antigens (HLA) on chromosome 6 has been sought for numerous diseases, especially when an immunological basis has been entertained. The TNF-α gene, discussed above, is located in this region. Moreover, the locus encoding a steroidogenic enzyme, *CYP21*, also maps within the HLA region. The fact that mutations in *CYP21* which cause late onset or cryptic 21-hydroxylase deficiency are associated with PCOS has encouraged investigators to search for association and/or linkage of PCOS with the HLA region.

Human leukocyte antigens

A small study conducted by Mandel et al. (1983) involving four families in which at least two siblings had PCOS verified by elevated serum androgen and LH levels found no linkage between PCOS and HLA. However, larger studies have yielded conflicting results. Hague et al. (1990) found an increased frequency of HLA DRW6 and a reduced frequency of HLA DR7 in a study of 99 subjects with polycystic ovary morphology on ultrasound compared to 110 control females. However, no linkage between HLA and PCOS was noted in a study of 16 families. Ober et al. (1992) reported an association between DQA1*0501 and PCOS in 19 women affected with PCOS including hirsutism and elevated plasma androgen levels compared to 46 controls. Homozygosity for this allele was also increased among the PCOS women, leading the authors to suggest that PCOS susceptibility allele is linked to HLA and that this allele is recessive.

What needs to be done?

A more complete understanding of the genetics of PCOS will require studies of two kinds: determination of the prevalence of PCOS in relatives (usually sisters) of an index case, and studies to test for linkage between PCOS and candidate genes, or possibly throughout the genome.

Reliable estimation of prevalence in relatives requires *unbiased* surveys of families. These can establish the prevalence in close female relatives (offspring and sisters) of an 'index' case. It is difficult to eliminate bias towards increased prevalence in sisters, since most surveys tend to ascertain preferentially families with multiple affected women. Furthermore, in a disease like PCOS, where female fertility is reduced, it is very difficult to interpret data on prevalence in mothers of cases, since mothers who reproduce may have the putative genes, but be in part a selected non-penetrant group. Looking 'down' the pedigree, it is possible to estimate prevalence in offspring (daughters) of affected women with greater confidence; however, such studies usually require extensive follow-up, making them very difficult in practice. In general, it is easier to estimate the prevalence in sisters of an index case, or equivalently a relative risk (relative to prevalence in the general population). This risk ratio figure is important because, in principle, it gives an upper limit for the degree of familial aggregation to be explained by particular genes. As individual genes believed to confer susceptibility are identified, it is essential to evaluate their contribution to the total familial risk, for instance by the methods of Risch (1990).

A different kind of family study is needed for analysis of possible linkage to candidate genes. In contrast to a prevalence study where families with multiple affected members are found only in proportion to their presence in the population, linkage studies for PCOS will usually *require* families with multiple affected sisters (see below for an exception). The approach used to test for linkage is the 'affected sib-pair' (ASP) method (Lander and Schork, 1994). Because several or many genes will be tested in such a study, findings that meet the criterion for statistical significance for one of these genes may be obtained by chance ('false positive') more easily than if only one gene is tested. One solution to this problem is to increase sample size (number of families). When this is done, extreme levels of significance are possible in the case of truly linked genes, reducing the likelihood of false-positive conclusions. But if only modest evidence for linkage is found, replication in an independent series of families is always required, and the ultimate confirmation must come from identifying the causative genetic variant, not just a linked marker.

There is an alternative design for linkage studies, which requires only one affected offspring per family. The rationale for this approach is the possibility that a marker tested for linkage will be so close to the causative variant in the candidate gene that there will be linkage disequilibrium, a tendency for the disease variant and some marker allele to appear on the same chromosome more often that expected by chance. The standard method for detecting this phenomenon is the transmission/disequilibrium test (TDT) (Spielman, McGinnis and Ewens, 1993), referred to above. The TDT is a valid test for linkage regardless of the number of affected offspring per sibship, so the same families analysed by ASP methods can also be tested by the TDT. The 'trios' of parents and affected daughter needed for the TDT are much easier to ascertain than the multiple-sister families needed for ASP methods, so it is tempting to focus on studying just the former. However, it is important to note that a disease-predisposing gene may be detectable by ASP methods and not by TDT (or vice versa), so both methods should be used (Spielman and Ewens, 1996).

In view of the uncertainty about the male phenotype (if any) corresponding to PCOS, it seems prudent to restrict all analyses to affected women, and exclude male phenotypes from all analyses at present. If strong evidence for linkage is found in analysis of women, it will be immediately possible to re-evaluate the phenotype of men in the same families, taking into consideration the alleles shared with the affected women. This procedure will eventually put the choice and analysis of the male phenotype on a firm footing.

Conclusions

The existing literature provides a strong basis for arguing that PCOS clusters in families and that there is a gene or collection of genes that are linked to PCOS susceptibility. The mode of inheritance of the disorder is still uncertain, although the majority of studies are consistent with an autosomal dominant pattern, modified perhaps by environmental factors. However, this is far from being firmly established.

Although several genetic loci have been proposed to be linked to PCOS, including *CYP11A*, the insulin gene and follistatin, the evidence substantiating linkage is weak. This should not be disheartening news because the continued exploration of candidate genes will eventually shine light on loci that are worthy of intensive investigation while also diminishing interest in other genes. This will, we believe, ultimately lead us to those loci that are indeed major determinants of PCOS susceptibility.

Acknowledgements

The authors thank Ms Judith Wood for assistance in the preparation of the manuscript of this chapter. Studies on PCOS in the authors' laboratories have been supported by the National Cooperative Program in Infertility Research (U54 HD34449).

REFERENCES

Almahbobi, G. and Trounson, A.O. (1996). The role of intraovarian regulators in the aetiology of polycystic ovarian syndrome. *Reproductive Medicine Review* 5, 151–68.

Barbieri, R.L., Makris, A., Randall, R.W. et al. (1986). Insulin stimulates androgen accumulation in incubations of ovarian stroma obtained from women with hyperandrogenism. *Journal of Clinical Endocrinology and Metabolism* 62, 904–10.

Bishun, N.P. and Morton, W.R.M. (1964). Chromosome mosaicism in Stein–Leventhal syndrome. *British Medical Journal* 7, 1200.

Carey, A.H., Waterworth, D., Patel, K. et al. (1994). Polycystic ovaries and premature male pattern baldness are associated with the allele of the steroid-metabolism gene CYP17. *Human Molecular Genetics* 3, 1873–6.

Carmina, E. and Lobo, R.A. (1999). Do hyperandrogenic women with normal menses have poly-cystic ovary syndrome? *Fertility and Sterility* 71, 319–22.

Conway, G.S., Avey, C. and Rumsby, G. (1994). The tyrosine kinase domain of the insulin recep-tor gene is normal in women with hyperinsulinemia and polycystic ovary syndrome. *Human Reproduction* 9, 1681–3.

Dunaif, A. (1997) Insulin resistance and polycystic ovary syndrome: mechanisms and implica-tions for pathogenesis. *Endrocrine Review* 18, 774–800.

Elter, K., Erel, C.T., Cine, N. et al. (1999). Role of the mutations Trp8→Arg and Ile15→Thr of the human luteinizing hormone beta-subunit in women with polycystic ovary syndrome. *Fertility and Sterility* 71, 425–30.

Franks, S. (1997). The 17α-hydroxylase/17,20 lyase (CYP17) and polycystic ovary syndrome. *Clinical Endocrinology* 46, 135–6.

Franks, S., Gharani, N., Waterworth, D. et al. (1997). The genetic basis of polycystic ovary syn-drome. *Human Reproduction* 12, 2641–8.

Gharani, N., Waterworth, D.M., Batty, S. et al. (1997). Association of the steroid synthesis gene CYP11a with polycystic ovary syndrome and hyperandrogenism. *Human Molecular Genetics* 6, 397–402.

Gilling-Smith, C., Story, H., Rogers, Y. and Franks, S. (1997). Evidence for a primary abnormal-ity of thecal cell steroidogenesis in the polycystic ovary syndrome. *Clinical Endocrinology* 47, 93–9.

Gilling-Smith, C., Willis, D.S., Beard, R.W. and Franks, S. (1994). Hypersecretion of androste-nedione by isolated thecal cells from polycystic ovaries. *Journal of Clinical Endocrinology and Metabolism* 79, 1158–65.

Guo, Q., Kumar, T.R., Woodruff, T. et al. (1998). Overexpression of mouse follistatin causes reproductive defects in transgenic mice. *Molecular Endocrinology* 12, 96–106.

Hague, W.M., Adams, J., Algar, V. et al. (1990). HLA associations in patients with polycystic ovaries with congenital adrenal hyperplasia caused by 21-hydroxylase deficiency. *Clinical Endocrinology* 32, 407–15.

Jakubiczka, S., Quaisr, A., Nickel, I., Kleinstein, J., and Wieacker, P. (1997). Molecular genetic studies at the androgen receptor-gene in female patients with PCO syndrome. *Geburtshilfe Frauenheilkunde* 57, 545–8.

Kahsar-Miller, M., Boots, I.R. and Azziz, R. (1999). Dopamine D3 receptor polymorphism is not associated with polycystic ovary syndrome. *Fertility and Sterility* 71, 436–8.

Knorr, K., Knorr-Gartner, H. and Webele-Kallhardt, B. (1969). Chromosome analysis findings in the Stein–Leventhal syndrome (etiology of the Stein–Leventhal syndrome). *Endokrinologie* 54, 364–73.

Lander, E.S. and Schork, N.J. (1994). Genetic dissection of complex traits. *Science* 265, 2037–48.

Legro, R.S., Dietz, G.W., Comings, D.E., Lobo, R.A. and Kovacs, B.W. (1994). Association of dop-amine D2 receptor gene haplotypes with anovulation and fecundity in female Hispanics. *Human Reproduction* 9, 1271–5.

Legro, R.S., Driscoll, D., Strauss, III J.F., Fox, J. and Dunaif, A. (1998a). Evidence for a genetic basis for hyperandrogenemia in polycystic ovary syndrome. *Proceedings of the National Academy of Sciences of the United States of America* 95, 14956–60.

Legro, R.S., Muhlman, D.R., Comings, D.E., Lobo, R.A. and Kovacs, B.W. (1995). A dopamine

D3 receptor genotype is associated with hyperandrogenic chronic anovulation and resistant to ovulation induction with chlomiphene citrate in female Hispanics. *Fertility and Sterility* **63**, 779–84.

Legro, R.S., Spielman, R., Urbanek, M. et al. (1998b). Phenotype and genotype in polycystic ovary syndrome. *Recent Progress in Hormone Research* **53**, 217–56.

Liovic, M., Prezelj, J., Kocijancic, A., Majdic, G. and Komel, R. (1997). CYP17 gene analysis in hyperandrogenized women with and without exaggerated 17-hydroxyprogesterone responses to ovarian stimulation. *Journal of Endocrinological Investigation* **20**, 189–93.

Mandel, F.P., Chang, R.J., Dupont, B. et al. (1983). HLA genotyping in family members and patients with polycystic ovarian disease. *Journal of Clinical Endocrinology and Metabolism* **54**, 862–4.

Mather, J.P., Moore, A. and Li, R. (1997). Activins, inhibins, follistatins: further thoughts on a growing family of regulators. *Proceedings of the Society for Experimental Biology and Medicine* **215**, 209–15.

McKeigue, P. and Wild, S. (1997). Association of insulin gene VNTR polymorphism with polycystc ovary syndrome. *Lancet* **349**, 1771–2.

Milner, C.R., Craig, J.E., Hussey, N.D. and Norman, R.J. (1999). No association between the −308 polymorphism in the tumour necrosis factor α (TNFα) promoter region and polycystic ovaries. *Molecular Human Reproduction*, **5**, 5–9.

Moghrabi, N., Hughes, I.A., Dunaif, A. and Andersson, S. (1998). Deleterious missense mutations and a silent polymorphism in human 17β-hydroxysteroid dehydrogenase 3 gene (HSD17B3). *Journal of Clinical Endocrinology and Metabolism* **83**, 2855–60.

Moller, D.E., Choen, O., Yamaguchi, Y. et al. (1994). Prevalence of mutations in the insulin receptor gene in subjects with features of the type A syndrome of insulin resistance. *Diabetes* **43**, 247–55.

Moller, D.E. and Flier, J.S. (1988). Detection of an alteration in the insulin receptor gene in a patient with insulin resistance, acanthosis nigricans and polycystic ovary syndrome. *New England Journal of Medicine* **319**, 1526–9.

Nelson, V.L., Legro, R.S., Strauss, III J.F. and McAllister, J.M. (1999). Augmented androgen production is a stable steroidogenic phenotype of propagated theca cells from polycystic ovaries. *Molecular Endocrinology* **13**, 946–57.

Netter, A., Bloch-Michel, H., Salomon, Y. et al. (1961). Study of karyotypes in Stein–Leventhal syndrome. *Annals of Endocrinology* (Paris) **22**, 841–9.

Nur, J., Grewal, M.S., Guron, C.J., and Buckshee, K. (1987). C-band polymorphism of chromosome No. 1 in patients with polycystic ovary disease. *Asia-Oceania Journal of Obstetrics and Gynecology* **13**, 75–8.

Ober, C., Weil, S., Steck, T. et al. (1992). Increased risk for polycystic ovary syndrome associated with human leukocyte antigen DQA1*0501. *American Journal of Obstetrics and Gynecology* **167**, 1803–6.

Rajkhowa, M., Talbot, J.A. and Jones, P.W. (1995). Prevalence of an immunological LH beta-subunit variant in a UK population of healthy women and women with polycystic ovary syndrome. *Clinical Endocrinology* **43**, 297–303.

Rajkhowa, M., Talbot, J.A., Jones, P.W. and Clayton, R.N. (1996). Polymorphism of glycogen synthetase gene in polycystic ovary syndrome. *Clinical Endocrinology* **44**, 85–90.

Risch, N. (1990). Linkage strategies for genetically complex traits. II. The power of affected relative pairs. *American Journal of Human Genetics* **46**, 229–41.

Rojanasakul, A., Gustavson, K.H., Lithell, H. and Nillius, S.J. (1985). Tetraploidy in two sisters with the polycystic ovary syndrome. *Clinical Genetics* **27**, 167–74.

Rosenfield, R.L., Barnes, R.B. and Ehrmann, D.A. (1994). Studies of the nature of 17-hydroxyprogesterone hyperresponsiveness to gonadotropin-releasing-hormone agonist challenge in functional ovarian hyperandrogenism. *Journal of Clinical Endocrinology and Metabolism* **79**, 1686–92.

Sorbara, L.R, Tang, Z., Cama, A. et al. (1994). Absence of insulin receptor gene mutations in three insulin-resistant women with polycystic ovary syndrome. *Metabolism* **43**, 1568–74.

Spielman, R.S. and Ewens, W.J. (1996). The TDT and other family-based tests for linkage disequilibrium and association. *American Journal of Human Genetics* **59**, 983–9.

Spielman, R.S., McGinnis, R.E. and Ewens, W.J. (1993). Transmission test for linkage disequilibrium: the insulin gene region and insulin-dependent diabetes mellitus. *American Journal of Human Genetics* **52**, 506–16.

Stenchever, M.A., Macintyre, M.N., Jarvis, J.A. and Hempel, J.M. (1968). Cytogenic evaluation of 41 patients with Stein–Leventhal syndrome. *Obstetrics and Gynecology* **32**, 794–801.

Talbot, J.A., Bicknell, E.J., Rajkhowa, M. et al. (1996). Molecular scanning of the insulin receptor gene in women with polycystic ovary syndrome. *Journal of Clinical Endocrinology and Metabolism* **81**, 1979–83.

Taylor, S.I., Cana, A., Accili, D. et al. (1992). Mutations in the insulin receptor gene. *Endocrine Review* **13**, 566–95.

Techatraisak, K., Conway, G.S. and Rumsby, G. (1997). Frequency of a polymorphism in the regulatory region of the 17α-hydroxylase-17,20-lyase (CYP17) gene in hyperandrogenic states. *Clinical Endocrinology* **46**, 131–4.

Urbanek, M., Legro, R.S., Driscoll, D.A. et al. (1999). Thirty-seven candidate genes for polycystic ovary syndrome: strongest evidence for linkage is with follistatin. *Proceedings of the National Academy of Sciences, USA* **96**, 8573–8.

Virkamaki, A., Ueki, K. and Kahn, K.R. (1999). Protein–protein interaction in insulin signaling and the molecular mechanisms of insulin resistance. *Journal of Clinical Investigation* **103**, 931–43.

Waterworth, D.M., Bennett, S.T., Gharani, N. et al. (1997). Linkage and association of insulin gene VNTR regulatory polymorphism with polycystic ovary syndrome. *Lancet* **349**, 986–90.

Willis, D. and Franks, S. (1995). Insulin action in human granulosa cells from normal and polycystic ovaries is mediated by the insulin receptor and not the type-I insulin-like growth factor receptor. *Journal of Clinical Endocrinology and Metabolism* **80**, 3788–90.

Willis, D., Mason, H., Gilling-Smith, C. and Franks, S. (1996). Modulation by insulin of follicle-stimulating hormone and luteinizing hormone actions in human granulosa cells of normal and polycystic ovaries. *Journal of Clinical Endocrinology and Metabolism* **81**, 302–9.

Witchel, S.F., Lee, P.A., Suda-Hartman, M. Smith, R. and Hoffman, E.P. (1998). 17α-hydroxylase/17,20-lyase disregulation is not caused by mutations in the coding regions of CYP17. *Journal of Pediatric and Adolescent Gynecology* **11**, 133–7.

Zhang, Y., Word, R.A., Fesmire, S., Carr, B.R. and Rainey, W.E. (1996). Human ovarian expression of 17β-hydroxysteroid dehydrogenase types 1, 2, and 3. *Journal of Clinical Endocrinology and Metabolism* **81**, 3594–8.

5

The pathology of polycystic ovary syndrome

Andrew G. Östör

Introduction

Although the condition of polycystic ovaries has been known for a long time (see Chapter 2), it achieved prominence as a result of the seminal article by Stein and Leventhal in 1935 and for many years was referred to as the Stein–Leventhal syndrome. Given the efflux of time and a concerted effort to discourage eponyms (Östör and Phillips, 1999), the condition became known as polycystic ovary syndrome (PCOS).

Polycystic ovary syndrome is a clinicopathological syndrome characterized by anovulation or infrequent ovulation, obesity, hirsutism, and numerous follicular cysts in both ovaries, which are usually enlarged (Yen, 1980; Scully, Young and Clement, 1998). The finding of polycystic ovaries (PCO), however, does not, *per se*, warrant such a diagnosis. Polycystic ovaries are, in fact, more common in otherwise normal women without the syndrome (unpublished observation). This contention is supported by ultrasonographic studies which have revealed an overlap between women with PCOS and overt clinical manifestations of the syndrome and those with multiple follicular cysts associated with menstrual irregularity or evidence of hyperandrogenism so minor that they considered themselves normal (Adams, Polson and Franks, 1986). In other studies of 'normal' women, more than 20% had polycystic ovaries on ultrasound (Polson et al., 1988; Clayton et al., 1992). Thus, the boundary between the clinical syndrome associated with PCO and normality is blurred.

Macroscopic features

Typically, both ovaries, rarely one (Futterweit, 1985), are rounded and enlarged. In one study the ovarian volume of women with PCOS was three times that of controls (Delahunt et al. 1975; Lunde, Hoel and Sandvik, 1988). Occasionally, the ovaries are of normal size (Smith, Steinberger and Perloff, 1965). Classically, the surface of the ovaries is oyster-white, giving the appearance of a true capsule (Fig.

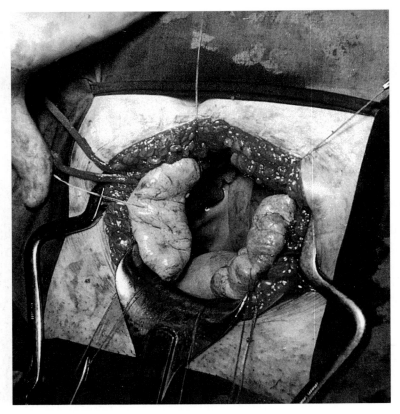

Fig. 5.1   Intraoperative photograph showing enlarged, rounded ovaries with an oyster-white appearance.

5.1). Small cysts are visible under the surface, where they appear as sago-like bodies. Sectioning reveals a thickened, white, superficial cortex and the presence of numerous cystic follicles, usually less than 10 mm in size (Fig. 5.2), near the surface, while the central portion consists of homogenous stroma with only rare or no stigmata of ovulation, e.g. corpora lutea or albicantes (Green and Goldzieher, 1965; Biggs, 1981).

Microscopic features

The thickened cortex is hypocellular, fibrotic, sclerosed and contains primordial follicles which appear 'entrapped'. The latter, however, are normal in number and morphology (Fig. 5.3). Thick-walled blood vessels may also be seen (Goldzieher and Green, 1962; Hughesdon, 1982). Tongues of similarly fibrotic stroma may extend into the deeper cortex. The cystic follicles are typically lined by several layers

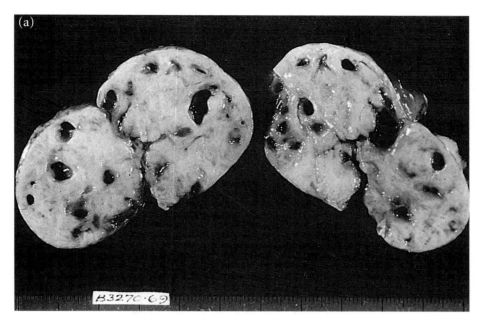

Figs 5.2a   The cut surface of the ovary displays numerous, small peripheral cysts set in a fibrous stroma. The cortex is thickened and appears sclerosed.

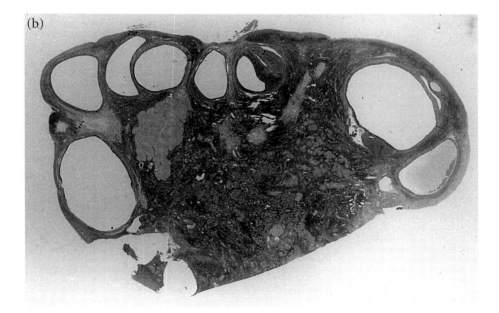

Fig. 5.2b   Whole-mount section of a polycystic ovary showing numerous follicular cysts. (Note the absence of a corpus luteum; the presence of a corpus albicans is unusual.)

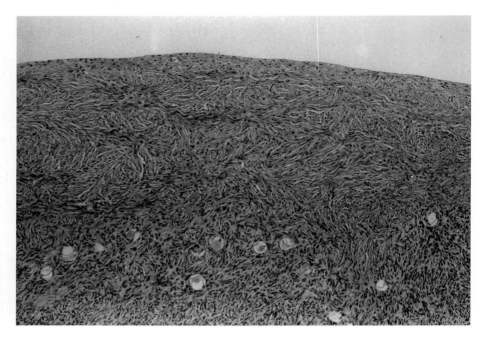

Fig. 5.3   Microphotograph showing a thickened and sclerosed cortical stroma containing 'entrapped' primordial follicles.

of non-luteinized granulosa cells (Fig. 5.4) that may have focally exfoliated. An outer layer of luteinized theca interna cells is sometimes referred to as 'follicular hyperthecosis'. It should be stressed that cystic follicles in patients with PCOS differ from those in normal women only in their increased number (Green and Goldzieher, 1965; Lunde et al., 1988). In fact, a doubling of ripening follicles and subsequent atretic follicles are generally seen.

It may be appropriate to define the various forms of follicular development at this point. The terms *primordial*, *primary*, *secondary* and *tertiary follicle* refer respectively to follicles with a single layer of flat granulosa cells, a single layer of cuboidal granulosa cells, two or more layers of granulosa cells without an antrum, and the same with an antrum, regardless of size. The terms *tertiary*, *antral* and *graafian* follicles are used interchangeably, whilst a *cystic follicle* refers to macroscopically visible forms without implying abnormality (Hughesdon, 1982). The deeper cortical and medullary stroma may have up to a five-fold increase in volume and may contain luteinized stromal cells and foci of smooth muscle. Nests of hilus (Leydig) cells may be more numerous in patients with PCOS than in age-matched controls (Hughesdon, 1982). As noted, stigmata of prior ovulation are typically absent, but corpora lutea have been reported in up to 30% of cases in some series

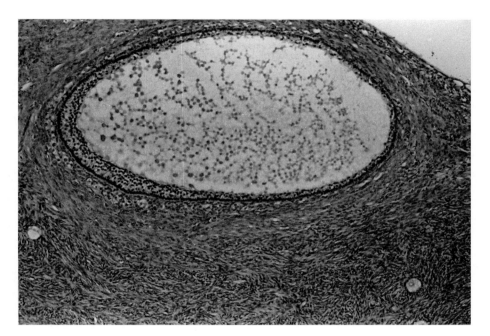

Fig. 5.4   Microphotograph of the lining of a follicular cyst. Note that the wall is composed of an inner layer of non-luteinized granulosa cells and an outer layer of luteinized theca cells.

(Green and Goldzieher, 1965; Hughesdon, 1982). Examination of only a few sections of wedge biopsies often fails to reveal diagnostic features.

The endometrium in patients with PCOS may show weakly proliferative features, simple hyperplasia, atypical hyperplasia or, in less than 5 per cent of cases, adenocarcinoma, which is almost always low grade (Case Records of the Massachusetts General Hospital, Case 23, 1966; Coulam, Annegers and Krans, 1983).

Differential diagnosis

Polycystic ovaries may be encountered in prepubertal children, in otherwise normal girls in the first few years after the onset of puberty (Merrill, 1963), in girls in the second decade with primary hypothyroidism (Lindsay, Voorhess and Macgillivray, 1980), adrenal hyperplasia (Benedict et al., 1962; Goldzieher,1981; Chrousos et al., 1982), autoimmune oophoritis (Bannatyne, Russell and Shearman, 1990), after long-term use of oral contraceptives (Plate, 1967), in association with peri-ovarian adhesions (Quan, Charles and Craig, 1963) and after long-term androgen therapy in female to male transsexuals (Pache et al., 1991). It seems likely, however, that these conditions are coincidental.

Another condition to be considered in the differential diagnosis is stromal hyperthecosis, which some authorities feel represents one end of the spectrum of PCOS (Givens, 1977). In this disorder, luteinized cells are scattered singly and in small nests or nodules throughout a typically hyperplastic ovarian stroma (Scully et al., 1998). Although there is a fair degree of overlap clinically between the two, the pathological features are sufficiently different not to pose a major diagnostic difficulty.

REFERENCES

Adams, J., Polson, D.W. and Franks, S. (1986). Prevalence of polycystic ovaries in women with anovulation and idiopathic hirsutism. *British Medical Journal* **293**, 355–9.

Bannatyne, P., Russell, P. and Shearman, R.P. (1990). Autoimmune oophoritis: a clinicopathologic assessment of 12 cases. *International Journal of Gynecological Pathology* **9**, 191–207.

Benedict, P.H., Cohen, R., Cope, O. et al. (1962). Ovarian and adrenal morphology in cases of hirsutism or virilism and Stein–Leventhal syndrome. *Fertility and Sterility* **13**, 380–95.

Biggs, J.S.G. (1981). Polycystic ovarian disease – current concepts. *Australian and New Zealand Journal of Obstetrics and Gynaecology* **21**, 26–36.

Case Records of the Massachusetts General Hospital, Case 23 (1966). *New England Journal of Medicine* **274**, 1139–45.

Chrousos, G.P., Loriaux, L., Mann, D.L. et al. (1982). Late onset 21-hydroxylase deficiency mimicking idiopathic hirsutism or polycystic ovarian disease. *Annals of Internal Medicine* **96**, 143–8.

Clayton, R.N., Ogden, V., Hodgkinson, J. et al. (1992). How common are polycystic ovaries in normal women and what is their significance for the fertility of the population? *Clinical Endocrinology* **37**, 127–34.

Coulam, C.B., Annegers, J.F. and Kranz, J.S. (1983). Chronic anovulation syndrome and associated neoplasia. *Obstetrics and Gynecology* **61**, 403–7.

Delahunt, J.W., Clements, R.V., Ramsay, I.D. et al. (1975). The monocystic ovary syndrome. *British Medical Journal* **4**, 621–2.

Futterweit, W. (1985). *Polycystic Ovarian Disease. Clinical Perspectives in Obstetrics and Gynecology.* New York: Springer-Verlag.

Givens, J.R. (1977). Polycystic ovarian disease. In *Gynecologic Endocrinology*, ed. J.R. Givens, pp. 127–42. Chicago: Year Book.

Goldzieher, J.W. (1981). Polycystic ovarian disease. *Fertility and Sterility* **35**, 371–94.

Goldzieher, J.W. and Green, J.A. (1962). The polycystic ovary. I. Clinical and histologic features. *Journal of Clinical Endocrinology and Metabolism* **22**, 325–38.

Green, J.A. and Goldzieher, J.W. (1965). The polycystic ovary. IV. Light and electron microscope studies. *American Journal of Obstetrics and Gynecology* **91**, 173–81.

Hughesdon, P.E. (1982). Morphology and morphogenesis of the Stein–Leventhal ovary and of so-called 'hyperthecosis'. *Obstetrical and Gynecological Survey* **37**, 59–77.

Lindsay, A.N., Voorhess, M.L. and MacGillivray, M.H. (1980). Multicystic ovaries detected by sonography in children with hypothyroidism. *American Journal of Diseases of Children* **134**, 588–92.

Lunde, O., Hoel, P.S. and Sandvik, L. (1988). Ovarian morphology in patients with polycystic ovaries and in an age-matched reference material. *Gynecologic Obstetric Investigation* **25**, 192–201.

Merrill, J.A. (1963). The morphology of the prepubertal ovary: relationship to the polycystic ovary syndrome. *Southern Medical Journal* **56**, 225–31.

Östör, A.G. and Phillips, G.E. (1999). Immortal women: essays in medical eponyms: *American Journal of Surgical Pathology* **23**, 495–501.

Pache, T.D., Chadha, S., Gooren, L.J.G. et al. (1991). Ovarian morphology in long-term androgen-treated female to male transsexuals. A human model for the study of polycystic ovarian syndrome? *Histopathology* **19**, 445–52.

Plate, W.P. (1967). Ovarian changes after long-term oral contraception. *Acta Endocrinologica* **55**, 71–7.

Polson, D.W., Wadsworth, J., Adams, J. et al. (1988). Polycystic ovaries – a common finding in normal women. *Lancet* **ii**, 870–2.

Quan, A., Charles, D. and Craig, J.M. (1963). Histologic and functional consequences of peri-ovarian adhesions. *Obstetrics and Gynecology* **22**, 96–101.

Scully, R.E., Young, R.H. and Clement, P.B. (1998). Tumors of the ovary, maldeveloped gonads, fallopian tube, and broad ligament. In *Atlas of Tumor Pathology*, Third Series, Fascicle 23, pp. 409–50. Washington DC: Armed Forces Institute of Pathology.

Smith, K.D., Steinberger, E. and Perloff, W.H. (1965). Polycystic ovarian disease: a report of 301 patients. *American Journal of Obstetrics and Gynecology* **93**, 994–1001.

Stein, I.F. and Leventhal, M.L. (1935). Amenorrhea associated with bilateral polycystic ovaries. *American Journal of Obstetrics and Gynecology* **29**, 181–91.

Yen, S.S.C. (1980). The polycystic ovary syndrome. *Clinical Endocrinology* **12**, 177–207.

6

Imaging polycystic ovaries

Yann Robert, Yves Ardaens and Didier Dewailly

Introduction

In clinical practice, ultrasonography has replaced the laparoscopic evaluation of polycystic ovaries (PCO). With the advent of transvaginal endosonography, not only the size and the shape of ovaries are visualizable but also their internal structure, namely follicles and stroma. It is now possible to get pictures that have a definition close to anatomical cuts.

The main histological features of PCO are presented in Table 6.1: the volume of PCO is often exaggerated and the ovaries tend to be spherical instead of ovoidal. This is due to the increased thickness of the ovarian cortex, whose stroma is hyperplastic and fibrotic, and whose number of antral follicles (2–6 mm in diameter) is excessive (Goldzieher and Green, 1962).

Ultrasonography

The transabdominal versus the transvaginal route

Our opinion is that the transabdominal route should always be the first step of pelvic sonographic examination, followed by the transvaginal route, except in virgin and in those refusing the transvaginal route. The main advantage of this route is that it offers a panoramic view of the pelvic cavity. Therefore, it allows the exclusion of associated uterine or ovarian abnormalities with an abdominal development. Indeed, lesions with cranial growth could be missed by using the transvaginal approach exclusively. A sagittal examination allows for the location of the uterus and measurement of its length and thickness. A transverse examination from the cervix to the fundus allows for measurement of its width. A probe translation is then laterally performed from the top of the uterine cavity to the iliac vessels, searching for the ovaries. A full bladder is required for visualization of the ovaries. However, one should be aware that an overfilled bladder can compress the ovaries, yielding a falsely increased length. This emphasizes the need for assessing the ovarian size by measuring the area or the volume (see below) and by repeating

Table 6.1. Histological features of polycystic ovary syndrome

Whole ovarian hypertrophy
Thickened capsule ($>100\ \mu$)
Increased number of subcapsular follicle cysts
Scarcity of corporea lutea or albicantia
Hyperplasia and fibrosis of the ovarian stroma
Decreased thickness of the granulosa layer
Atretic pattern of the granulosa layer
Increased thickness of the theca interna
Premature luteinization of theca cells

Source: From Goldzieher and Green (1962).

the measurement after partial micturition. If not found between the uterus and the iliac vessels, the ovaries must be searched for upwards, in the iliac fossa more or less close to the abdominal wall, or downwards and backwards in the pouch of Douglas. Locating the ovaries before transvaginal examination is always helpful and makes the examination easier.

The major drawback of the transabdominal route is the poor spatial resolution of the low-frequency probes (3–4 MHz), making it difficult to assess the inner echostructure of the ovaries (presence of small follicles, number and size), especially in patients with a fatty abdominal wall. Indeed, the transvaginal approach gives a more accurate view of the internal structure, avoiding apparently homogeneous ovaries as seen with transabdominal scans, particularly in obese patients. With the transvaginal route, high-frequency probes (>6 MHz) with a better spatial resolution but less examination depth can be used because the ovaries are close to the vagina and/or the uterus and because the presence of fatty tissue is usually less of a problem (except when very abundant). Hull (1989) found that transabdominal sonography was inadequate for the diagnosis of PCO in 40% of cases, whereas the transvaginal approach greatly improved the accuracy, allowing the number and size of the follicles to be estimated.

How polycystic ovaries differ from normal and multifollicular ovaries

Multifollicular ovaries (MFO) are encountered in different physiological and pathological situations, such as mid-late normal puberty, central precocious puberty, hypothalamic anovulation, hyperprolactinaemia and, most importantly, the early normal follicular phase in adult women before one follicle among the cohort becomes dominant. They represent an important ultrasonographic differential diagnosis for PCO (Adams et al., 1985). Theoretically, PCO differ from normal ovaries and from MFO by being larger, more follicular and having a stromal

Table 6.2. Ultrasonic criteria used for the diagnosis of polycystic ovary syndrome

External morphological signs
Increased ovarian area or volume
Increased roundness index (ovarian width/ovarian length ratio)
Decreased uterine width/ovarian length ratio (U/O)

Internal morphological signs
Number of small echoless regions < 10 mm in size per ovary (microcysts)
Peripheral repartition of microcysts
Increased echogenicity of ovarian stroma
Increased surface of the ovarian stroma on a cross-sectional cut (by computerized measure)

Note:
See Ardaens et al. (1991) and Robert et al. (1995) for critical review of threshold and diagnostic values.

hypertrophy (Table 6.2). However, in practice, these differences were more or less clear, mainly for technical reasons.

In the early stages of its use in the 1970s, the weak resolution of ultrasonography only enabled it to detect the external morphological signs of PCO:

The length, the upper limit of which is 4 cm, is the simplest criterion, but this uni-dimensional approach may lead false-positive results when a full bladder compresses the ovary (with the transabdominal route) or false-negative results when the ovaries are spherical, with a relatively short length.

Because of the increased ovarian size and the normal uterine width, the uterine width: ovarian length ratio is decreased (<1) in PCOS.

PCOS often display a more spherical shape. This morphological change can be evaluated by the sphericity index (ovarian width:ovarian length), which is more than 0.7 in PCO.

These parameters are less used nowadays because of their low sensitivity (Ardaens et al., 1991).

The ovarian area is still used and has the advantage of being a physical entity which can be measured in real-time conditions. However, evaluation of the ovarian size via the transvaginal approach is difficult. To be most accurate, it requires careful selection of the picture in which the ovary appears longest and widest. This picture must then be frozen. Two means can be proposed for calculating the ovarian area: either fitting an ellipse to the ovary, the area calculation being done by the machine, or outlining the ovary by hand and automatically calculating the outlined area. This last technique is preferable in cases of non-ellipsoid ovaries, as sometimes observed. In the authors' experience with a large control group, the sum of the areas of both ovaries area is less than 11 cm^2 in normal women and in MFO

(Dewailly et al., 1994). Beyond this threshold, the diagnosis of PCO can be suggested. Measurement of the volume is another approach. The volume of the ovaries can be estimated after measurement of the length, width and thickness and use of the classical formula $L \times W \times T \times 0.523$. However, the ovaries have to be studied in three orthogonal planes, which are not easy to obtain: are the planes definitely orthogonals? From the recent experience of others (Fauser and van Santbrink, 1996), the normal ovarian volume is now considered to be 4–11 cm³. However, the use of ovarian hypertrophy (either increased area or volume) as a diagnostic sign for PCOS yielded varying results, for several reasons. First, the accuracy of this method depends on the skill and the accuracy of the ultrasonographer. The main difficulty is in obtaining strictly longitudinal ovarian cuts, which is an absolute condition for accurate measurement of the ovarian axis (length, width, thickness). The inaccuracy results from selection of an inadequate plane (not the longest and the widest) and the difficulty in outlining the ovarian shape. Second, the upper normal threshold was different from one study to another, depending on the size and selection of the control population used for normative data (Table 6.3). As an example, the ovarian area was previously considered as normal up to 10 cm² (Orsini, Venturoli and Lorusso, 1985; El Tabbakh et al., 1986; Table 6.3), whereas our more recent experience with a large control group has led us to reassess this figure, making it almost two times lower (5.5 cm²) (Robert et al., 1995) (see below). Likewise, the upper normal limit of the ovarian volume suffers from some variability in the literature (Pache et al., 1992; Yeh, Futterweit and Thornton, 1987; Fauser and van Santbrink, 1996; Table 6.3). Lastly, the prevalence of ovarian hypertrophy might have been overestimated in some series in which the most typical cases of PCOS were preferentially included. With the improved resolution of transvaginal ultrasonography in the 1980s, it became possible to analyse reliably the internal structure of PCO (see Table 6.2).

The polyfollicular pattern (i.e. excessive number of small echoless regions less than 10 mm in diameter) is strongly suggestive, because it is in perfect accord with the name of the syndrome (i.e. 'polycystic'). In PCOS, the follicle distribution is predominantly peripheral, with typically an echoless peripheral array, as initially described by Adams et al. (1985; Figs. 6.1 and 6.2). In some studies (Bataglia et al., 1998), younger patients displayed this peripheral distribution more often, whereas a more generalized pattern, with small cysts in the central part of the ovary, was noticed in older women. By definition, the polyfollicular pattern is also observed in MFO. Therefore, there is a significant risk of false-positive results when only the polyfollicular pattern is taken in account. Theoretically, the polyfollicular pattern is different in PCO and MFO. In the former, the follicle number per ovarian cut is higher, but there is considerable controversy about the cut-off value between MFO and PCO (>5?, >10?, >15?). In MFO, follicles seem to be randomly scattered

Table 6.3. Summary of the results of some ultrasound studies in the literature

References	Ultrasound route[a]	Ultrasonic criteria	Criteria indicative of PCO when:	Patients with clinical PCOS phenotype having the criteria (%)	Controls having the criteria (%)	Number of studied patients	Number of studied controls
Yeh et al. (1987)	TA	Ovarian volume	>10 cm³	70	0	108	25
		Number of follicles 5–8 mm in size	>5	74	11	68	18
		Roundness index (ovarian width/ovarian length)	>1	7	6	100	24
Pache et al. (1992)	TV	Ovarian volume	>8 cm³	About 70	0	52	29
		Number of follicles >6 mm	>11	About 50	0	52	29
		Mean follicular size	<4	About 70	7	52	29
		Increased echogenicity of ovarian stroma	Present	94	10	52	29
Robert et al. (1995)	TV	Increased stromal area (by computerized measure)	>7.6 cm² (sum of both ovaries)	61	4	69	48
		Increased total ovarian area	>10.8 cm² (sum of both ovaries)	55	2	69	48

Notes:

[a] TA, transabdominal route; TV, transvaginal route.

The table illustrates the difficulty of making comparisons about some criteria whose thresholds were different (e.g. number of follicles). Likewise, the observation of an abnormal ovarian stroma was purely visual in one study (Pache et al., 1992), whereas it was quantified in another (Robert et al., 1995). Furthermore, patient and control populations were not similarly recruited.

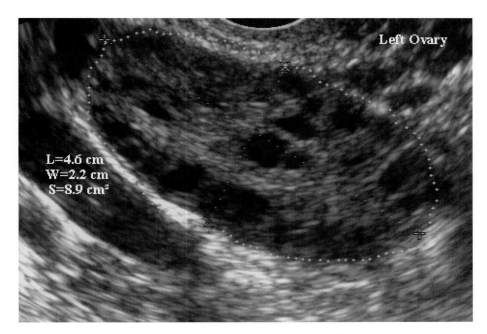

Fig. 6.1   Polycystic ovary (B mode). The ovarian length (4.6 cm) and width (2.2 cm) are increased as well as the ovarian area (8.9 cm²). The follicle number, with a diameter between 2 and 5 mm, is more than ten. The distribution within the ovary is mainly peripheral, but some follicles can be seen in the central part of the ovary.

throughout the ovaries. However, this analysis is purely qualitative. In many cases, the estimation of the polyfollicular pattern is confusing and does not permit clear differentiation between MFO and PCO. Furthermore, its reproducibility and operator dependency have never been determined.

The increased stroma helps to differentiate PCO from MFO. Stromal hypertrophy is characterized by an increased component of the ovarian central part, which is somewhat hyperechoic (Fig. 6.2). In our (Ardaens et al., 1991; Dewailly et al., 1994) and in others' opinion (Pache et al., 1992), stromal hypertrophy and hyperechogenicity are the most reliable ultrasonographic signs to distinguish between PCO and MFO because these features are specific to the former (see below). However, the estimation of hyperechogenicity is considered to be highly subjective, mainly because it depends on the settings of the ultrasound machine. Likewise, in the absence of a precise quantification, stromal hypertrophy is also a subjective sign. This prompted us to design a computerized quantification of ovarian stroma, allowing selective calculation of the stromal area by subtraction of the cyst area from the total ovarian area on a longitudinal ovarian cut (Dewailly et al., 1994; Robert et al., 1995). By this means, it was possible to set the upper normal

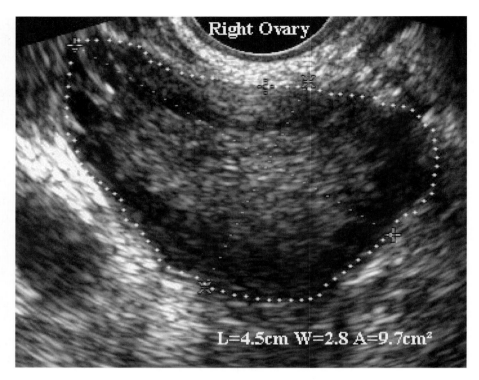

Fig. 6.2   Polycystic ovary (B mode). The ovarian length (4.5 cm) and width (2.8 cm) and the outlined area (9.7 cm²) are increased. The small follicles (2–4 mm) display a typical peripheral pattern, around the hyperechoic stroma.

limit of the stromal area (i.e. 95th percentile of a large control group of 48 normal women) at 380 mm² per ovary. In this study, the diagnostic value of the total ovarian area was also reconsidered. Providing a precise outlining of the ovarian shape on a strictly longitudinal cut of the ovaries, it appeared that it was highly correlated to the stromal area, and values above 5.5 cm² (95th percentile of controls) for at least one ovarian area were found exclusively in patients with the clinical phenotype of PCOS. Therefore, it is not necessary to computerize the ultrasonographic data for clinical practice; we would recommend the use of the total ovarian area, which can be easily and reliably recorded either by the transabdominal or transvaginal route as many ultrasound machines now contain software to determine the area of an outlined structure (Fig. 6.2).

Sensitivity and specificity of ultrasonographic features of polycystic ovaries

Using ultrasonography, the percentages of patients with a clinical phenotype of PCOS and polycystic ovaries have varied between 50% and 100%. Differences in technical procedures and non-consensual use of ultrasound criteria for PCO mainly explain this variability in the results. The stringency of the latter has been variable and they did not always rely on quantitative measures. Differences in the definition of the clinical and/or biological phenotypes of PCOS may also explain the discrepancies concerning the prevalence of morphological features of PCO in the syndrome. Conversely, in a large series of ultrasonographically selected patients, clinical and endocrine features of PCOS were heterogeneous and inconsistent (Conway, Honour and Jacobs, 1989). However, no major difference was found between the clinical and hormonal data from patient populations selected either by ultrasound alone or without sonographic data (Franks, 1995). Comparison between morphological and ultrasonographic features of PCO is scarce in the literature (Saxton et al., 1990; Takahashi et al., 1994) for the obvious reasons that ovarian biopsies are now regarded as useless and, more importantly, unethical because they expose patients to the risk of pelvic adhesions. As a consequence, no gold standard is available to assess the specificity and sensitivity of ultra-sonography.

To address this complicated issue, we designed a biomathematical protocol using cluster analysis (this should not be confused with the cluster methods that have been used for the analysis of luteinizing hormone (LH) pulsatility) (Dewailly et al., 1993). This biomathematical procedure differs from the classical statistical methods in that it does not require grouping of patients according to arbitrarily chosen parameters, whose thresholds are set arbitrarily. This method helped us to recognize PCOS in a mixed population of women with different causes of anovu-lation and/or hyperandrogenism (i.e. PCOS, hyperprolactinaemia, hypothalamic anovulation, idiopathic hirsutism and miscellaneous aetiologies). Among a set of hormonal and ultrasonographic signs of PCOS, increased ovarian stroma appeared to be the most potent parameter for grouping patients in biomathematically homo-geneous clusters. Its grouping potency exceeded those of elevated serum testo-sterone and androstenedione levels as well as of polyfollicular pattern, which gave intermediate results, while the elevated serum basal LH was a much weaker group-ing parameter. In this analysis, the polyfollicular pattern was found in 31% of the patients who were grouped by the computer in a 'non-PCOS' group. Retrospective analysis revealed that this group was mainly constituted of patients with hyper-prolactinaemia and hypothalamic anovulation. An increased ovarian stroma was found in 61% of the patients with a clinical phenotype of PCOS and in any patient with MFO in relation with a hypothalamic anovulation (Robert et al., 1995). These data emphasize the necessity of choosing specific ultrasound signs (e.g. abnormal ovarian stroma), even if their sensitivity is not optimal, rather than to more sensi-tive signs with less specificity that can be observed in other diseases (e.g. polyfollic-ular pattern, which actually applies to MFO as well as to PCO). In practice, measurement of the ovarian area or volume is a good alternative to the quantification of the stroma (see above), providing that normal data are thoroughly established.

Magnetic resonance imaging

Data about magnetic resonance imaging (MRI) for PCO are still scarce in the literature (Maubon et al., 1993; Kimura et al., 1996; Woodward and Gilfeather, 1998). This techique allows a multiplanar approach to the pelvic cavity, which helps to localize the ovaries. Imaging quality is improved by the use of a pelvic-dedicated phased-array coil receiver. The most useful planes are the transverse and coronal views. The T2-weighted sequence is best suited to the ovarian morphology. With this sequence, the follicular fluid displays a hypersignal (white) and the solid component (stroma) a low signal (black). T1-weighted sequences offer less information, but the gadolinium injection allows one to study the stromal vascularization. The fat saturation technique increases the contrast obtained after the medium uptake by the vascularized areas.

The external signs of PCO (see above) are easy to analyse on MRI transverse sections (Fig. 6.3). In addition, the T2-weighted sequence displays the excessive number of follicles, but their detection and numbering are less easy than with ultrasonography, because of the poor spatial resolution of MRI, unless high magnetic fields are used (1 to 1.5 Tesla). As with ultrasonography, stromal hypertrophy remains a subjective observation, although it is obvious in many cases. After gadolinium injection, there is a high uptake by the stroma, suggesting that it is highly vascularized in PCO.

In most cases, in practice, MRI does not provide more information than ultrasonography for the imaging of PCO (Kimura et al., 1996). It is only helpful in difficult situations such as severe hyperandrogenism, when ultrasonography is either not possible or unhelpful (virgin or obese patients, respectively). Its main role is to exclude a virilizing ovarian tumour, which should be suspected when the ovarian volume is not symmetrical and/or when there is a circumscribed signal abnormality, either before or after gadolinium injection. PCO associated with an ovarian tumour might be a pitfall.

Other techniques and future developments

Three-dimensional approach

To avoid the difficulties and pitfalls in outlining or measuring ovarian shape, three-dimensional ultrasonography has been proposed using a dedicated volumic probe or a manual survey of the ovary (Kyei-Mensah, Zaidi and Campbell, 1996; Wu et

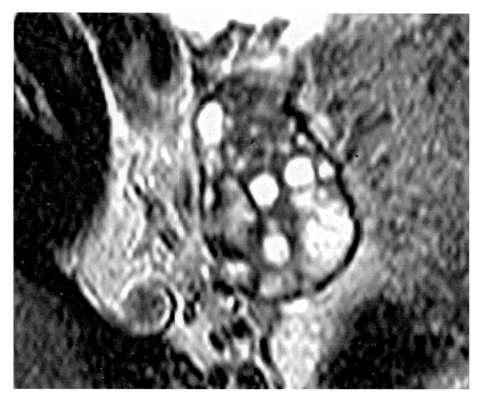

Fig. 6.3   Polycystic ovary syndrome: magnetic resonance after gadolinium injection.

al., 1998). From the stored data, the scanned ovarian volume is displayed on the screen in three adjustable orthogonal planes, allowing the three dimensions and subsequently the volume to be more accurately evaluated.

Doppler ultrasonography

The assessment of uterine arteries is not addressed in this chapter, which is exclusively devoted to PCO imaging. Colour (or power) Doppler allows detection of the vascularization network within the ovarian stroma. Power Doppler is more sensitive to the slow flows and shows more vascular signals within the ovaries, but it does not discriminate between arteries and veins (Fig. 6.4). Moreover, the sensitivity of different machines is variable. The pulsed Doppler focuses on the hilum or internal ovarian arteries and offers a more objective approach. Because of the slow flows, the pulse repetition frequency is at minimum (400 Hz) with the lowest frequency filter (50 Hz) (Fig. 6.5).

The study of ovarian vascularization by these techniques is still highly subjective. The blood flow is more frequently visualized in PCOS (88%) than in normal

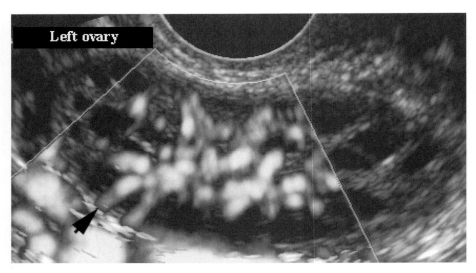

Fig. 6.4   Polycystic ovary: power Doppler. The high sensitivity of power Doppler allows depiction of flow in small vessels, magnifying the increased vascularization in the stroma. In this case, a radiating pattern was observed, with vessels between the small follicles.

patients (50%) in the early follicular phase and seems to be increased (Bataglia et al., 1996). No significant difference was found between obese and lean women with PCOS, but the stroma was less vascularized in patients displaying a general cystic pattern than in those with peripheral cysts. In the latter, the pulsatility index (PI) values were significantly lower and inversely correlated to the follicle stimulating hormone (FSH)/LH ratio. In another study (Aleem and Predanic, 1996), the resistive index (RI) and PI were significantly lower in PCOS (RI = 0.55 ± 0.01 and PI = 0.89 ± 0.04) than in normal patients (RI = $0.78 + 0.06$ and PI = $1.87 + 0.38$) and the peak systolic velocity was greater in PCOS ($11.9 + 3.2$) than in normal women ($9.6 + 2.1$). No correlation was found between the number of follicles and the ovarian volume, but there was a positive correlation between LH levels and increased peak systolic velocity. In Zaidi et al.'s (1995) study, no significant difference in PI values was found between the normal and PCOS groups, while the ovarian flow, as reflected by the peak systolic velocity, was increased in the former.

To summarize, the increased stroma component in PCOS seems to be accompanied by a higher visualization, as reflected by an increased peak systolic velocity and a decreased PI. However, in all these different studies, values in PCOS patients overlapped widely with those of the normal patients. No data so far support any diagnostic usefulness of Doppler ultrasonography in PCO. However, recent data indicate that it could have some value in predicting the risk for ovarian hyperstimulation during gonadotrophin treatment (Agrawal et al., 1998).

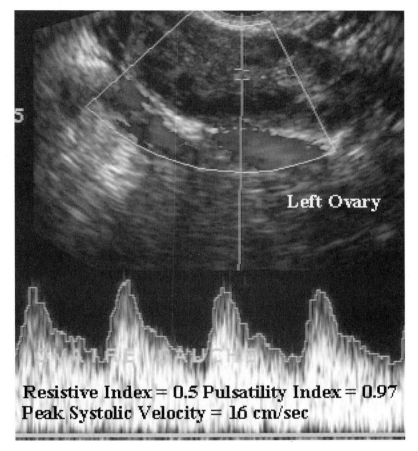

Left Ovary

Resistive Index = 0.5 Pulsatility Index = 0.97
Peak Systolic Velocity = 16 cm/sec

Fig. 6.5   Polycystic ovary: colour and pulsed Doppler. The arterial flow is more easily depicted in
PCOS than in normal ovary, displaying low resistance indexes.

Conclusions

The ultrasonographic study of PCOS has now left its era of artistic haziness. It must
be viewed as a diagnostic tool which requires the same quality controls as a biological one, such as the plasma LH assay. This supposes that its results are expressed as
quantitative variables rather than as purely descriptive data. This also requires that
the normal ranges of these variables are thoroughly established from a carefully
sized and selected control population. Lastly, it can be used by the clinician only if
the ultrasonographer is sufficiently trained and his or her results are reproducible.
By its sensitivity (providing that enough specificity is guaranteed), ultrasonography has widened the clinical spectrum of PCOS, a good number of cases being

almost asymptomatic and detected by chance. Widening this spectrum has also reduced the number of cases of idiopathic hirsutism and idiopathic anovulation.

REFERENCES

Adams, J.M., Polson, D.W., Abulwadi, N. et al. (1985). Multifollicular ovaries: clinical and endocrine features and response to pulsatile gonadotropin-releasing hormone. *Lancet* 2, 1375–8.

Agrawal, R., Conway, G., Sladkevicius, P. et al. (1998). Serum vascular endothelial growth factor and Doppler blood flow velocities in in vitro fertilization: relevance to ovarian hyperstimulation syndrome and polycystic ovaries. *Fertility and Sterility* 70, 651–8.

Aleem, F.A. and Predanic, M.P. (1996). Transvaginal color Doppler determination of the ovarian and uterine blood flow characteristics in polycystic ovary disease. *Fertility and Sterility* 65, 510–16.

Ardaens, Y., Robert, Y., Lemaitre, L., Fossati, P. and Dewailly, D. (1991). Polycystic ovarian disease: contribution of vaginal endosonography and reassessment of ultrasonic diagnosis. *Fertility and Sterility* 55, 1062–8.

Bataglia, C., Artini, P.G., Genazzani, A.D. et al. (1996). Color Doppler analysis in lean and obese women with polycystic ovaries. *Ultrasound in Gynaecology and Obstetrics* 7, 342–6.

Bataglia, C., Artini, P.G., Salvatori, M. et al. (1998). Ultrasonographic pattern of polycystic ovaries: color Doppler and hormonal correlations. *Ultrasound in Gynaecology and Obstetrics* 11, 332–6.

Conway, G.S., Honour, J.W. and Jacobs, H.S. (1989). Heterogeneity of the polycystic ovary syndrome: clinical, endocrine and ultrasound features in 556 patients. *Clinical Endocrinology* 30, 459–70.

Dewailly, D., Duhamel, A., Robert, Y. et al. (1993). Interrelationship between ultrasonography and biology in the diagnosis of polycystic ovarian disease. *Annals of New York Academy of Sciences* 687, 206–16.

Dewailly, D., Robert, Y., Helin, I. et al. (1994). Ovarian stromal hypertrophy in hyperandrogenic women. *Clinical Endocrinology* 41, 557–62.

El Tabbakh, G. H., Lotfy, I., Azab, I. et al. (1986). Correlation of the ultrasonic appearance of the ovaries in polycystic ovarian disease and the clinical, hormonal, and laparoscopic findings. *American Journal of Obstetrics and Gynecology* 154, 892–5.

Fauser, B.C.J.M. and van Santbrink, E.J.P. (1996). Sonographic characteristics of PCO: sensitivity and specificity. In *The Ovary: Regulation, Dysfunction and Treatment*, ed. M. Filicori and C.Flamigni, pp. 303–9. Amsterdam: Elsevier Science.

Franks, S. (1995). Polycystic ovary syndrome. *New England Journal of Medicine* 333, 853–61.

Goldzieher, M.W. and Green, J. A. (1962). The polycystic ovary. I. Clinical and histologic features. *Journal of Clinical Endocrinology and Metabolism* 22, 325–38.

Hull, M.G.R. (1989). Polycystic ovary disease: clinical aspects and prevalence. *Research Clinical Forums* 11, 21–34.

Kimura, I., Togashi, K., Kawakami, S. et al. (1996). Polycystic ovaries: implications of diagnosis with MR imaging. *Radiology* 201, 549–52.

Kyei-Mensah, A., Zaidi, J. and Campbell, S. (1996). Ultrasound diagnosis of polycystic ovary syndrome. *Baillières Clinical Endocrinology and Metabolism* 10, 249–62.

Maubon, A., Courtieu, C., Vivens, F. et al. (1993). Magnetic resonance imaging of normal and polycystic ovaries. Preliminary results. *Annals of New York Academy of Sciences* 687, 224–9.

Orsini, L.F., Venturoli, S. and Lorusso, R. (1985). Ultrasonic findings in polycystic ovarian disease. *Fertility and Sterility* 43, 709–14.

Pache, T.D., Wladimiroff, J.W., Hop, W.C.J. and Fauser, B.C.J.M. (1992). How to discriminate between normal and polycystic ovaries: transvaginal US study. *Radiology* 183, 421–3.

Robert, Y., Dubrulle, F., Gaillandre, G. et al. (1995). Ultrasound assessment of ovarian stroma hypertrophy in hyperandrogenism and ovulation disorders: visual analysis versus computerized quantification. *Fertility and Sterility* 64, 307–12.

Saxton, D.W., Farquhar, C.M., Rae, T. et al. (1990). Accuracy of ultrasound measurements of female pelvic organs. *British Journal of Obstetrics and Gynaecology* 97, 695–9.

Takahashi, K., Eda, Y., Abu-Masa, A. et al. (1994). Transvaginal ultrasound imaging, histopathology and endocrinopathy in patients with polycystic ovarian syndrome. *Human Reproduction* 9, 1231–6.

Woodward, P.J. and Gilfeather, M. (1998). Magnetic resonance imaging of the female pelvis. *Seminars in Ultrasound, CT and MR* 19, 90–103.

Wu, M-H., Tang, H-H., Hsu, C-C., Wang, S-T. and Huang, K-E. (1998). The role of three-dimensional ultrasonographic imaging in ovarian measurment. *Fertility and Sterility* 69, 1152–5.

Yeh, H.C., Futterweit, W. and Thornton, J.C. (1987). Polycystic ovarian disease: US features in 104 patients. *Radiology* 163, 111–16.

Zaidi, J., Campbell, S., Pittrof, R. et al. (1995). Ovarian stromal blood flow in women with polycystic ovaries: a possible new marker for diagnosis? *Human Reproduction* 10, 1992–6.

7

Long-term health implications for women with polycystic ovary syndrome

Eva Dahlgren and Per Olof Janson

Introduction

Polycystic ovary syndrome (PCOS) is a heterogeneous clinical entity affecting 5–10% of premenopausal women. It is defined as the association of hyperandrogenism with chronic anovulation without specific underlying diseases of the adrenal and pituitary glands and it is frequently associated with insulin resistance. It is known to be a familial disorder, but in spite of exciting recent reports on the association with PCOS of specific genes encoding cholesterol side-chain cleavage (Gharani et al., 1997) and the role of the insulin gene *VNTR* (Waterworth et al., 1997), the mode of inheritance and the molecular genetic factors are still largely unknown (Legro, 1995; Franks et al., 1997).

In recent years increasing attention has been paid to aspects of PCOS other than those related to anovulatory infertility. The long-term impact of the metabolic disturbances associated with the disorder on women's health has focused considerable interest on follow-up studies and intervention studies. Such studies are, however, so far sparse. This chapter gives a brief review of the long-term implications of PCOS on women's reproductive health, hormonal balance, clinical expressions such as hirsutism and obesity, bone metabolism, risks of cancer, and cardiovascular risk. The discussions of primary prevention of all those issues are mostly speculative because of the present lack of firm evidence.

Reproductive health

Menstruation

According to our retrospective follow-up study involving 33 women who were wedge resected during 1956 to 1965, there was no difference from controls in the age of menarche (Dahlgren et al., 1992b). Twenty per cent of the PCOS cases had a history of regular cycles during a period of ten years after the menarche and 20% reported that their periods became regular following the wedge resection. Twenty-eight per cent of the PCOS cohort reported irregular menstruations during the entire fertile period. Most of the women who became pregnant resumed regular cycles after the pregnancy. Women with PCOS appeared to enter the menopause later than referents, as assessed by follicle-stimulating hormone (FSH) levels in the study. Thus, when dividing women with PCOS and age-matched and weight-matched referents into two subgroups according to whether they presented FSH values of more or less than 50 U/L, 60% of the referents and 27% of the women with PCOS presented values of more than 50 U/L.

Fecundity

In our follow-up study (Dahlgren et al., 1992b), 75% of the women with PCOS were married, which at that time (1956–65) was a prerequisite for infertility treatment. Out of the 70% of the PCOS cohort of women who wanted to become pregnant, only 24% remained nulliparous. Also, today, with the availability of ovulation induction, compounds like clomiphene, recombinant gonadotrophins, gonadotrophin-releasing hormone (GnRH), with and without adjuvant treatment with GnRH analogue downregulation, dexamethasone, metformin and invasive techniques like ovarian drilling and in-vitro fertilization (IVF), the 'difficult responders' are still a challenge. Aspiration of immature oocytes followed by in-vitro maturation in conjunction with IVF may in the future help to optimize infertility treatment in women with PCOS.

Hysterectomy

Bleeding irregularities with menorrhagia are indications for hysterectomy worldwide. In our retrospective cohort follow-up study (Dahlgren et al., 1992b), women with PCOS had undergone hysterectomy on benign indications three times more often than the referents (21% vs 7%, $p < 0.05$). An increased incidence of previous hysterectomy in New Zealand women with PCOS was also reported by Birdsall, Farquhar and White (1997).

Hirsutism

About 60% of women with PCOS show hirsutism, varying from growth of some coarse hair on the upper lip and chin to excessive coarse hair on the face, trunk and thighs. In general, the hirsutism develops some years after menarche and is typically progressive, with weight gain, possibly due to increased serum insulin levels and reduced serum concentrations of sex hormone binding globulin (SHBG). Hirsutism which is unrelated to Cushing's disease or ovarian and adrenal tumours is not a challenge to health in itself, but for many women it causes serious problems in their social life, threatening their self-esteem and affecting their quality of life.

Those women who cannot accept their excessive hair growth will often be subjected to attempts at treatment with anti-androgens and/or oral contraceptives which raise serum SHBG levels, and in serious cases destruction of hair follicles with cautery or laser may be employed. It seems reasonable to intervene early in life with anti-androgen treatment to stop further progression of hirsutism. Also in the perimeno-pause, when oestrogen levels normally decrease, women with PCOS may benefit from hormonal replacement therapy to balance the decreasing levels of SHBG.

Treatment with oral contraceptives and/or cyproterone acetate is quite widely used, at least in the Scandinavian countries, often offering a satisfactory control of the growth rate of excessive hair. However, this treatment has been shown to disturb carbohydrate metabolism, indicating that this type of intervention should be regarded with caution in insulin-resistant women. There are different opinions about whether treatment with GnRH analogue alone is effective in reducing hirsutism (Falsetti, Pasinetti and Ceruti, 1994; Carmino and Lobo, 1997). However, in a recent study it has been shown to improve both hirsutism and insulin sensitivity in peripheral tissue (Dahlgren et al., 1998).

Obesity

The average woman has been shown to increase her body weight by 4 kg during perimenopause (Björkelund et al., 1997). In a cohort study (Dahlgren et al., 1992b), follow-up was performed for three years for the women with PCOS and their referents. The women with PCOS decreased in weight, by an average of about 2 kg, but retained their upper body obesity, with a constant waist:hip ratio (WHR) of 0.81 ± 0.07. In contrast, the referents gained an average of 2 kg but their WHR decreased significantly (0.83 ± 0.08 to 0.78 ± 0.06; $p < 0.001$). Thus, women with PCOS appear to remain centrally obese when approaching the menopause. Whereas obesity is not an overall risk factor of cardiovascular disease, central–visceral obesity is highly correlated to insulin resistance and atherogenic lipopro-tein patterns (Björntorp, 1991). It is therefore likely that, even with advancing age, women with PCOS are still at risk of developing cardiovascular disease. However, more research needs to be performed, especially concerning PCOS women in the post-menopausal years, because there is still a paucity of good longitudinal studies concerning obesity. In view of the possibility of an increased cardiovascular risk in ageing women with PCO, it is reasonable to advise continued attention to measurements of blood pressure, serum lipids and insulin as well as considering prevention by hormone replacement therapy.

The classical pattern of PCOS, with hyperandrogenism, increased serum lutein-izing hormone (LH)/FSH ratio, normal oestradiol and increased oestrone levels as well as increased insulin and triglyceride concentrations, is also found in women with PCOS in the perimenopause. However, in our study, the aberrations were found to be less pronounced during this period than earlier in life. Interestingly, as mentioned previously, we also demonstrated that, compared to age-matched and weight-matched referents, significantly fewer women with PCOS had reached the menopause (Dahlgren et al., 1992b).

Bone metabolism

There has been concern about the bone mineral density in oligomenorrhoeic and amenorrhoeic women with PCOS because osteopenia is a common feature in amenorrhoea of of hypothalamic origin. However, published data show a normal (Dixon et al., 1989; Di Carlo et al., 1992) or even supernormal mineralization of the skeleton (Dagogo-Jack, al-Ali and Qurttom, 1997) in women with PCOS and a positive correlation between androgen levels and bone mineral density (Adami et al., 1998).

Different GnRH analogue treatments have, however, been found to decrease mineralization of the spine and hip (Falsetti et al., 1994; Lupoli et al., 1997), if not combined with hormone replacement therapy (Simberg et al., 1996) or oral contraceptives (Castelo Branco et al., 1997).

Risks of cancer

Endometrial cancer

Endometrial cancer in women under 40 years of age is rare, with a reported incidence of 1–8%. There are numerous case reports in the literature on the association of PCOS with the development of endometrial cancer in young women (Gregorini, Lespi and Alvarez, 1997). In the Göteborg area, comprising one-fifth of the female population in Sweden, 77 women aged 31–45 and 99 women aged 46–65 years with endometrial cancer were investigated. When comparing these women with 1746 referents, 39–65 years of age, it was found that increased body mass index, hirsutism and hypertension were significantly more common in both groups of women with endometrial cancer, indicating that untreated ovarian dysfunction, found for instance in individuals with PCOS, is associated with an increased risk of endometrial cancer (Dahlgren et al., 1991).

Breast cancer

There are currently no data supporting the hypothesis that PCOS in itself is a risk factor of breast cancer. Conversely, Gammon and Thompson (1991) reported from a multicentre population-based study an inverse relationship between physician-diagnosed PCOS and breast cancer.

Ovarian cancer

Schildkraut et al. (1996) reported a 2.5-fold (95% confidence interval (CI) = 1.1–5.9) increased risk of epithelial ovarian cancer among women with PCOS in a population-based, case-control study involving 426 cancer cases and 4081 controls. The association was found to be stronger among women who never used oral contraceptives. Taken together, these data support the so-called gonadotrophin theory for the development of ovarian cancer. Although more studies need to be done to verify the findings of Schildkraut et al. (1996), the relative protection afforded by oral contraceptives against ovarian cancer must be taken into consideration when advising women with PCOS with no immediate infertility problem.

Cardiovascular risk

In 1921, Achard and Thiers described the bearded diabetic, but it was not until 1980 that more systematic research focused on the relation between hyperandrogenism and hyperinsulinism (Burghen, Givens and Kitabchi, 1980). Women with PCOS are clinically characterized by obesity, hirsutism, oligomenorrhoea and infertility. Apart from hormonal abberations, i.e. hyperandrogenism and increased LH:FSH ratio, increased serum triglycerides and decreased high density lipoprotein (HDL)-cholesterol levels were also found. These findings led to the proposal of possible cardiovascular risk (Mattsson et al., 1984; Wild et al., 1990).

Obesity was thought to be the cause of hyperinsulinaemia in women with PCOS until Chang and coworkers (1983) reported that women with PCOS are markedly more insulin resistant and show enhanced insulin secretion on glucose stimulation compared to weight-matched controls. Since then, there has accumulated an overwhelming amount of documentation on the correlation between hyperandrogenism and hyperinsulinaemia, but there is still no consensus about whether hyperinsulinaemia is the cause or the result of hyperandrogenism. On the other hand, it is now well accepted that hyperinsulinaemia is involved in the so-called metabolic syndrome, characterized by obesity, in particular central obesity, elevated serum levels of triglycerides, cholesterol, and insulin resistance in the tissues (Reaven, 1988). Both men and women showing features of the metabolic syndrome have an increased risk of developing hypertension and diabetes mellitus. Indeed, an increased prevalence of hypertension (see, for instance, Dahlgren et al., 1992b; Conway et al., 1992) and diabetes mellitus (Dunaif et al., 1987; Dahlgren et al., 1992a) has been found in women with PCOS. Conway et al. (1992), comparing lean and obese women with PCOS with respect to three cardiac risk factors – hyperinsulinaemia, fasting serum lipid concentrations, and raised blood pressure – presented evidence that hyperinsulinaemic women with PCOS have an increased risk of developing cardiovascular disease.

When applying a risk factor model for myocardial infarction, involving increased waist-to-hip ratio (WHR), increased serum triglycerides, diabetes mellitus, hypertension and age, in a retrospective cohort follow-up study of women diagnosed as having the Stein–Leventhal syndrome at wedge resection up to 30 years before the study, there was an estimated seven-fold increased risk of developing myocardial infarction in the whole cohort between the ages of 40 and 61 years (Dahlgren et al., 1992a).

There are numerous other reports in the literature of a higher prevalence of the above-mentioned risk factors in different studies on PCOS (see, for instance, Palmer, Rosenberg and Shapiro, 1992; Schildkraut et al., 1996; La Vecchia et al. 1997). Recently, in a long-term follow-up study in the UK to assess cardiovascular mortality among women diagnosed as having PCOS between 1930 and 1979, the women did not have a significantly increased mortality rate from circulatory disease compared to controls (Pierpoint et al., 1998). An explanation of this unexpected finding is pointed out by the authors, namely that the endocrine profile of women with PCOS may protect against circulatory disease.

In view of the lack of solid data on the effects of therapeutic interventions on cardiovascular risk, we can only speculate on the most appropriate treatment for women with PCOS. It has been shown (Pasquali et al., 1983, 1986; Kiddy et al., 1989; Holte et al., 1995) that weight reduction will restore hormonal and carbohydrate variables in overweight women with PCOS. This approach has been shown to be effective on a short-term basis in the treatment of anovulatory infertility. The problem, however, is to achieve a permanent weight reduction. Experience shows that life-style changes with exercise and reduced calorie intake only result in temporary effects. One explanation as to why many women with PCOS easily regain weight may be that they have a low postprandial thermogenesis (Franks, Robinson and Willis, 1996) as well as a rapid insulin surge on glucose administration (Holte et al., 1994).

Treatment with insulin-sensitizing drugs (metformin, troglitazone) has shown promising results in preliminary studies (Velazquez, Acosta and Mendoza, 1997; Morin-Papunen et al., 1998; Diamanti-Kandarakis et al., 1998), including reinstated menstrual periods, improved metabolic variables and reduced hyperandrogenicity. However, this type of pharmacological treatment has not yet become everyday practice. Thus, in addition to ovulation induction, oral contraceptives with or without androgen receptor blockers, GnRH analogues with oestrogen add-back, and possibly hormone replacement therapy in the perimenopause, recommendations of mild to moderate exercise with diet restrictions, as well as taking part in programmes aimed at stopping smoking remain the treatments we can offer these patients at the present moment.

Acknowledgements

This chapter was supported by research grants from The Swedish Medical Research Council and The Faculty of Medicine, Göteborg University, Göteborg, Sweden.

REFERENCES

Achard, M. C. and Thiers, M. J. (1921). Le virilism pilaire et son association a l'Ìnsuffisance gly-colytique (diabète des femmes a barbe). *Bulletin Academie National Medicine (Paris)* **86**, 51–66.

Adami, S., Zamberlan, N., Castello, R. et al. (1998). Effect of hyperandrogenism and menstrual cycle abnormalities on bone mass and bone turnover in young women. *Clinical Endocrinology (Oxford)* **48**, 169–73.

Birdsall, M.A., Farquhar, C.M. and White, H.D. (1997). Association between polycystic ovaries and extent of coronary heart disease in women having cardiac catheterization. *Annals of Internal Medicine* **26** (1), 32–5.

Björkelund, C., Hulten, B., Lissner, L. et al. (1997). New height and weight standards for the middle aged and aged. Weight increases more than height. *Journal of the Swedish Medical Association (Läkartidningen)* **94**, 332–5.

Björntorp, P. (1991). Hypothesis on visceral fat accumulation: the missing link between psycho-social factors and cardiovascular disease? *International Journal of Obesity* **230**, 195–201.

Burghen, G.A., Givens, J.R. and Kitabchi, A.E. (1980). Correlation of hyperandrogenism and hyperinsulinism in polycystic ovarian disease. *Journal of Clinical Endocrinology and Metabolism* **50**, 113–16.

Carmino, E. and Lobo, R.A. (1997). Gonadotropin-releasing hormone agonist therapy for hir-sutism is as effective as high dose cyproterone acetate but results in longer remission. *Human Reproduction* **12**, 663–6.

Castelo Branco, C., Martinez de Osaba, M.J., Pons, F. and Fortuny, A. (1997). Gonadotropin-releasing hormone analogue plus an oral contraceptive containing desogestrel in women with severe hirsutism: effects on hair, bone and hormonal profile after 1 year use. *Metabolism* **46**, 437–40.

Chang, R.J., Nakamura, R.M., Judd, H.L. and Kaplan, S.A. (1983). Insulin resistance in non-obese patients with polycystic ovarian disease. *Journal of Clinical Endocrinology and Metabolism* **57**, 356–9.

Conway, G.S., Agrawal, R., Betteridge, D.J. and Jacobs, H.S. (1992). Risk factors for coronary artery disease in lean and obese women with the polycystic ovary syndrome. *Clinical Endocrinology* **37**, 119–25.

Dagogo-Jack, S., al-Ali, N. and Qurttom, M. (1997). Augmentation of bone mineral density in hirsute women. *Journal of Clinical Endocrinology and Metabolism* **82**, 2821–5.

Dahlgren E., Friberg L.G., Johansson, S. et al. (1991). Endometrial carcinoma; ovarian dysfunc-tion – a risk factor in young women. *European Journal of Obstetrics, Gynecology and Reproductive Biology* **41**, 143–50.

Dahlgren, E., Johansson, S., Lapidus, L., Odén, A. and Janson, P-O. (1992a). Polycystic ovary syndrome and risk for myocardial infarction – evaluation from a risk factor model based on a prospective population study of women. *Acta Obstetricia et Gynecologica Scandinavica* **71**, 599–604.

Dahlgren, E., Johansson, S., Lindstedt, G. et al. (1992b). Women with polycystic ovary syndrome wedge resected in 1956 to 65: a long term follow up focusing on natural history and circulating hormones. *Fertility and Sterility* **57**, 505–13.

Dahlgren, E., Landin, K., Krotkiewski, M., Holm, G. and Janson, P.O. (1998). Effects of two anti-androgen treatments on hirsutism and insulin sensitivity in women with polycystic ovary syndrome. *Human Reproduction* **13**, 2706–11.

Diamanti-Kandarakis, E., Kouli, C., Tsianateli, T. and Bergiele, A. (1998). Therapeutic effects of metformin on insulin resistance and hyperandrogenism in polycystic ovary syndrome. *European Journal of Endocrinology* **138**, 269–74.

Di Carlo, C., Shoham, Z., MacDougall, J. et al. (1992). Polycystic ovaries as a relative protective factor for bone mineral loss in young women with amenorrhea. *Fertility and Sterility* **57**, 314–19.

Dixon, J. E., Rodin, A., Murby, B., Chapman, M.G. and Fogelman, I. (1989). Bone mass in hirsute women with androgen excess. *Clinical Endocrinology (Oxford)* **30**, 271–8.

Dunaif, A., Graf, M., Mandeli, J., Laumas, V. and Dobrjanska, A. (1987). Characterization of groups of hyperandrogenic women with acanthosis nigricans, impaired glucose tolerance and/or hyperinsulinemia. *Journal of Clinical Endocrinology and Metabolism* **65**, 499–507.

Falsetti, L., Pasinetti, E. and Ceruti, D. (1994). Gonadotropin-releasing hormone agonist (GnRH-A) in hirsutism. *Acta Europaea Fertilitatis* **25**, 303–6.

Franks, S., Robinson, S. and Willis, D.S. (1996). Nutrition, insulin and polycystic ovary syndrome. *Reviews of Reproduction* **1**, 47–53.

Franks, S., Gharani, N., Waterworth, D. et al. (1997). The genetic basis of polycystic ovary syndrome. *Human Reproduction* **12**, 2641–8.

Gammon, M.D. and Thompson, W.D. (1991). Polycystic ovaries and the risk of breast cancer. *American Journal of Epidemiology* **134** (8), 818–24.

Gharani, N., Waterworth, D.M., Batty, S. et al. (1997). Association of the steroid synthesis gene CYP11a with polycystic ovary syndrome and hyperandrogenism. *Human Molecular Genetics* **6**, 397–402.

Gregorini, S.D., Lespi, P.J. and Alvarez, G.R. (1997). Endometrial carcinoma with polycystic ovaries. Report of two cases in women younger than 40 years old. *Medicina (Buonas Aires)* **57** (2), 209–12.

Holte, J., Bergh, T., Berne, C., Berglund, L. and Lithell, H. (1994). Enhanced insulin response to glucose in relation to insulin resistance in women with polycystic ovary syndrome and normal glucose tolerance. *Journal of Clinical Endocrinology and Metabolism* **78**, 1052–8.

Holte, J., Bergh, T., Berne, C., Wide, L. and Lithell, H. (1995). Restored insulin sensitivity but persistently increased early insulin secretion after weight loss in obese women with polycystic ovary syndrome. *Journal of Clinical Endocrinology and Metabolism* **80**, 2586–93.

Kiddy, D. S., Hamilton-Fairley, D., Seppälä, M. et al. (1989). Diet-induced changes in sex hormone binding globulin and free testosterone in women with normal or polycystic ovaries:

correlation with serum insulin and insulin-like growth factor-I. *Clinical Endocrinology (Oxford)* **31**, 757–63.

La Vecchia, C., Decarli, A., Franseschi, S. et al. (1997). Menstrual and reproductive factors and the risk of myocardial infarction in women under fifty-five years of age. *American Journal of Obstetrics and Gynecology* **157** (5), 1108–12.

Legro R. (1995). The genetics of polycystic ovary syndrome (Commentary). *American Journal of Medicine* **98** (**Suppl. 1A**), 9S–16S.

Lupoli, G., Di Carlo, C., Nuzzo, V. et al. (1997). Gonadotropin-releasing hormone agonists administration in polycystic ovary syndrome. Effects on bone mass. *Journal of Endocrinological Investigation* **20**, 493–6.

Mattsson, L-Å., Cullberg, G., Hamberger, L., Samsioe, G. and Silfverstolpe, G. (1984). Lipid metabolism in women with polycystic ovary syndrome: possible implications for increased risk of coronary heart disease. *Fertility and Sterility* **42**, 579–84.

Morin-Papunen, L.C., Koivunen, R.M., Ruokonen, A. and Martikainen, H.K. (1998). Metformin therapy improves the menstrual pattern with minimal endocrine and metabolic effects in women with polycystic ovary syndrome. *Fertility and Sterility* **69**, 691–6.

Palmer, J.R., Rosenberg, L. and Shapiro, S. (1992). Reproductive factors and risk of myocardial infarction. *American Journal of Epidemiology* B (4), 408–16.

Pasquali, R., Casimirri, F., Venturoli, S. et al. (1983). Insulin resistance in patients with polycystic ovaries: its relationship to body weight and androgen levels. *Acta Endocrinologica* **104**, 110–16.

Pasquali, R., Fabbri, R., Venturoli, S. et al. (1986). Effect of weight loss and antiandrogenic therapy on sex hormone blood levels and insulin resistance in the obese patients with polycystic ovaries. *American Journal of Obstetrics and Gynecology* **154**, 139–144.

Pierpoint, T., McKeigue, P.M., Isaacs, A.J., Wild, S.H. and Jacobs, H.S. (1998). Mortality of women with polycystic ovary syndrome at long term follow up. *Journal of Clinical Epidemiology* **51**, 581–6.

Reaven, G. M. (1988). Role of insulin resistance in human disease. *Diabetes* **37**, 1595–607.

Schildkraut, J.M., Schwingl, P.J., Bastos, E., Evanoff, A. and Huges, C. (1996). Epithelial ovarian cancer risk among women with polycystic ovary syndrome. *Obstetrics and Gynecology* **88**, 554–9.

Simberg, N., Tiitinen, A., Silfvast, A., Viinikka, L. and Ylikorkala, O. (1996). High bone density in hyperandrogenic women: effect of gonadotropin-releasing hormone agonist alone or in conjunction with estrogen–progestin replacement. *Journal of Clinical Endocrinology and Metabolism* **81**, 646–51.

Velazquez, E., Acosta, A. and Mendoza, S. G. (1997). Menstrual cyclicity after metformin therapy in polycystic ovary syndrome. *Obstetrics and Gynecology* **90**, 392–5.

Waterworth, D.M., Bennett, S.T., Gharani, N. et al. (1997). Linkage and association of the insulin gene VNTR regulatory polymorphism with polycystic ovary syndrome. *Lancet* **349**, 986–90.

Wild, R.A., Grubb, B., Hartz, A. et al. (1990). Clinical signs of androgen excess as risk factors for coronary artery disease. *Fertility and Sterility* **54**, 255–9.

8

Skin manifestations of polycystic ovary syndrome

Jack Green and Rodney Sinclair

Introduction

Hirsutism, androgenetic alopecia, seborrhoea and acne are all skin manifestations of androgen excess and may all occur in the context of polycystic ovary syndrome (PCOS) (Table 8.1). Acanthosis nigricans is a cutaneous marker of insulin resistance that is also associated with PCOS. The pilosebaceous unit consists of the hair follicle and associated sebaceous and apocrine glands and is the main cutaneous target of circulating androgens.

Physiology of the sebaceous gland

Sebaceous glands occur on all parts of the skin except on the glabrous skin of the palms and soles. They are most numerous on the face, scalp and back, occurring at a concentration of between 400 and 900 glands per cm². Each of the several lobes of the gland has a duct lined with keratinizing squamous epithelium, and these join to form a main duct which enters the follicular canal. Glandular cells, which divide at the periphery, move towards the centre of the glands, becoming increasingly filled with sebaceous material. During this process, the cells undergo complete dissolution and thus the sebaceous gland's secretion is considered holocrine. The lipid composition of this secretion differs from epidermal lipid in that it contains wax esters and squalene, which the former does not, although there is a similar percentage of glycerides (Cunliffe and Simpson, 1998).

Acne

Definition

Acne is a chronic inflammatory disorder of the pilosebaceous units.

Incidence

It is usually first evident in the early adolescent years and has a peak incidence in the later teenage years, affecting up to 80% of school children. Although the incidence

Table 8.1. Dermatological features of PCOS diagnosed by direct ovarian visualization, ultrasound or histologically

	Balen et al. (1995)	Conway et al. (1989)	Franks (1988)	Goldzieher and Axelrod (1963)
	Ultrasound diagnosis			Histological diagnosis
Number of patients	1741	556	300	1079
Hirsuties (%)	66.2	61	64	69
Acne (%)	34.7	24	27	
Alopecia (%)		8	3	
Acanthosis nigricans (%)	2.5	2	1	

Source: Modified from Simpson and Barth (1997).

decreases in the third and subsequent decades, a minority of patients have persistence of lesions into middle age.

Pathogenesis

Pathogenic factors involved in acne include increased sebum production, abnormal keratinization of the pilosebaceous duct, abnormal microbial flora, in particular relating to increased *Priopionibacterium acnes*, and inflammation (Cunliffe and Simpson, 1998). The presumed sequence of events is that androgens enlarge sebaceous glands, which are themselves responsible for converting androgens into more active metabolites, causing further sebaceous gland enlargement. These enlarged glands subsequently produce more sebum, which promotes increased *P. acnes* colonies within the hair follicle as these bacteria thrive in a sebaceous environment. The *P. acnes* digest the sebum, making it more viscous as well as producing inflammatory by-products. Subsequent hyperkeratosis in response to the inflammation, as well as the increased sebum viscosity, lead to follicular plugging and subsequent formation of comedones, the initial lesion of acne. If the follicular structure is then disrupted, the release of inflammatory mediators into the surrounding dermis will lead to papule, pustule and cyst formation.

Association with polycystic ovary syndrome

Acne is seen in approximately one-third of PCOS patients (Franks, 1988; Conway, Honour and Jacobs, 1989; Balen et al., 1995) and, conversely, a majority of women with severe or resistant acne have PCOS (Betti et al., 1990; Eden, 1991). It is increased sebaceous secretion (Burton and Shuster, 1971; Holmes, Williams and Cunliffe, 1972) that is principally associated with PCOS and this correlates with the

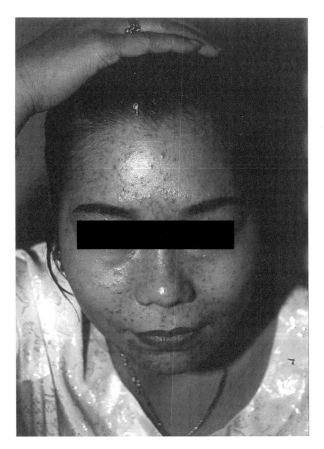

Fig. 8.1   Moderately severe acne.

severity of acne (Burton and Shuster, 1971). While some studies have demonstrated an association between acne incidence and androgen levels (Darley et al., 1980, 1982; Held et al., 1984; Lucky et al., 1994), others have demonstrated no such relationship (Levell et al., 1989). Androgen excess has also been associated with more severe acne (Marynick et al., 1983).

Clinical features

Acne primarily affects the face and, less often, the back and chest. Lesions are grouped into non-inflammatory and inflammatory. Comedones are non-inflamed lesions and are either open comedones, or blackheads (the black colour is due to melanin), or closed comedones, also known as whiteheads. Inflammatory lesions are either superficial, papules or pustules, or deeper, deep pustules, nodules and cysts. The lesions are usually tender (Cunliffe and Simpson, 1998; Fig. 8.1).

The lesions of acne are not static and often evolve from one type to another.

Resultant scarring is common, but significant in only a minority of acne patients. Icepick-like depressed scars most often occur on the cheeks, whereas hypertrophic scars occur most commonly on the trunk.

Treatment

Mild acne can be treated topically with keratolytics such as azaleic acid, retinoids, or with antibacterials such as benzoyl peroxide, clindamycin 1% lotion and erythromycin 2% gel (Cunliffe and Simpson, 1998). More severe forms generally require oral antibiotics such as the tetracyclines, erythromycin and trimethoprim.

Anti-androgens such as spironolactone and cyproterone acetate are indicated in women with a marked premenstrual accentuation of acne or when antibiotic treatments have failed. The choice of oral contraceptive for women with acne is important as some can cause an exacerbation. In general, oral contraceptives which are higher in oestrogen and lower in progestogen are preferred. There is also a preference for combinations containing cyproterone acetate, desogestrel or norethisterone as the progestogen.

For severe cases, isotretinoin is prescribed and produces long-term remission in more than 70% of patients. Isotretinoin is teratogenic, and adequate contraceptive measures need to be taken during treatment and for one month afterwards (Cunliffe and Simpson, 1998).

Physiology of the hair follicle

The average person is said to have two million hair follicles on the body, of which only 100000 are on the scalp. The two predominant hair types that exist are vellus and terminal hairs. Vellus hairs are fine, lightly pigmented, cosmetically imperceptible hairs that are present over most of the body and are produced by smaller hair follicles. Terminal hairs are larger, pigmented, cosmetically significant hairs that are found on the scalp, eyebrows and eyelashes prior to puberty in all people and are produced by larger hair follicles. In addition, some children will have noticeable terminal hairs on their forearms and shins. Following puberty, terminal hairs appear in the axillae, pubic area and male beard. In addition, terminal hairs become more abundant on the forearms and legs of women. In men, hairs also appear on the chest, shoulders and back.

Human hair follicles have a growth cycle consisting of three phases. The growing phase, called anagen, generally lasts several months on the body and two to five years on the scalp. It is the main determinant of hair length. Anagen is followed by a short catagen phase, lasting around two weeks, during which the hair stops growing and the lower portion of the hair follicle involutes. The third phase is telogen, a resting phase, which lasts approximately three months. At the end of the third month, the hair is extruded from the follicle and the lower portion of the hair follicle regenerates as it re-enters the anagen phase. At any given time different hairs will be at different stages of the cycle as hair growth on the body and scalp is not synchronized. This is in contrast to animals, in which synchronized hair growth is seen, culminating in seasonal moulting.

Transformation from vellus to terminal hairs at puberty in the axillae, pubic and male beard area is driven by systemic androgens. Transformation from terminal to vellus hairs on the scalp in the context of androgenetic alopecia is also driven by the same androgens. How these androgens can have opposite effects on hair growth is not understood and it remains a paradox (Simpson and Barth, 1997).

Hirsutism

Definition

Hirsuties may be defined as the growth of terminal hair on the body of a woman in the same patterns and sequence as that which develop in the normal post-pubertal male (Simpson and Barth, 1997). As the number of hair follicles remains constant from birth until death, hirsuties is not characterized by an increase in the number of hairs but rather by the quality, size, degree of pigmentation as well as the length of the hairs produced by the individual follicles.

Incidence

Cultural norms and fashion determine the amount of hair that is seen as acceptable on the female face and body. Deviations from these norms, real or perceived, can be a source of anxiety and low self-esteem in susceptible individuals. Allowing for these cultural and personal influences on the definition of hirsuties, approximately 9% of the young female population are considered to be hirsute (McKnight, 1964). It is important to distinguish hirsuties from hypertrichosis, which refers to non-androgen-dependent, excessive hair growth (Dawber, de Berker and Wojnarowska, 1998).

Pathogenesis

Dihydrotestosterone is thought to be the predominant androgen involved in the development of hirsuties. The dermal papilla has been shown to express androgen receptors, and interactions of dihydrotestosterone with the androgen receptors in the dermal papilla are thought to directly influence the size of the hair follicle and, consequently, the hair produced by that follicle.

Association with polycystic ovaries

Polycystic ovary disease is the most commonly diagnosed ovarian cause of hirsutism (Bailey-Pridham and Sanfilippo, 1989; Sperling and Heimer, 1993). Even in the

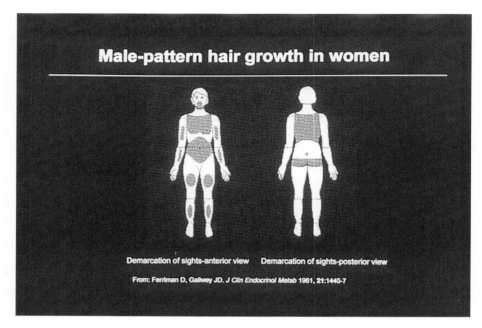

Fig. 8.2   Diagram of the areas of male-pattern hair growth in women. (Reproduced with permission from Oxford Clinical Communications.)

context of regular menstrual cycles, ultrasonic investigation will demonstrate a high rate of polycystic ovaries in hirsute patients (Adams, Polson and Franks, 1986; O'Driscoll et al., 1994).

The incidence of hirsutism in women diagnosed with PCOS is of the order of 60–70% amongst Caucasians (Goldzieher and Axelrod, 1963; Franks, 1988; Conway et al., 1989; Balen et al., 1995) and approximately 30% amongst Japanese women (Lobo, 1991). The Japanese women with PCOS are less likely to develop hirsuties than their counterparts from America or Italy, even when controlled for differences in androgen status and insulin resistance, which suggests that there is also a racial influence on the prevalence of hirsuties.

Clinical features

Clinically, one sees variable amounts of terminal hairs on sites associated with male secondary sexual development. The extent and severity of this terminal hair growth can be graded. The standard grading system was described by Ferriman and Gallwey (1961; Fig. 8.2). They scored nine 'hormonal sites' on a scale of 1 to 4 according to the degree of terminal hair growth. The scores were then added and used for comparison. Other methods that assess the degree of terminal hair growth on the upper lip, chin, lower abdomen and thighs have also been described and used in clinical trials (Derksen, et al., 1993), but the Ferriman and Gallwey scale remains the most popular.

The main differential diagnosis is hypertrichosis, which tends to have an earlier onset and is not responsive to anti-androgen medication.

Treatment

Psychological

This aspect of treatment is easily overlooked, but is important given the significant psychological morbidity that may accompany hirsutism. A simple explanation of the problem and education regarding attainable goals of treatment are important (Conn and Jacobs, 1998), as is awareness of when psychiatric referral is required.

Physical methods of hair removal

There are several physical methods that are employed in the removal of unwanted hair. These include bleaching, shaving, plucking, depilatory creams, electrolysis and laser.

Bleaching of the hair with hydrogen peroxide is used to disguise pigmented facial hairs. For many women the cosmetic result is sufficient for this method to be used first. Occasionally, bleaching leads to discolouration of the skin or an artificial yellow hue to the hair.

Shaving is a common method for controlling unwanted hair and, contrary to common belief, does not affect the rate or duration of the anagen (growing phase) of the hair cycle, nor the hair diameter (Trotter, 1923). Side-effects include irritation and pseudofolliculitis. Some women might find it unacceptable to shave their facial hair as the act of shaving itself may reinforce feelings of being masculinized (Conn and Jacobs, 1998).

Epilation is simple and perhaps the most commonly used method of hair removal. Repetitive plucking may lead to permanent hair follicle matrix damage, resulting in finer, thinner hairs (Hamilton and Potten, 1974). Side-effects include post-inflammatory hyperpigmentation, folliculitis, pseudofolliculitis and, rarely, scarring (Olsen, 1999).

Chemical depilatories are usually thioglycates that disrupt the disulphide bonds of the hair shaft. They are spread on an area of unwanted hair for up to 15 minutes and then wiped away with the destroyed hair. Skin irritation is common and, whilst useful for bikini lines, they are less well tolerated in the axilla and on the face.

Electrolysis is a proven method of permanent hair removal (Dawber, 1998). Two forms exist, galvanic (direct current electrolysis) and thermolysis (alternate current electrolysis). It works by cauterizing the dermal papilla of the hair follicle. Several treatments may be necessary. The procedure is very operator dependent. Poor results are common and folliculitis, hyperpigmention and scarring are not uncommon sequelae.

Lasers produce monochromatic light which is absorbed by specific chromophores in the skin and converted into thermal energy. This leads to vaporization of the target tissue. Lasers currently in use for hair removal include the ruby laser, the alexandrite laser and the semiconductor diode laser, which all target melanin in the hair bulb, and the YAG laser, which works via absorbance of carbon particles in a topical paste that is massaged into the skin prior to its use and thus falls into the follicular tracts. The Epilight, which is an intense pulsed light system, is not a laser because the light generated is not monochromatic. It is also used for hair removal (Olsen, 1999). Side-effects of these treatments include erythema, hyperpigmentation and hypopigmentation, blistering and pain. Usually, several treatments are required to improve efficacy, but none of the presently utilized lasers has been proven to destroy hair permanently (Olsen, 1999).

Weight loss

There is an increased frequency of hirsutism in obese as compared with thin women with PCOS (Kiddy, et al., 1990). This is associated with a rise in the concentration of sex hormone binding globulin (SHBG) and a fall in concentration of free testosterone. Weight loss by obese, hirsute women both with and without polycystic ovaries usually leads to a reduction in body hair growth (Ruutiainen et al., 1988; Kiddy et al., 1992; Piacquadio et al., 1994).

Pharmacological

Prior to the commencement of treatment, patients should understand that any effect on hair growth will take several months to become apparent and, in general, only partial improvement may be expected. The drugs currently available are only suppressive and will need to be taken long term (Dawber et al., 1998). As there is the potential to feminize a male fetus, women should be advised not to become pregnant whilst on treatment.

Oral contraceptives

Oral contraceptives work by suppression of ovarian androgen production and elevation of SHBG, thereby reducing free testosterone. They can be used alone or in combination with other anti-androgens such as cyproterone acetate or spironolactone. Diane35ED® (Falsetti and Galbignani, 1990), containing 2 mg cyproterone acetate and 35 μg of ethinyl oestrodiol, and Marvelon®, containing desogestrel, have been shown to be effective in the treatment of hirsutes (Ruutiainen, 1986). Certain oral contraceptive pills, in particular those containing increased doses of norethisterone and levonorgesterol, will exacerbate hirsuties and should be avoided.

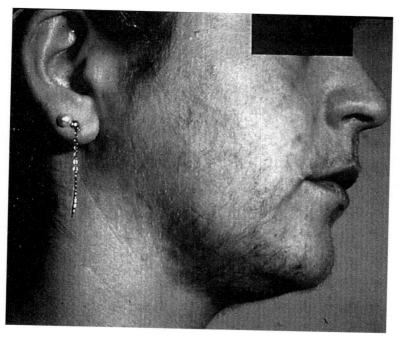

Fig. 8.3   Facial hirsuties. (Reproduced with permission from Oxford Clinical Communications.)

Cyproterone acetate

Cyproterone acetate has a dual mode of action. It antagonizes the androgen receptor in the skin and also acts as a weak progestagen that inhibits gonadotrophin secretion, thereby decreasing ovarian androgen production (Figs. 8.3 and 8.4).

It is normally administered with cyclical oestrogens, both to facilitate regular menstruation and also to prevent conception due to the risk of emasculating the male fetus. Dosage recommendations are 50–100 mg on days 5–15 of the menstrual cycle. There are several dose ranging studies that suggest that there is no difference in efficacy with different doses (Barth, Cherry and Wojnarowska, 1991).

Potential side-effects include loss of libido, weight gain, fatigue, breast tenderness, gastrointestinal upset, headaches, lowered mood, as well as the teratogenesis to male fetuses. As cyproterone acetate is lipophilic, conception is best avoided for three months after the drug is ceased.

Spironolactone

Spironolactone is an oral aldosterone antagonist with anti-androgenic properties. It reduces the bioavailability of testosterone by interfering with its production, increasing its metabolic clearance and reducing cutaneous 5α-reductase activity. It

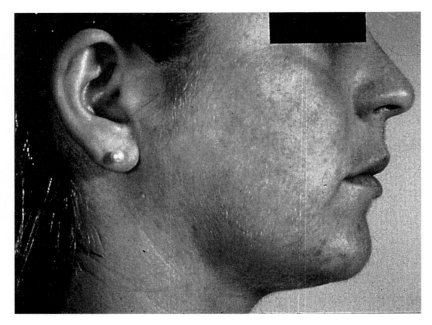

Fig. 8.4   The same patient as in Fig. 8.3 after treatment with cyproterone acetate. (Reproduced with permission from Oxford Clinical Communications.)

also complexes with the intracellular androgen receptor, forming a biologically inactive compound. The usual dose is 100–200 mg daily.

The potential side-effects include menstrual irregularities, breast tenderness, gastrointestinal disturbance, headache and dizziness. Due to its potassium-sparing diuretic effect, hyperkalaemia is a risk if it is combined with potassium-sparing diuretics or angiotensin-converting enzyme inhibitors or used in patients with renal failure. The patients' electrolytes should be checked while they are taking this medication. A contraceptive pill is not always recommended in conjunction with this medication, but adequate contraceptive measures should be taken when using spironolactone.

Flutamide

Flutamide is a non-steroidal pure anti-androgen. It has no glucocorticoid, progestational, androgenic or oestrogenic activity. It works by binding to androgen receptors, but has no effect on gonadotrophin secretion. Studies have demonstrated its efficacy and tolerability (Cusan et al., 1990; Falsetti et al., 1997). Side-effects include dry skin, menstrual disturbance, fatigue, lowered libido and gastric upset; hepatotoxicity is an infrequent but significant adverse reaction that develops in the first few weeks of therapy.

Finasteride

Finasteride is a type II 5α-reductase inhibitor which has been demonstrated to reduce hirsutism with minimal side-effects in patients with PCOS (Castello et al., 1996; Tolino et al., 1996). However, due to the potential risk of emasculation of the fetus, it should be used in conjunction with a contraceptive in women of child-bearing potential.

Androgenetic alopecia

Definition

Androgenetic alopecia is a progressive, non-scarring, patterned loss of scalp terminal hairs. It requires both a hereditary predisposition and sufficient androgens to realize this genetic potential.

Incidence

It is common in females, with the onset of hair loss beginning in the second to fourth decades, and approximately 50% of affected women will have significant hair loss by the age of 60.

Pathogenesis

In males, the normal levels of circulating androgens are thought to be sufficient for full expression of a genetic predisposition to baldness. In contrast, in females, the degree of alopecia is in part related to circulating androgen levels (Miller et al., 1982; DeVillez and Dunn, 1986). Both adrenal and ovarian dehydroepiandrosterone and testosterone are implicated in the pathogenesis of female balding (DeVillez and Dunn, 1986). In particular, dihydroxytestosterone, a reduction metabolite of testosterone, is thought to be the principal androgen responsible for androgenetic alopecia.

Association with polycystic ovary syndrome

A number of women with PCOS suffer with baldness (Franks, 1988; Conway et al., 1989) and PCOS sufferers make up a sizable fraction of women with alopecia (Futterweit et al., 1988). Androgenetic alopecia, in particular early androgenetic alopecia, is commonly underdiagnosed. The incidence of 8% reported by Conway and Jacobs (1990) almost certainly underestimates the true incidence.

Clinical features

The usual pattern of hair loss is different from that of men and has been described by Ludwig (1977; Fig. 8.5). There is diffuse hair loss over the crown, with preservation of the frontal hair line (Fig. 8.6). Widening of the hair parting is an early sign

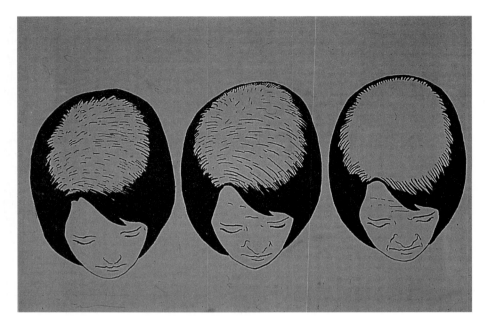

Fig. 8.5   Ludwig stages I, II and III of androgenetic alopecia.

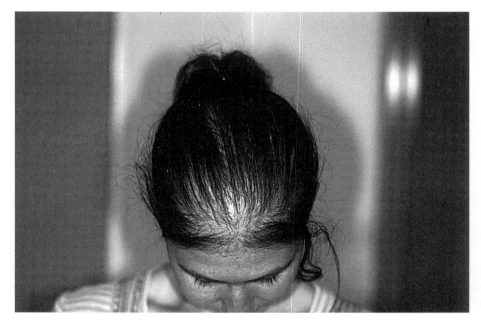

Fig. 8.6   Diffuse alopecia predominantly over the vertex of the scalp.

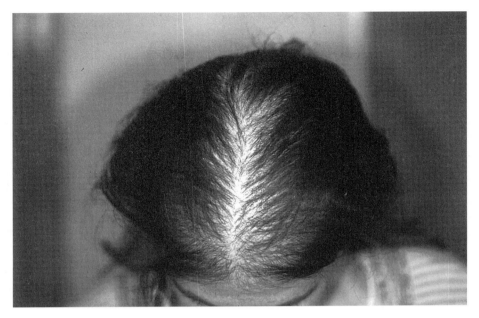

Fig. 8.7   Widening of the hair parting in the same patient as in Fig. 8.6.

of androgenetic alopecia (Fig. 8.7). In affected areas, one sees hairs which are either indeterminate or vellus in that they have lighter pigmentation, are shorter and finer in diameter than terminal hairs. A minority of women with this disorder display the Hamilton pattern of alopecia.

Treatment

Non-pharmacological

As for hirsutism, it is important to address psychological sequelae of alopecia as well as educating patients about both the cause of the hair loss and realistic goals regarding treatment efficacy. Some studies have shown that weight loss benefits patients with androgenetic alopecia, possibly by being associated with decreased androgen production (Piacquadio et al., 1994).

Appropriate hair styling and camouflage can greatly improve the appearance and diminish morbidity in androgenetic alopecia. Wigs are appropriate for women with more extensive hair loss. Hair transplantation may also be appropriate for some women.

Pharmacological

Minoxidil

Minoxidil is a piperidinopyrimidine derivative that causes vasodilation and prolongs anagen. It is used topically on the scalp and is available as a 2% and a 5% solution. One millilitre is applied to the scalp twice daily and massaged in. It should be applied both to the bald areas and to the vulnerable areas, and the hair should not be wetted for an hour after application. Several months of treatment are needed before loss of shedding and then subsequent hair regrowth are observed, but sometimes regrowth is not seen until 12 months of treatment has been completed. Most women notice decreased hair shedding and some regrowth of non-vellus hairs; however, many of these hairs are indeterminate rather than terminal hairs and are thus not cosmetically significant (DeVilez et al., 1994). Side-effects include hypertrichosis, erythema, pruritus and dry scalp.

Cyproterone acetate, spironolactone and finasteride

Cyproterone acetate, as well as being useful in hirsutism, is used to treat androgenetic alopecia. The dose is the same as that for hirsutism, 50–100 mg daily for ten days of each cycle. A contraceptive pill should also be used concomitantly. Although hair shedding can be diminished, there is usually no, or very mild, hair regrowth observed. No effect is usually noticed for a period of three to six months.

Spironolactone is also used to treat androgenetic alopecia at the same doses as for hirsutism, 100–200 mg daily. An oral contraceptive is not required, but renal function should be checked as there is a risk of hyperkalaemia. Again, a period of at least three to six months is required before any response to therapy will be noticed by the patient.

Finasteride is only infrequently prescribed for androgenetic alopecia in females and usually only in post-menopausal women. More studies are required to demonstrate its efficacy in female androgenetic alopecia and to determine the optimal dose.

A major problem in the treatment of androgenetic alopecia is the difficulty for both the patient and the clinician of assessing treatment efficacy. This is compounded by the fact that a major goal of treatment is to arrest any further hair loss, with regrowth of hair being seen as a welcome but less likely outcome of treatment. The interpretation of clinical photographs has been difficult because of the problems of obtaining consistent lighting, camera focal length and angle of photography. However, the recent advent of the combination of digital clinical photography with stereotactic stabilizing devices has significantly improved the accuracy of assessing the response to treatment. Currently, this is only available in specialized centres, but

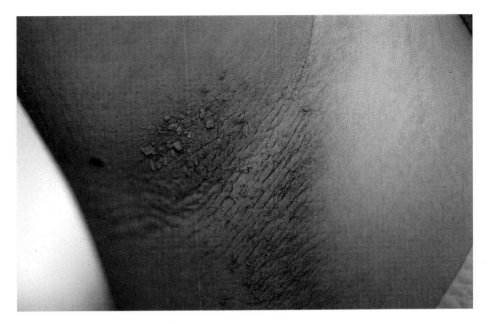

Fig. 8.8   Acanthosis nigricans of the axilla.

ultimately it is hoped that it will be more widely accessible, which will help facilitate patient compliance with medication by being an accurate measure of efficacy.

Acanthosis nigricans

Acanthosis nigricans is a mucocutaneous eruption characterized by hyperkeratosis, papillomatosis and increased pigmentation. It occurs in up to 5% of women with PCOS (Dunaif et al., 1985; Franks, 1988; Conway et al., 1989; Balen et al., 1995). The papillomatosis gives the skin a velvety contour (Fig. 8.8). Plaques most often occur in the axillae, the nape of the neck, under the breasts and in the flexures (Schwartz, 1994). Various clinical subtypes of acanthosis nigricans have been described. The variety associated with PCOS is the benign acanthosis nigricans. When women with this benign subtype have had their ovarian morphology identified, polycystic ovaries have been an almost universal finding (Rendon et al., 1989; Conway and Jacobs, 1990).

The term HAIR-AN syndrome has been coined to describe the constellation of symptoms of *h*yper*a*ndrogenism, *i*nsulin *r*esistance and *a*canthosis *n*igricans (Dunaif et al., 1985; Corenblum and Baylis, 1990; Simpson and Barth, 1991).

Conclusion

Dermatological manifestations are common in women with PCOS. Approximately 30% get acne, 60–70% get hirsutism and at least 8% develop androgenetic alopecia. Acanthosis nigricans is less common.

Hormonal manipulation will control many of those conditions. However, there are many adjunct treatments that are also beneficial and which may be used in conjunction or as alternatives. When the skin problems are severe or causing concern to the patient, a combined approach between the gynaecologist, dermatologist and general practitioner is appropriate.

REFERENCES

Adams, J., Polson, D. and Franks, S. (1986). Prevalence of polycystic ovaries in women with anovulation and idiopathic hirsutism. *British Medical Journal* **293**, 355–8.

Bailey-Pridham, D. and Sanfilippo, J. (1989). Hirsutism in the adolescent female. *Pediatric Clinics* **36**, 581–99.

Balen, A., Conway, G., Kaltsas, G., Techatraisak, K. and Manning, P. (1995). Polycystic ovary syndrome: the spectrum of the disorder in 1741 patients. *Human Reproduction* **10**, 2107–11.

Barth, J., Cherry, C. and Wojnarowska, F. (1991). Cyproterone acetate for severe hirsutism: results of a double-blind dose-ranging study. *Journal of Clinical Endocrinology and Metabolism* **35**, 5–10.

Betti, R., Bencini, P., Lodi, A. et al. (1990). Incidence of polycystic ovaries in patients with late-onset or persistent acne: hormonal reports. *Dermatologica* **181**, 109–11.

Burton, J. and Shuster, S. (1971). The relationship between seborrhoea and acne vulgaris. *British Journal of Dermatology* **84**, 600–2.

Castello, R. Tosi, F., Perrone, F. et al. (1996). Outcome of long-term treatment with 5α-reductase inhibitor finasteride in idiopathic hirsutism: clinical and hormonal effects during a 1-year course of therapy and 1-year follow up. *Fertility and Sterility* **66** (5), 734–40.

Conn, J. and Jacobs, H. (1998). Managing hirsutism in gynaecological practice. *British Journal of Obstetrics and Gynaecology* **105**, 687–96.

Conway, G., Honour, J. and Jacobs, H. (1989). Heterogeneity of the polycystic ovary syndrome: clinical endocrine and ultrasound features in 556 patients. *Clinical Endocrinology* **30**, 459–70.

Conway, G. and Jacobs, H. (1990). Acanthosis nigricans in obese women with the polycystic ovary syndrome: disease spectrum not distinct entity. *Postgraduate Medical Journal* **66**, 536–8.

Corenblum, B. and Baylis, B. (1990). Medical therapy for the syndrome of familial virilization, insulin, resistance, and acanthosis nigricans. *Fertility and Sterility* **53**, 421–5.

Cunliffe, W. and Simpson, N. (1998). *Disorders of sebaceous glands*. In *Rook/Wilkinson/Ebling Textbook of Dermatology*, ed. R. Champion, J. Burton, D. Burns and S. Breathnach, pp. 1927–84. Oxford: Blackwell Science.

Cusan, L., Dupont, A., Belanger, A. et al. (1990). Treatment of hirsutism with the pure anti-androgen flutamide. *Journal of the American Academy of Dermatology* 23, 462–9.

Darley, C., Kirby, J., Besser, G. et al. (1982). Circulating testosterone, sex hormone binding globulin and prolactin in women with late onset or persistent acne vulgaris. *British Journal of Dermatology* 106, 517–22.

Darley, C., Moore, J., Besser, G. and Munro, D. (1980). Androgen status in women with acne vulgaris. *British Journal of Dermatology* 103, (Suppl. 18), 17.

Dawber, R. (1998). Facial and body hair. In *Cosmetic Dermatology*, ed. R. Baran and H. Maibach, pp. 201–4. London: Martin Dunitz.

Dawber, R., de Berker, D. and Wojnarowska, F. (1998). Disorders of hair. In *Textbook of Dermatology*, ed. R. Champion, J. Burton, D. Burns and S. Breathnach, pp. 2869–73. Oxford: Blackwell Science.

Derksen, J. Moolenaar, A., van Seters, A. and Kock, D. (1993). Semiquantitative assessment of hirsutism in Dutch women. *British Journal of Dermatology* 128, 259–63.

DeVillez, R. and Dunn, J. (1986). Female androgenic alopecia. *Archives of Dermatology* 122, 1011–15.

DeVillez, R. Jacobs, F. Szpunar, C. and Warner, M. (1994). Androgenetic alopecia in the female. Treatment with 2% topical minoxidil solution. *Archives of Dermatology* 130, 303–7.

Dunaif, A., Hoffman, A., Scully, R. et al. (1985). Clinical, biochemical and ovarian morphologic features in women with acanthosis nigricans and masculinization. *Obstetrics and Gynecology* 66, 545–52.

Eden, J. (1991). The polycystic ovary syndrome presenting as resistant acne successfully treated with cyproterone acetate. *Medical Journal of Australia* 155, 677–80.

Falsetti, L., De Fusco, D., Elefherioiu, G. and Rosina, B. (1997). Treatment of hirsutism by finasteride and flutamide in women with polycystic ovary syndrome. *Gynecological Endocrinology* 11, 251–7.

Falsetti, L. and Galbignani, E. (1990). Long-term treatment with the combination ethinylestradiol and cyproterone acetate of polycystic ovary syndrome. *Contraception* 42, 611–19.

Ferriman, D. and Gallwey, J. (1961). Clinical assessment of body hair growth in women. *Journal of Clinical Endocrinology* 21, 1440–7.

Franks, S. (1988). Polycystic ovary syndrome: a changing perspective. *Clinical Endocrinology* 31, 87–118.

Futterweit, W., Dunaif, A., Yeh, H.-C. and Kingsley, P. (1988). The prevalence of hyperandrogenism in 109 consecutive female patients with diffuse alopecia. *Journal of the American Academy of Dermatology* 19, 831–6.

Goldzieher, J. and Axelrod, L. (1963). Clinical and biochemical features of polycystic ovarian disease. *Fertility and Sterility* 14, 631.

Hamilton, E. and Potten, C. (1974). The effect of repeated plucking on mouse skin cell kinetics. *Journal of Investigative Dermatology* 62, 560–2.

Held, B., Nader, S., Rodriguez-Rigau, L., Smith, K. and Steinberger, E. (1984). Acne and hyperandrogenism. *Journal of the American Academy of Dermatology* 10, 223–6.

Holmes, R., Williams, M. and Cunliffe, W. (1972). Pilo-sebaceous duct obstruction and acne. *British Journal of Dermatology* 87, 327–32.

Kiddy, D., Hamilton-Fairley, D., Bush, A. et al. (1992). Improvement in endocrine and ovarian function during dietary treatment of obese women with polycystic ovary syndrome. *Clinical Endocrinology* **36**, 105–11.

Kiddy, D., Sharp, D., White, D. et al. (1990). Difference in clinical and endocrine features between obese and non-obese subjects with polycystic ovary syndrome: an analysis of 263 consecutive cases. *Clinical Endocrinology* **32**, 213–20.

Levell, M. Cawood, M., Burke, B. and Cunliffe, W. (1989). Acne is not associated with abnormal plasma androgens. *British Journal of Dermatology* **120**, 649–54.

Lobo, R. (1991). Hirsutism in polycystic ovary syndrome: current concepts. *Clinical Obstetrics and Gynecology* **34**, 817–26.

Lucky, A., Biro, F., Huster, G. et al. (1994). Acne vulgaris in premenarchal girls. *Archives of Dermatology* **130**, 308–14.

Ludwig, E. (1977). Classification of the types of androgenetic alopecia (common baldness) occurring in the female sex. *British Journal of Dermatology* **97**, 247–54.

Marynick, S., Chakmakjian, Z., McCaffree, D. and Herndon, J. (1983). Androgen excess in cystic acne. *New England Journal of Medicine* **308**, 981–6.

McKnight, E. (1964). The prevalence of 'hirsutism' in young women. *Lancet*, **I**, 410–13.

Miller, J., Darley, C., Karkavitsas, K., Kirby, J. and Munro, D. (1982). Low sex-hormone binding globulin levels in young women with diffuse hair loss. *British Journal of Dermatology* **106**, 331–6.

O'Driscoll, J., Mamtora, H., Higginson, J. et al. (1994). A prospective study of the prevalence of clear-cut endocrine disorders and polycystic ovaries in 350 patients presenting with hirsutism or androgenic alopecia. *Clinical Endocrinology* **41**, 231–6.

Olsen, E. (1999). Methods of hair removal. *Journal of the American Academy of Dermatology* **40**, 143–57.

Piacquadio, D., Rad, F., Spellman, M. and Hollenbach, K. (1994). Obesity and female androgenic alopecia: a cause and effect? *Journal of the American Academy of Dermatology* **30**, 1028–30.

Rendon, M., Cruz, P., Sontheimer, R. and Bergstresser, P. (1989). Acanthosis nigricans: a cutaneous marker of tissue resistance to insulin. *Journal of the American Academy of Dermatology* **21**, 461–9.

Ruutiainen, K. (1986). The effect of an oral contraceptive containing ethinylestradiol and desogestrel on hair growth and hormonal parameters of hirsute women. *International Journal of Gynaecology and Obstetrics* **24**, 361–8.

Ruutiainen, K., Erkkola, R. Gronroos, M. and Irjala, K. (1988). Influence of body mass index and age on the grade of hair growth in hirsute women of reproductive ages. *Fertility and Sterility* **50**, 260–5.

Schwartz, R. (1994). Acanthosis nigricans. *Journal of the American Academy of Dermatology* **31**, 1–19.

Simpson, N. and Barth, J. (1991). *Hair patterns: hirsuties and baldness*. In *Diseases of the Hair and Scalp*. ed. R. Rook and R. Dawber, pp. 71–136. Oxford: Blackwell Science.

Simpson, N. and Barth J. (1997). *Hair patterns: hirsuties and androgenetic alopecia*. In *Diseases of the Hair and Scalp*. ed. R. Dawber, pp. 67–122. Oxford: Blackwell Science.

Sperling, L. and Heimer, W. (1993). Androgen biology as a basis for the diagnosis and treatment of androgenic disorders in women. I. *Journal of the American Academy of Dermatoloty* **28**, 669–81.

Tolino, A., Petrone, A., Sarnacchiaro, F. et al. (1996). Finasteride in the treatment of hirsutism: new therapeutic perspectives. *Fertility and Sterility*, **66** (1), 61–5.

Trotter, M. (1923). The resistance of hair to certain supposed growth stimulants. *Archives of Dermatology and Syphology* 7, 93–8.

9

Lifestyle factors in the aetiology and management of polycystic ovary syndrome

Robert J. Norman and Anne M. Clark

Introduction

Polycystic ovary syndrome (PCOS) is thought to arise from a combination of familial and environmental factors that interact to cause the characteristic menstrual and metabolic disturbances. It is our contention that alteration of the environmental components of this condition is fundamental to the management of the condition and that pharmaceutical treatment (including clomiphene citrate, gonadotrophins and insulin-sensitizing agents) should only be used after adequate counselling and action relating to lifestyle alterations. Weight loss, altered diet and exercise are important aspects to discuss with the patient, as are stopping smoking and improving psychological attitudes. Because of the importance of obesity in the majority of women with this condition, much of this chapter concentrates on obesity in polycystic ovary syndrome.

Obesity and disease

Obesity is a costly and increasingly prevalent condition in Western society. In the USA, 33% of Americans are obese, with women (34%), blacks (49%) and Hispanics (47%) showing the highest rates of obesity. In Australia, 37% of the population are overweight or obese according to recent Australian Bureau of Statistics data. The prevalence of overweight/obesity increases in Australian women as they age, with 34% of all women between 20 and 69 years having a body mass index (BMI) over 25 kg/m^2 and 12% having a BMI over 30 kg/m^2. In the Reproductive Medicine Unit at the University of Adelaide, 39.8% of women have a BMI over 25 kg/m^2 and 17.4% a BMI >30 kg/m^2 based on over 5000 patients presenting between 1991 and 1997.

Obesity is associated in women with an increased risk of diabetes mellitus, osteoarthritis, cardiovascular disease, sleep apnoea, breast and uterine cancer and reproductive disorders. Whereas women have increased body fat as an essential requirement for reproductive efficiency in pregnancy (Frisch, 1985, 1987), fat in excess of normal can lead to menstrual abnormality, infertility, miscarriage and difficulties in performing assisted reproduction. Observational and theoretical considerations indicate that body weight has an inverted 'U' effect on reproduction whereby low and high body mass contributes to infertility, menstrual disorders and poor reproductive outcome (Correa and Jacoby, 1978).

The most commonly used index of obesity is the BMI – weight in kg/height in m^2 – which correlates reasonably well with body fat, although at height extremes there is less association. Total body fat has been assessed by physical methods (such as skinfold thickness, underwater weighing, DEXA densitometry, magnetic resonance imaging and infrared spectroscopy (Pasquali and Casimirri, 1993). The distribution of fat is also thought to be important and can be assessed by these methods, although the waist to hip ratio (WHR) or, simply, the waist circumference is the easiest clinical method. The reproductive literature is largely based on weight or BMI, with few data available on body composition or distribution. However, the general medical literature does contain evidence that even peripheral (non-central) obesity is highly significant in poor health outcomes and the absence of information on fat distribution relating to reproductive factors may not be essential to an understanding of the importance of obesity.

Women have greater fat reserves than men but fat distribution is more likely to be peripheral (gynaecoid) than abdominal (android). Obese and overweight women are over-represented in gynaecological and reproductive medicine clinics. BMI ranges are usually defined as follows: underweight (<19 kg/m^2), normal weight (19.1–24.9 kg/m^2), overweight (25–29.9 kg/m^2) and obese (>30 kg/m^2). Central or peripheral obesity is usually divided at WHRs of 0.82–0.85.

Metabolic activity of fat tissue

Adipose tissue is an important site of active steroid production and metabolism (Pasquali and Casimirri, 1993). It is able to convert androgens to oestrogens (aromatase activity) oestradiol to oestrone and dehydroepiandrosterone to androstenediol (17β-hydroxy-steroid dehydrogenase activity). Aromatase is found in bone, the hypothalamus, liver, muscle, kidney and adipose tissue in the breast, abdomen, omentum and marrow. Within adipose tissue, aromatase activity has been identified in the cells of peri-adipocyte fibrovascular stroma and may differ between various depots of adipose tissue. Whereas in 'simple' obesity, blood levels of androgens do not appear to differ from those of non-obese controls, production and clearance rates are significantly different (Pasquali and Casimirri, 1993). Abdominal fat distribution also significantly influences androgen and oestrogen metabolism. In hyperandrogenic obesity, such as PCOS, increased production rates of androgens are associated with menstrual irregularities. The amount of androstenedione converted to oestrone varies depending on the total body weight, with women in the following groups showing the conversion rates in brackets: 49–63 kg (1.0%), 63.1–91 kg (1.5%), >91 kg (2.3%). Other mechanisms that influence the adipose tissue as an endocrine organ are:

1. metabolism of oestrogens to 2-hydroxy oestrogen (relatively inactive) or to 16-hydroxylated oestrogen (active in obesity);
2. the storage of steroid hormones in fat; and
3. the effects of adiposity on insulin secretion from the pancreas and hence the levels of sex hormone-binding globulin (SHBG).

Leptin is the product of the *ob* gene, a protein produced in fat cells that signals the magnitude of the energy stores to the brain and has significant effects on the reproductive system of rodents. Absence of the full-length *ob* gene, or its receptor, leads to obesity and reproductive dysfunction. Replacement of leptin in *ob/ob* mice restores fertility. Administration of recombinant leptin to rodents induces puberty earlier than in control animals, indicating important effects, directly or indirectly, on ovarian function. Zachow and Magoffin (1997) have shown that leptin directly affects insulin-like growth factor-induced oestradiol production in the rodent ovary in the presence of follicle-stimulating hormone (FSH).

Initial reports suggested that leptin was increased in a significant proportion of women with anovulation, specifically with PCOS. Subsequently, this has not been confirmed (Chapman, Wittert and Norman, 1997) and leptin does not alter in women who are given insulin-sensitizing agents such as troglitazone (Mantzoros, Dunaif and Flier, 1997) or gonadotrophin-reducing drugs such as the oral contraceptive pill (Nader, Riad Gabriel and Saad, 1997). The true role of leptin in influencing ovarian function therefore remains unclear. This hormone may have an effect on ovarian function directly via actions on the ovary or, alternatively, through the hypothalamic–pituitary–ovarian axis. Whereas the exact role of leptin remains unclear in PCOS, current techniques for intervention by weight loss or drugs have little impact on concentrations of leptin other than by reduction of body fat.

Obesity, polycystic ovary syndrome and menstruation

The original description of what is now known as the polycystic ovary syndrome associated obesity and anovulation with infertility. Classical studies by Mitchell and Rogers (1953) and Hartz et al. (1979) confirmed these findings in much larger groups of women. The former group reported that obesity was present at a four times higher rate in women with menstrual disturbances than in women with normal cycles. Forty-five per cent of amenorrhoeic women were obese, while only 9–13% of women with normal periods were overweight. Hartz et al. (1979) studied

26 638 women by questionnaire and noted that anovulation was strongly associated with obesity. Grossly obese women had a rate of menstrual disturbance 3.1 times more frequent than women in the normal weight range. In their study, teenage obesity was positively correlated with menstrual irregularity later in life, and obesity was correlated with abnormal and long cycles, heavy flow and hirsutism. However, this study was selective in that volunteers were recruited from a weight control organization, data were self-reported and only one-third of all subjects were suitable for analysis. Lake and colleagues (Lake, Power and Cole, 1997) studied nearly 5800 women who were born in 1958 and seen at ages 7, 11, 16, 23 and 33 years. Obesity in childhood and the early twenties increased the risk of menstrual problems (odds ratio, OR, 1.75 and 1.59 respectively). Women who were overweight at 23 years (BMI 23.9–28.6 kg/m²) were 1.32 times more likely and if obese (>28.6 kg/m²) 1.75 times more likely to have menstrual difficulties. Interestingly, in view of the association between overweight and early menarche, girls with menarche at 9, 10 or 11 years were more likely to have menstrual problems at 16.5 years (OR 1.45 for mild and 1.94 for severe menstrual abnormality), but this was not reflected at age 33 years. Balen and colleagues (1995) in London have also shown a close relationship between weight and menstrual disorders. Of 1741 subjects with PCOS, 70% had menstrual disturbances and only 22% had normal menstrual function if their BMI was over 30 kg/m². Similar results were reported by Kiddy et al. (1990): obese subjects with PCOS had a 88% chance of menstrual disturbance compared to 72% in non-obese subjects with PCOS.

It is likely that obesity and overweight do contribute to a significant proportion of menstrual dysfunction. There is little in the literature to separate predisposing or associated features such as PCOS from so-called 'simple' obesity, although there are suggestions that women with polycystic ovaries suffer more from weight-related menstrual dysfunction than those with normal ovaries (Hartz et al., 1979).

Obesity, polycystic ovary syndrome and infertility

Many multiparous women are obese and, indeed, most obese women are able to conceive readily. Initial study of the literature suggests that several excellent investigators have not been able to confirm the adverse effect of weight on reproductive performance. The Oxford Family Planning Study (Howe et al., 1985) did not show any relationship between conception rates and weight or BMI in women stopping contraception, but those women were a selected group of largely parous subjects. Similar criticism applies to a well-conducted prospective study on fecundity in volunteer women who were followed for six months to examine the effect of environmental agents on reproduction.

Hartz et al. (1979) found in a very large study that obesity in the teenage years was more common among married women who never became pregnant than for married women who did become pregnant. In the Nurses' Health Study, which involved 2527 married infertile nurses, the risk of ovulatory infertility increased from a RR of 1.3, (1.2–1.6) in the group with a BMI as low as 24 kg/m^2 to a rate of 2.7 (2.0–3.7) in women with a BMI over 32 kg/m^2 (Rich Edwards et al., 1994). In the same year, Grodstein and colleagues (Grodstein, Goldman and Cramer, 1994) showed that anovulatory infertility in 1880 infertile women and 4023 controls was higher in those with a BMI of >26.9 kg/m^2 (relative risk, RR, 3.1, 2.2–4.4), with a smaller non-significant risk of 1.2 (0.8–1.9) in those with BMI of 25–26.9 kg/m^2. So, even high-normal to slightly overweight levels may have an effect on fertility.

Lake et al. (1997) studied a cohort of women born in 1958 and followed up at 7, 11, 16, 23 and 33 years. They showed that weight during childhood did not predict subsequent fecundity, but weight at 23 years did predict fecundity if the woman was obese (OR 0.69, 0.56–0.87). Results relating BMI at 33 years were weaker but consistent with those for 23 years. Obese women at 23 years were less likely to become pregnant within 12 months than women of normal weight (infertility rates = obese 33.6% vs normal weight 18.6%). Zaadstra et al. (1993) found that the upper quartile of BMI (33.1 kg/m2) in a group of apparently normal women who were undergoing donor insemination had a reduced chance of pregnancy (OR 0.43). This was a particularly significant study because few of the women required medication to stimulate ovulation. Balen et al. (1995) in the UK also found that obese women had higher infertility rates. In 204 North American women studied by Green, Weiss and Daling (1988) there was a reduced fertility rate among women with more than 20% of ideal body weight (OR 2.1) – this did not apply to women who had previously been pregnant.

The literature is therefore quite clear in associating increased body mass with a higher incidence of infertility. Most of the studies do not clearly classify women as having PCOS or normal ovaries, but a large percentage of the obese female population is likely to have this condition.

Obesity, polycystic ovary syndrome and miscarriage

Weight excess is associated with an increased risk of miscarriage. In a study of over 13 000 women seeking their first spontaneous pregnancy (Hamilton-Fairley et al., 1992), 11% of women with a BMI 19–24.9 kg/m^2, 14% with BMI 25–27.9 kg/m^2 and 15% of those >28 kg/m^2 miscarried (OR 1, 1.26 and 1.37 respectively). Women over 82 kg are more likely to miscarry than thinner women after ovulation induction (Bohrer and Kemmann, 1987) (OR 2.7 for 82–95 kg and 3.4 for >95 kg), while even a mild increase in BMI (25–28 kg/m^2) leads to a significant risk of pregnancy loss (OR 1.37, 1.18–1.60) in some series (Hamilton-Fairley et al., 1992; Pettigrew and Hamilton-Fairley, 1997) but not in others (McClure et al., 1992). It has been generally claimed that women with PCOS are more likely to miscarry than those without PCOS. This has been attributed, at least in part, to higher luteinizing hormone (LH) concentrations in PCOS that may lead to impaired oocyte and embryo quality.

Obesity, polycystic ovary syndrome and pregnancy

Since the 1940s, there have been many articles on the effect of obesity on pregnancy and obstetric outcome. Some of the American studies detail results on massively obese women indicating much higher health risks and increased costs to the health system. Studies from Europe (Galtier Dereure et al., 1995) confirm that high pre-pregnancy weight is associated with an increased risk in pregnancy of hypertension, toxaemia, gestational diabetes, urinary infection, macrosomia, Caesarean section, increased hospitalization and cost. Despite this, overall neonatal outcome appears to be satisfactory.

Obesity, polycystic ovary syndrome and glucose intolerance

There is abundant evidence associating increasing BMI with diabetes mellitus. Subjects with PCOS have a substantial added risk of glucose intolerance. In a study from Adelaide, 18% of all women over BMI 30 kg/m^2 in their twenties and thirties had impairment of glucose metabolism, while 15% of women with PCOS who had normal glucose tolerance when initially studied showed conversion to impaired glucose tolerance or frank diabetes when restudied five to seven years later (Norman and Masters, unpublished). Conway et al. (1992) showed that 8% of lean and 11% of obese women with PCOS had abnormal glucose tolerance. In a recent prospective study, we have shown that women with PCOS convert from initially normal glucose tolerance to impaired glucose tolerance or diabetes mellitus at a rate of approximately 3% per year. Almost all of this change can be associated with increasing obesity, and prevention of weight gain would be expected to be beneficial in the minimization of abnormal glucose tolerance.

There is now evidence that women with PCOS are more likely to exhibit gestational diabetes when pregnant and that many women with glucose intolerance in pregnancy have features of PCOS. This makes it even more important that potential complications from PCOS should be sorted out before embarking on treatment to induce pregnancy.

Obesity, polycystic ovary syndrome and response to infertility treatment

Most studies show conclusive evidence that increasing BMI is associated with an increased requirement for clomiphene citrate. In several of these, large doses of clomiphene (up to 200 mg per day) were required to ensure ovulation in the heaviest women. If this drug is considered to have some association with ovarian cancer, it is probably undesirable for so much to be used per cycle of treatment. There does not, however, appear to be an association of body weight with poor conception rates in cycles of oral anti-oestrogens. In a study of 2841 cycles of clomiphene citrate, there was no association between body weight and pregnancy rate (Dickey et al., 1997) as previously suggested by Friedman and Kim (1985). Doses of gonadotrophins required to induce ovulation are also higher in anovulatory women and those requiring ovarian stimulation for any reason (McClure et al., 1992).

Recently, we have shown that the procedure of intrauterine insemination with gonadotrophins in women with normal menstrual cycles and unexplained infertility gives pregnancy rates up to BMI 30 kg/m^2 similar to those of women of normal weight (Fuh et al., 1997). Although women with a BMI >35 kg/m^2 have a lower pregnancy result, paradoxically this treatment was statistically more successful in women between BMI 30 and 34.9 kg/m^2, suggesting a subtle endocrine abnormality in this group of women.

The data relating to in-vitro fertilization (IVF) and other assisted reproduction are less certain. While Clark et al. (1995) found a poor success rate in IVF pregnancies for the very obese, other studies have not shown any difference for women with moderate to severe obesity (Lewis et al., 1990).

Fat distribution, polycystic ovary syndrome and reproduction

Obesity can be central or peripheral in distribution and there is evidence suggesting different hormonal and metabolic responses depending upon the distribution of fat. Women with central fat have high levels of LH, androstenedione, oestrone, insulin, triglycerides, very low-density lipoproteins and apolipoprotein β, and lower levels of high-density lipoprotein (Pettigrew and Hamilton-Fairley, 1997). Gynaecological effects of central adiposity are also significant. Zaadstra et al.(1993) showed that a WHR (central adiposity) was associated with a markedly lower conception rate in a donor insemination programme. The Iowa Women's Health Study also indicated that high WHRs were associated with more menstrual abnormalities and higher prevalence of infertility (Kaye et al., 1990). Norman et al. (1995a, 1995b) showed that high WHR was associated with greater disturbance in reproductive hormones, (particularly insulin) in PCOS, as subsequently confirmed by others (Hollmann, Runnebaum and Gerhard, 1997). Reproductive response to diet and infertility treatment is likely to be closely related to central fat, as indicated by the data of Clark et al. (1995, 1998) and Huber-Buchholz, Carey and Norman (1999).

Effect of weight loss on menstruation and infertility

There were several reports in the 1950s that indicated that weight loss induces menstrual regulation in a proportion of women with obesity and anovulation. Later, Bates and Whitworth (1982) were the first to show a reduction in plasma androgens with dieting and associated return of menstrual cycles. These endocrine and clinical observations have been confirmed by several studies, including those by Pasquali et al. (1989a, 1989b). Kiddy et al. (1989, 1990, 1992) and Pettigrew and Hamilton-Fairley (1997) revisited dietary manipulation of subjects with obesity and PCOS, showing that strict calorie restriction with a subsequent 5% or greater weight loss led to changes in insulin, insulin-like growth factor, SHBG and menstruation. Menstrual regularity and hirsutism improved, with some spontaneous pregnancies resulting. Since then, there have been several studies confirming that weight loss improves clinical and biochemical parameters that are disordered due to weight problems (Clark et al., 1995, 1998; Hollmann et al., 1997). All the above studies, while showing the principle that dietary control leads to favourable reproductive outcomes, fail to address the issue of long-term compliance in a clinical situation. The one exception is the work published in Adelaide which has shown how menstrual regularity and pregnancy can be restored by exercise and dietary advice without an emphasis on low calorie intake (Clark et al., 1995, 1998). More than 90% of obese, oligomenorrhoeic women showed a dramatic improvement in menstrual patterns, with a high spontaneous conception rate and a lower miscarriage rate than before treatment (Fig. 9.1). Even women with causes of infertility not related to anovulation (such as tubal blockage or a male partner with oligospermia) showed dramatic improvements in assisted reproduction pregnancies (Tables 9.1 and 9.2). Weight loss into the normal range is not required for a good clinical response, indicating that weight loss per se was not the main reason for success. Mitchell and Rogers in 1953 had made the observation that 'the onset of menses frequently precedes any marked loss of weight and occurs so soon after the start of the therapeutic regimen that the absolute degree of obesity cannot be the only factor involved'.

Several studies have reported that surgically induced weight loss (gastrojejunal anastomosis and gastric stapling) is successful in restoring menstruation and pregnancy, but these operations may have significant morbidity and very poor neonatal outcome. However, in one of these studies, the miscarriage rate was substantially reduced after the operation when compared to that before the operation (Bilenka et al., 1995).

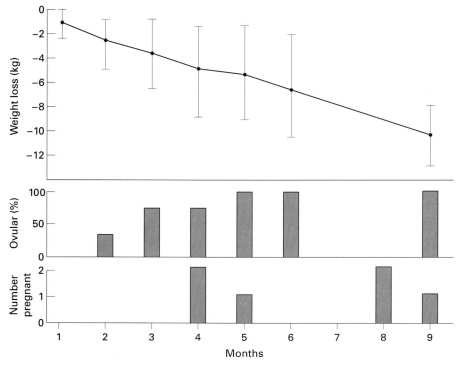

Fig. 9.1   Changes in weight and ovulation rates during the study period for those subjects who completed six months of trial. The number of spontaneous pregnancies is shown in the bottom panel.

Weight loss and exercise programmes in lifestyle modification

Clark has described how women have achieved sustained weight loss and alteration of reproductive function by being encouraged to join a group that meets weekly for six months. Having become frustrated by the lack of results when individual dietary advice was given by a dietician or medical practitioner, she pioneered the unique concept (at least in gynaecology) of lifestyle modification within groups of overweight women seeking to achieve a pregnancy (Fig. 9.2). Women were encouraged to agree to join a group for six months, during which time they understood they would not be given any fertility treatment. At the first meeting, they were encouraged to bring their partners, who were given the information about the group approach, and subsequently meetings were held every week for about two hours. At these meetings, exercise and dietary advice were combined with other activities such as fashion information for the overweight, supermarket trips and medical information on the pathophysiology of PCOS. The exercise component lasted

Table 9.1. Pregnancies per cycle after participation in the programme and occurring simultaneously in non-study patients

	Completed group ($n = 67$)	'Drop-out' group ($n = 20$) post-programme	Average pregnancy rate in the unit over same period, pregnancy rate (%)
OI	0/3 (0)	0/4 (0)	24
IUI	6/11 (55)	0/10 (0)	19
IVF	26/47 (55)	0/35 (0)	20

Notes:

OI = ovulation induction, IUI = intrauterine insemination, IVF = in-vitro fertilization.
Values in parentheses are percentages.

Table 9.2. Comparison between those who completed and those who did not complete the study

	Completed ($n = 67$)	'Drop-out' ($n = 20$)
Change in body mass index (kg/m^2)	-3.7 ± 1.6	-0.4 ± 1.4^a
Resumed spontaneous ovulation (%)	90	0.9[b]
Pregnancy (%)		
Spontaneous	27	0.0[b]
Treatment	53	0.0[b]
Miscarriage (%)	18	0.0
Total women pregnant (%)[c]	77.6	0.0[b]
Total women with live birth (%)	67	0.0

Notes:

[a] $p < 0.001$.

[b] $p < 0.001$.

[c] Nine (13%) avoiding treatment.

Source: From Clark et al. (1998).

about an hour, with gentle exercises such as stepping and walking, and was conducted by a keep-fit instructor who was aware of the problems of the overweight person. The exercise session was followed by a group session in which a lecture, seminar or discussion concentrated on subjects of interest to the women. Initially, a dietician gave advice on healthy eating patterns without seeking to get women to follow a low-calorie diet. No attempt was made to induce massive caloric reduction, slow weight loss being the preferred option. Initially, many of the women expected diet sheets and advice similar to those obtained from commercial

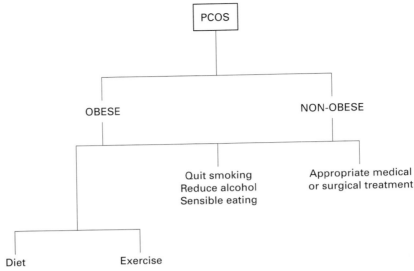

Fig. 9.2   Approach to polycystic ovary syndrome: lifestyle modification.

1. Information about role of weight and body composition in reproductive disorders.
2. Agreement to seek lifestyle changes for at least 6 months.
3. Group meeting with partners to explain the course.
4. Weekly meetings for 2–2½ hours with women.
5. Gentle aerobic exercises for 1 hour (walking, stepping etc.).
6. Lecture/seminar for 1 hour (good eating, psychological aspects, medical information etc.).
7. Put into practice for next 6 months.
8. If return of periods, pregnancy etc., no further medical treatment.
9. If disorder persists after 6 months, offer appropriate medical treatment.

Fig. 9.3   The Fertility Fitness© programme.

weight-loss companies, but in time they realized that sustained weight loss can only be achieved by a life-long alteration in eating patterns and not by crash diets (Fig. 9.3).

Re-distribution of fat and weight is the first obvious sign before weight loss in this programme. Menstrual regularity can be induced without any weight loss provided the dietary retraining and exercise are taken seriously. Even 2–5% weight change can be effective in restoring ovulation. In 1995, Clark et al. reported on a study of anovulatory women with PCOS: 12 of 13 ovulated by the end of six months and the majority became pregnant within a year, most spontaneously. In a subsequent report (Clark et al., 1998), this success rate was extended to all women with obesity who had a range of infertility conditions and showed the efficacy of this approach. In most of the women, weight loss has been sustained and it is likely that long-term health benefits will result. Our philosophy is that alteration of lifestyle, particularly weight, will lead to benefits in the short, medium and long term. Menstruation can be restored, fertility promoted naturally or by assisted reproduction with better results, the risks of diabetes mellitus, cardiovascular disease and hyperlipidaemia ameliorated, and the musculoskeletal and metabolic side-effects reduced (Fig. 9.4). Retraining of diet and exercise patterns can have life-long benefits and alter health outcomes significantly.

Reasons for weight-related menstrual problems

Infertile, anovulatory obese women have higher plasma androgens, insulin and LH concentrations and lower SHBG levels when compared to normal-weight women or obese subjects with regular periods. It is possible that the increased oestrogen production from peripheral tissues leads to a disorder of the hypothalamic–pituitary–ovarian axis. Insulin resistance is common in anovulatory women and, together with reduced hepatic clearance of insulin and increased sensitivity of the beta cells to secretory stimuli, is thought to be the major cause of hyperinsulinaemia. Insulin in turn can induce androgen secretion from an ovary that is polycystic or genetically prone to excess androgen production. Current hypotheses suggest that hyperinsulinaemia is a result of genetic or environmentally induced insulin resistance from peripheral tissues and this leads to increased androgen production from ovaries that are not resistant to the action of insulin. Reduction of hyperinsulinaemia should lead to reduction of hyperandrogenaemia and restoration of reproduction function. This hypothesis is clearly supported by the experimental observations by a number of investigators.

We have followed women participating in a weight-loss programme and have shown that return of ovulation coincides with a reduction in insulin resistance and a fall in central adiposity. In a group of anovulatory subjects who returned to ovulation with exercise and dietary restraint, waist circumference, central fat, LH and insulin fell more than in those who remained anovulatory throughout (Huber-Buchholz et al., 1999). In a less extensive, previous study Clark et al. (1995) had shown that fasting insulin was significantly reduced by weight loss in anovulatory women who became ovulatory. While there is convincing evidence that insulin sensitivity can be restored in overweight women with PCOS who lose weight (Holte et al., 1994, 1995; Holte, 1996), first phase insulin release remains significantly abnormal, indicating an underlying problem in pancreatic secretion in these subjects. Other investigators have disputed this observation. The return to ovulation

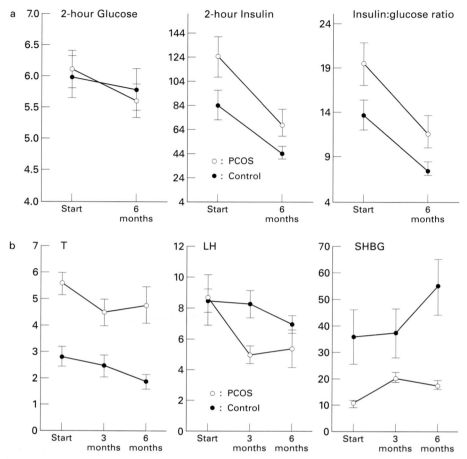

Fig. 9.4   Hormone changes in serum or plasma concentrations over the course of the study. (a) Glucose and insulin response to glucose. (b) Hormones at three time points of the study. T: testosterone (nmol/l); LH: luteinizing hormone (IU/l); PCOS: polycystic ovary syndrome; SHBG: sex hormone binding globulin (nmol/l); 2-hour glucose: post 75G glucose tolerance test (mmol/l); insulin: post 75G glucose tolerance test (mIU/l).

associated with a reduction in insulin reinforces studies with insulin-sensitizing agents such as troglitazone where improved insulin sensitivity without weight loss promotes ovulation and fertility (Dunaif et al., 1996; Ehrmann et al., 1997).

Luteinizing hormone pulse frequency and amplitude do not appear to alter during weight loss in obese subjects (Guzick et al., 1994), although absolute values of LH do decrease significantly in responders to diet, as judged by ovulation.

Other factors involved may include androgens, hypothalamic endorphins and leptin, all of which are increased in anovulatory overweight women. While leptin is increased in obese PCOS subjects, there is no increase over obesity not associated with PCOS, and return of ovulation is not associated with a reduction in leptin concentrations prior to the return of periods (Huber-Buchholz et al., 1999).

Depression is frequent in women with PCOS and infertility, as shown by assessments performed in Adelaide women. Participation in the programme was associated with an improvement in well-being and psychological parameters, which may indicate that restoration of reproductive potential is closely tied in with psychological changes (Galletly et al., 1996a, 1996b). These psychological factors may have an effect through the endorphin system and other neurotransmitters in the hypothalamic–pituitary axis.

Smoking

Many women with PCOS choose to smoke in response to stress or the desire to prevent further weight gain. The authors' experience shows that 40% of women in the unit in Adelaide who have PCOS are also smokers. There are convincing data that, apart from the well-known health hazards of smoking with respect to the cardiovascular and respiratory systems, there are effects associated with reduction of fertility potential (Table 9.3).

Studies show that the time to conception is increased by 30% for smokers and there is a twofold to threefold increased risk of failing to conceive by one year of attempting pregnancy. Augood, Duckitt and Templeton (1998) have recently published a systematic review and meta-analysis of the effects of smoking on fertility and concluded that the risk of infertility in smokers versus non-smokers was 1.60 (95% confidence interval 1.34–1.91). Women who subsequently went through a cycle of assisted reproduction were found to have an odds ratio of 0.66 (0.49–0.88) for pregnancies per number of attempts when comparing smokers and non-smokers (Table 9.3). This does not appear to be attributable to smoking in the male partner when the female partner's smoking status is taken into consideration.

Maternal smoking does not appear to affect the risk of spontaneous abortion, but may alter the rate of abnormal placentation, abruptio placentae and perinatal death after antepartum bleeding (Werler, 1997). Growth of the fetus is definitely altered by smoking, with birthweight reduced by an average of 200 g. There is a dose–response effect where birthweight decreases as the number of cigarettes smoked increases. Perinatal mortality rates are increased by about 30% due to excesses in low birthweight, prematurity and abnormal placentation.

All women with PCOS who try to become pregnant should be strongly advised to reduce or eliminate their smoking habit prior to therapeutic attempts at inducing ovulation with drugs. While this may require considerable effort, including the

Table 9.3. Meta-analysis of 12 studies of smoking exposure and female infertility

	Infertility cases (n) in smokers (N) n/N	Infertility cases (n) in non-smokers (N) n/N	OR (95%CI)	Weight (%)	OR (95%CI)
Cohort studies					
Baird-Wilcox 1985	11/135	13/543	—•—	3.3	3.62 [1.58, 8.26]
de Mouzon 1998	8/387	31/1500	—•—	3.5	1.00 [0.46, 2.19]
Spinelli 1997	29/203	41/410	—•—	5.9	1.54 [0.92, 2.55]
Alderet 1995	51/554	66/787	—•—	7.4	1.11 [0.76, 1.62]
Suonio 1990	96/521	198/1677	—•—	9.0	1.69 [1.29, 2.20]
Laurent 1992	241/1179	242/1535	—•—	9.8	1.37 [1.13, 1.67]
Bolumar (1) 1996	298/1341	312/1837	—•—	10.1	1.40 [1.17, 1.67]
Bolumar (2) 1996	358/1347	502/2642	—•—	10.3	1.54 [1.32, 1.80]
Joffe 1994b	331/1323	452/2129	—•—	10.2	1.24 [1.05, 1.46]
Subtotal (95% CI)	1423/6990	1857/13069	◆	69.5	1.42 [1.27, 1.58]
Chi-square 12.97 (dft = 8) Z = 6.13					
Case control studies					
Tzounou 1993	24/84	14/168	—•—	3.9	4.40 [2.13, 9.07]
Daling 1985	60/159	25/159	—•—	5.6	3.25 [1.90, 5.54]
Joesoef 1993	509/1815	261/1760	—•—	10.2	2.24 [1.89, 2.64]
Cramer 1985	900/1880	1833/4023	—•—	10.7	1.10 [0.98, 1.22]
Subtotal (95% CI)	1493/3938	2133/6110	◆	30.5	2.27 [1.28, 4.02]
Chi-square 68.5 (df = 3) Z = 2.82					
Total (95% CI)	2916/10928	3990/19179	◆	100.0	1.60 [1.34, 1.91]
Chi-square 81.47 (dt = 12) Z = 5.16					

Note:
The odds ratio (OR) and 95% confidence intervals (CI) are shown on a logarithmic scale. *Source:* From Augood, Duckitt and Templeton (1998)

use of nicotine patches and hypnotherapy, the end results are well justified in terms of improved pregnancy rates, perinatal mortality and health outcomes.

Conclusion

While the attending doctor may be tempted or pressurized to use fertility drugs for subjects with PCOS, lifestyle changes are critically important in these women, not only for successful management but also for long-term health.

REFERENCES

Augood, C., Duckitt, K. and Templeton, A.A. (1998). Smoking and female infertility: a systematic review and meta-analysis. *Human Reproduction* 13, 1532–9.

Balen, A.H., Conway, G.S., Kaltsas, G. et al. (1995). Polycystic ovary syndrome: the spectrum of the disorder in 1741 patients. *Human Reproduction* 10, 2107–11.

Bates, G.W. and Whitworth, N.S. (1982). Effect of body weight reduction on plasma androgens in obese, infertile women. *Fertility and Sterility* 38, 406–9.

Bilenka, B., Ben Shlomo, I., Cozacov, C., Gold, C.H. and Zohar, S. (1995). Fertility, miscarriage and pregnancy after vertical banded gastroplasty operation for morbid obesity. *Acta Obstetricia et Gynecologica Scandinavica* 74, 42–4.

Bohrer, M. and Kemmann, E. (1987). Risk factors for spontaneous abortion in menotropin-treated women. *Fertility and Sterility* 48, 571–5.

Chapman, I.M., Wittert, G.A. and Norman, R.J. (1997). Circulating leptin concentrations in polycystic ovary syndrome: relation to anthropometric and metabolic parameters. *Clinical Endocrinology (Oxford)* 46, 175–81.

Clark, A.M., Ledger, W., Galletly, C. et al. (1995). Weight loss results in significant improvement in pregnancy and ovulation rates in anovulatory obese women. *Human Reproduction* 10, 2705–12.

Clark, A.M., Thornley, B., Tomlinson, L., Galletley, C. and Norman, R.J. (1998). Weight loss in obese infertile women results in improvement in reproductive outcome for all forms of fertility treatment. *Human Reproduction* 13, 1502–5.

Conway, G.S., Agrawal, R., Betteridge, D.J. and Jacobs, H.S. (1992). Risk factors for coronary artery disease in lean and obese women with the polycystic ovary syndrome. *Clinical Endocrinology (Oxford)* 37, 119–25.

Correa, H. and Jacoby, J. (1978). Nutrition and fertility: some iconoclastic results. *American Journal of Clinical Nutrition* 31, 1431–6.

Dickey, R.P., Taylor, S.N., Curole, D.N. et al. (1997). Relationship of clomiphene dose and patient weight to successful treatment. *Human Reproduction* 12, 449–53.

Dunaif, A., Scott, D., Finegood, D., Quintana, B. and Whitcomb, R. (1996). The insulin-sensitizing agent troglitazone improves metabolic and reproductive abnormalities in the polycystic ovary syndrome. *Journal of Clinical Endocrinology and Metabolism* 81, 3299–306.

Ehrmann, D.A., Schneider, D.J., Sobel, B.E. et al. (1997). Troglitazone improves defects in insulin action, insulin secretion, ovarian steroidogenesis, and fibrinolysis in women with polycystic ovary syndrome. *Journal of Clinical Endocrinology and Metabolism* 82, 2108–16.

Friedman, C.I. and Kim, M.H. (1985). Obesity and its effect on reproductive function. *Clinical Obstetrics and Gynecology* 28, 645–63.

Frisch, R.E. (1985). Fatness, menarche, and female fertility. *Perspectives in Biology and Medicine* 28, 611–33.

Frisch, R.E. (1987). Body fat, menarche, fitness and fertility. *Human Reproduction* 2, 521–33.

Fuh, K.W., Wang, X., Tai, A., Wong, I. and Norman, R.J. (1997). Intrauterine insemination: effect of the temporal relationship between the LH surge, hCG administration and insemination on pregnancy rates. *Human Reproduction* 12, 2162–6.

Galletly, C., Clark, A., Tomlinson, L. and Blaney, F. (1996a). A group program for obese, infertile women: weight loss and improved psychological health. *Journal of Psychosomatic Obstetrics and Gynaecology* 17, 125–8.

Galletly, C., Clark, A., Tomlinson, L. and Blaney, F. (1996b). Improved pregnancy rates for obese, infertile women following a group treatment program. An open pilot study. *General Hospital Psychiatry* 18, 192–5.

Galtier Dereure, F., Montpeyroux, F., Boulot, P., Bringer, J. and Jaffiol, C. (1995). Weight excess before pregnancy: complications and cost. *International Journal of Obesity and Related Metabolic Disorders* 19, 443–8.

Green, B.B., Weiss, N.S. and Daling, J.R. (1988). Risk of ovulatory infertility in relation to body weight. *Fertility and Sterility* 50, 721–6.

Grodstein, F., Goldman, M.B. and Cramer, D.W. (1994). Body mass index and ovulatory infertility. *Epidemiology* 5, 247–50.

Guzick, D.S., Wing, R., Smith, D., Berga, S.L. and Winters, S.J. (1994). Endocrine consequences of weight loss in obese, hyperandrogenic, anovulatory women. *Fertility and Sterility* 61, 598–604.

Hamilton-Fairley, D., Kiddy, D., Watson, H., Paterson, C. and Franks, S. (1992). Association of moderate obesity with a poor pregnancy outcome in women with polycystic ovary syndrome treated with low dose gonadotrophin. *British Journal of Obstetrics and Gynaecology* 99, 128–31.

Hartz, A.J., Barboriak, P.N., Wong, A., Katayama, K.P. and Rimm, A.A. (1979). The association of obesity with infertility and related menstural abnormalities in women. *International Journal of Obesity* 3, 57–73.

Hollmann, M., Runnebaum, B. and Gerhard, I. (1997). Impact of waist-hip-ratio and body-mass-index on hormonal and metabolic parameters in young, obese women. *International Journal of Obesity and Related Metabolic Disorders* 21, 476–83.

Holte, J. (1996). Disturbances in insulin secretion and sensitivity in women with the polycystic ovary syndrome. *Baillière's Clinical Endocrinology and Metabolism* 10, 221–47.

Holte, J., Bergh, T., Berne, C., Berglund, L. and Lithell, H. (1994). Enhanced early insulin response to glucose in relation to insulin resistance in women with polycystic ovary syndrome and normal glucose tolerance. *Journal of Clinical Endocrinology and Metabolism* 78, 1052–8.

Holte, J., Bergh, T., Berne, C., Wide, L. and Lithell, H. (1995). Restored insulin sensitivity but persistently increased early insulin secretion after weight loss in obese women with polycystic ovary syndrome. *Journal of Clinical Endocrinology and Metabolism* **80**, 2586–93.

Howe, G., Westhoff, C., Vessey, M. and Yeates, D. (1985). Effects of age, cigarette smoking, and other factors on fertility: findings in a large prospective study. *British Medical Journal of Clinical and Research Education* **290**, 1697–700.

Huber-Buchholz, M.M., Carey, D.G.P. and Norman, R.J. (1999). Restoration of reproductive potential by lifestyle modification in obese polycystic ovary syndrome: role of insulin sensitivity and luteinizing hormone. *Journal of Clinical Endocrinology and Metabolism* **84**, 1470–4.

Kaye, S.A., Folsom, A.R., Prineas, R.J., Potter, J.D. and Gapstur, S.M. (1990). The association of body fat distribution with lifestyle and reproductive factors in a population study of postmenopausal women. *International Journal of Obesity* **14**, 583–91.

Kiddy, D.S., Hamilton-Fairley, D., Bush, A. et al. (1992). Improvement in endocrine and ovarian function during dietary treatment of obese women with polycystic ovary syndrome. *Clinical Endocrinology (Oxford)* **36**, 105–11.

Kiddy, D.S., Hamilton-Fairley, D., Seppala, M. et al. (1989). Diet-induced changes in sex hormone binding globulin and free testosterone in women with normal or polycystic ovaries: correlation with serum insulin and insulin-like growth factor-1. *Clinical Endocrinology (Oxford)* **31**, 757–63.

Kiddy, D.S., Sharp, P.S., White, D.M. et al. (1990). Differences in clinical and endocrine features between obese and non-obese subjects with polycystic ovary syndrome: an analysis of 263 consecutive cases. *Clinical Endocrinology (Oxford)* **32**, 213–20.

Lake, J.K., Power, C. and Cole, T.J. (1997). Women's reproductive health: the role of body mass index in early and adult life. *International Journal of Obesity and Related Metabolic Disorders* **21**, 432–8.

Lewis, C.G., Warnes, G.M., Wang, X.J. and Matthews, C.D. (1990). Failure of body mass index or body weight to influence markedly the response to ovarian hyperstimulation in normal cycling women. *Fertility and Sterility* **53**, 1097–9.

Mantzoros, C.S., Dunaif, A. and Flier, J.S. (1997). Leptin concentrations in the polycystic ovary syndrome [see comments]. *Journal of Clinical Endocrinology and Metabolism* **82**, 1687–91.

McClure, N., McQuinn, B., McDonald, J. et al. (1992). Body weight, body mass index, and age: predictors of menotropin dose and cycle outcome in polycystic ovarian syndrome? *Fertility and Sterility* **58**, 622–4.

Mitchell, G.W. and Rogers, J. (1953). The influence of weight reduction on amenorrhea in obese women. *New England Journal of Medicine* **249**, 835–7.

Nader, S., Riad Gabriel, M.G. and Saad, M.F. (1997). The effect of a desogestrel-containing oral contraceptive on glucose tolerance and leptin concentrations in hyperandrogenic women. *Journal of Clinical Endocrinology and Metabolism* **82**, 3074–7.

Norman, R.J., Hague, W.M., Masters, S.C. and Wang, X.J. (1995a). Subjects with polycystic ovaries without hyperandrogenaemia exhibit similar disturbances in insulin and lipid profiles as those with polycystic ovary syndrome. *Human Reproduction* **10**, 2258–61.

Norman, R.J., Masters, S.C., Hague, W. et al. (1995b). Metabolic approaches to the subclassification of polycystic ovary syndrome. *Fertility and Sterility* **63**, 329–35.

Pasquali, R., Antenucci, D., Casimirri, F. et al. (1989a). Clinical and hormonal characteristics of obese amenorrheic hyperandrogenic women before and after weight loss. *Journal of Clinical Endocrinology and Metabolism* **68**, 173–9.

Pasquali, R. and Casimirri, F. (1993). The impact of obesity on hyperandrogenism and polycystic ovary syndrome in premenopausal women. *Clinical Endocrinology (Oxford)* **39**, 1–16.

Pasquali, R., Casimirri, F., Colella, P. and Melchionda, N. (1989b). Body fat distribution and weight loss in obese women [letter]. *American Journal of Clinical Nutrition* **49**, 185–7.

Pettigrew, R. and Hamilton-Fairley, D. (1997). Obesity and female reproductive function. *British Medical Bulletin* **53**, 341–58.

Rich Edwards, J.W., Goldman, M.B., Willett, W.C. et al. (1994). Adolescent body mass index and infertility caused by ovulatory disorder. *American Journal of Obstetrics and Gynecology* **171**, 171–7.

Werler, M.M. (1997). Teratogen update: smoking and reproductive outcomes. *Teratology* **55**, 382–8.

Zaadstra, B.M., Seidell, J.C., Van Noord, P.A. et al. (1993). Fat and female fecundity: prospective study of effect of body fat distribution on conception rates [see comments]. *British Medical Journal* **306**, 484–7.

Zachow, R.J. and Magoffin, D.A. (1997). Direct intraovarian effects of leptin: impairment of the synergistic action of insulin-like growth factor-1 on follicle-stimulating hormone-dependent estradiol-17 beta production by rat ovarian granulosa cells. *Endocrinology* **138**, 847–50.

10

Ovulation induction for women with polycystic ovary syndrome

Adam Balen and Howard Jacobs

Introduction

The principle of the management of anovulatory infertility in women with poly-cystic ovary syndrome (PCOS) is to induce regular unifollicular ovulation, whilst minimizing the risks of ovarian hyperstimulation syndrome (OHSS) and multiple pregnancy.

The polycystic ovary syndrome is one of the most common endocrine disorders, although its aetiology remains unknown. This heterogeneous disorder may present, at one end of the spectrum, with the single finding of polycystic ovarian morphology as detected by pelvic ultrasound. At the other end of the spectrum, symptoms such as obesity, hyperandrogenism, menstrual cycle disturbance and infertility may occur, either singly or in combination. Endocrine and metabolic dis-turbances (elevated serum concentrations of luteinizing hormone (LH), testo-sterone, insulin and prolactin) are common and may have profound implications on the long-term health of women with PCOS (Balen, 1999).

We define PCOS as the presence of polycystic ovaries (PCO) detected by ultra-sound scan (enlarged ovaries with more than ten cysts of 2–8 mm) (Adams et al., 1985) plus symptoms of oligomenorrhoea/amenorrhoea, obesity and hyperandro-genism (acne, hirsutism) (Balen et al., 1995). Over 1800 women with PCO were studied at The Middlesex Hospital, London, and it was found that the original descriptive triad of amenorrhoea, obesity and hirsutism, Stein–Leventhal syn-drome) appears to be the extreme end of the spectrum of the disorder (Balen et al., 1995). Indeed, many women with PCO detected by ultrasound do not have symp-toms of PCOS, although symptoms may develop later, after a gain in weight, for example. Ovarian morphology appears to be the most sensitive marker for PCOS, compared with the classical endocrine features of a raised serum LH and/or testo-sterone concentration which were found in only 39.8% and 47.8% of our patients, respectively; the symptoms of obesity, hyperandrogenism (acne, hirsutism and alo-pecia) and menstrual cycle disturbances occurred in 38.4%, 70.3% and 66.2% of patients, respectively (Balen et al., 1995). We therefore prefer to make the diagnosis of PCOS when there are, in addition to the ultrasound finding of PCO, the associated symptoms (menstrual irregularity, hyperandrogenization, obesity) or endocrine abnormalities (raised serum LH and testosterone concentrations).

Factors that affect ovulation

Hypersecretion of LH is particularly associated with menstrual disturbances and infertility. Indeed, it is this endocrine feature that appears to result in reduced conception rates and increased rates of miscarriage in both natural and assisted conception (Balen, Tan and Jacobs, 1993a). The finding of a persistently elevated early to mid-follicular phase LH concentration (>10 IU/l with our assay) in a woman who is trying to conceive suggests the need to suppress LH levels by either pituitary desensitization, with a gonadotrophin-releasing hormone (GnRH) agonist, or laparoscopic ovarian diathermy. There are, however, no large prospectively randomized trials that demonstrate a therapeutic benefit from a reduction in serum LH concentrations during ovulation induction protocols.

We, and others, have found that the patient's body mass index (BMI) correlated with an increased rate of hirsutism, cycle disturbance and infertility (Kiddy et al., 1992; Balen et al., 1995). Obese women with PCOS hypersecrete insulin, which stimulates ovarian secretion of androgens and is associated with hirsutism, menstrual disturbance and infertility. It is seldom necessary to measure the serum insulin concentration, as this will not affect the management of the patient, but the prevalence of diabetes in obese women with PCOS is 11% (Conway, 1990) and so a measurement of glucose tolerance is important in these women. Obese women (BMI >30 kg/m2) should therefore be encouraged to lose weight. Weight loss improves the symptoms of PCOS and improves the patient's endocrine profile (Kiddy et al., 1992; Clark et al., 1995).

Pretreatment considerations

Whilst there is no doubt that a semen analysis should be performed before ovulation induction therapy is commenced, there is debate as to the appropriate time for testing tubal patency. Until recently, if there was no clear indication of the possibility of tubal damage (e.g. past history of pelvic infection, pelvic pain), a reasonable policy was to delay a test of tubal patency until there had been up to three or even six ovulatory cycles. In the light of recent evidence to suggest a possible link between ovulation induction therapy and a long-term risk of ovarian cancer (reviewed by Nugent et al., 1998), we should perhaps now be thinking about performing a complete assessment of every woman before choosing the appropriate therapy for her. Tubal patency should therefore be assessed by either hysterosalpingography or laparoscopy before embarking upon any form of ovulation induction therapy.

Ovulation induction strategies

Once the diagnosis of anovulatory infertility has been made, it is necessary to direct the patient to the appropriate therapy. It should be remembered, however, that the diagnosis is not absolute: amenorrhoeic women are anovulatory (although they may ovulate sporadically), whereas oligomenorrhoeic women may well ovulate erratically, albeit infrequently. Women with regular four-weekly cycles have the opportunity to conceive 13 times a year, and with less frequent ovulations the chances of conception over a given period of time obviously decline. It is therefore appropriate to treat oligo-ovulatory women, but sometimes difficult to provide a unifying diagnosis for use when comparing the results of different treatments.

Weight loss

An increasing BMI has been found to be correlated with an increased rate of hirsutism, cycle disturbance and infertility (Kiddy et al., 1990; Balen et al., 1995). Even moderate obesity (BMI > 27 kg/m^2) is associated with a reduced chance of ovulation (Grodstein, Goldman and Cramer, 1994), and a body fat distribution leading to an increased waist:hip ratio appears to have a more important effect than body weight alone (Zaadstra et al., 1993). Obese women (BMI > 30 kg/m^2) should therefore be encouraged to lose weight. Weight loss improves the endocrine profile (Kiddy et al., 1989, 1992), and the likelihood of ovulation and a healthy pregnancy. Achieving weight reduction is, however, extremely difficult, particularly as the metabolic status of the patient with PCOS conspires against weight loss (Nestler, Clore and Blackard, 1989; Michelmore et al., 1999).

A recent study by Clark et al. (1995) looked at the effect of a weight-loss and exercise programme on women with at least a two-year history of anovulatory infertility, clomiphene resistance and a BMI > 30 kg/m^2. The emphasis of the study was a realistic exercise schedule combined with positive reinforcement of a suitable eating programme over a six-month period of time. Thirteen out of the 18 women enrolled completed the study. Weight loss had a significant effect on endocrine function, ovulation and subsequent pregnancy. Fasting insulin and serum testosterone concentrations fell, and 12 of the 13 subjects resumed ovulation, 11 becoming pregnant (five spontaneously). Thus, with appropriate support, patients may ovulate spontaneously without medical therapy.

Weight loss should also be encouraged prior to ovulation induction treatments, as they appear to be less effective when the BMI is greater than 28–30 kg/m2 (Hamilton-Fairley et al., 1992; Filicori et al., 1994). Monitoring treatment is harder when the patient is obese and it may be difficult to see the ovaries clearly, thus risking multiple ovulation and multiple pregnancy. Furthermore, pregnancy carries greater risks in the obese (miscarriage, gestational diabetes, hypertension, problems with delivery) (Gjonnaess, 1984; Hamilton-Fairley et al., 1992), which is a further incentive to lose weight.

Weight reduction therapies

A number of agents have been used to aid weight loss, although there is really no substitute for a continued programme of exercise and diet. Appetite suppressants should be reserved for the extremely obese (BMI >35 kg/m^2), because of the potential for serious adverse effects (e.g. pulmonary hypertension), and close medical supervision is essential. Over the past 20 years or so it has become recognized increasingly that PCOS and hyperinsulinaemia are intimately related (Burghen, Givens and Kitabchi, 1980; Dunaif et al., 1989; Rajkhowa et al., 1994) with respect to pathogenesis, endocrine disturbances and molecular genetics (for reviews, see Conway, 1990; Rajkhowa and Clayton, 1995; Prelevic, 1997; Franks et al., 1997). Metformin inhibits the production of hepatic glucose and enhances the sensitivity of peripheral tissue to insulin, thereby decreasing insulin secretion (DeFronzo, Barzilai and Simonson, 1991). It has been shown that metformin ameliorates hyperandrogenism and abnormalities of gonadotrophin secretion in women with PCOS (Velasquez et al., 1994, 1997b; Nestler and Jakubowicz, 1996) and can restore menstrual cyclicity and fertility (Velasquez, Acosta and Mendoza, 1997a). Not all authors agree with these findings (Acbay and Gundogdu, 1996), particularly if there is no weight loss with metformin therapy (Ehrmann et al., 1997a). A recent study has evaluated the combination of metformin with clomiphene therapy with dramatic and rather surprising results (Nestler et al., 1998). We are currently performing a large, prospective, randomized, placebo-controlled study with, it is hoped, appropriate power to answer the questions concerning metformin and its potential benefits for reproductive function. The insulin-sensitizing agent troglitazone also appears significantly to improve the metabolic and reproductive abnormalities in PCOS (Dunaif et al., 1996; Ehrmann et al., 1997b), although this product has been withdrawn recently because of reports of deaths from hepatotoxicity. Newer insulin-sensitizing agents are currently being evaluated in phase 3 studies.

Medical therapies to induce ovulation

Clomiphene citrate/tamoxifen

Women with PCOS who are anovulatory have traditionally been treated with anti-oestrogens (clomiphene citrate or tamoxifen) as first-line therapy. Clomiphene citrate has been available for many years, is administered orally for five days (usually commencing on day 2 of a spontaneous or progestogen-induced bleed) and has tended not to have been closely monitored. It is now time to rethink this approach as there have been inadequate prospective, randomized studies comparing the efficacy of clomiphene citrate with other therapies.

Clomiphene citrate induces ovulation in approximately 70–85% of patients, although only 40–50% conceive (ESHRE, 1997). It has been suggested that the most important reason for reduced overall pregnancy rates with clomiphene citrate therapy is discontinuation of therapy, and that cumulative conception rates approach 100% after ten cycles, when corrected for those who discontinue therapy (which might be considered to be a rather biased way of analysing data) (Hammond, Halme and Talbert, 1983). Nonetheless, there is no doubt that the majority of cycles of clomiphene citrate treatment go unmonitored and it is recommended that at least the first cycle of treatment, if not all cycles, should be monitored with a combination of serial ultrasound scans and serum endocrinology (Balen and Jacobs, 1997; Balen, 1997). Kousta, White and Franks (1997) have recently reported their experience in the treatment of 167 patients and also found good cumulative conception rates (67.3% over six months in those who had no other subfertility factors), which continued to rise up to 12 cycles of therapy. They reported a multiple pregnancy rate of 11%, similar to that described in other series, and a miscarriage rate of 23.6%, with those who miscarried tending to have a higher serum LH concentration immediately after clomiphene administration. Recent reviews concerning the safety of clomiphene citrate with respect to congenital anomalies indicate that there is no increased risk (Shoham, Zosmer and Insler, 1991b; Venn and Lumley, 1994).

Shoham and colleagues (1990a) studied the hormonal profiles in a series of 41 women treated with clomiphene citrate, of whom 28 ovulated. In those who ovulated, 17 exhibited normal patterns of hormone secretion and five conceived, whilst 11 exhibited an abnormal response, characterized by significantly elevated serum concentrations of LH from day 9 until the LH surge, together with premature luteinization and higher E2 levels throughout the cycle – none of the patients with this abnormal response conceived. This strengthens the argument for careful monitoring of therapy and discontinuation if the response is abnormal.

It is therefore useful to measure serum LH levels in the mid-follicular phase (we aim for day 8 ± 1 day) and, if they are abnormally high (> 10 IU/l), the chance of success is reduced and the rate of miscarriage is raised. If there is an exuberant response to 50 mg, as in some women with PCOS, the dose can be decreased to 25 mg. Anti-oestrogen therapy should be discontinued if the patient is anovulatory after the dose has been increased in consecutive cycles (up to 100 mg for clomiphene citrate or 40 mg for tamoxifen). A daily dose of more than 100 mg rarely confers any benefit. If the patient is ovulating, it is not necessary to increase the dose as conception is expected to occur at a rate determined by factors such as the patient's age etc. Clomiphene, by its anti-oestrogenic action, can cause thickening of the cervical mucus (although this is a matter of some debate), which may impede passage of sperm through the cervix. A post-coital test should be considered when treatment is started.

It is thought by some that doses of 150 mg or more confer no benefit (Franks, 1992; Kousta et al., 1997) and only worsen the side-effects, particularly of a thickened cervical mucus, and might also have an anti-oestrogenic effect on the endometrium (Dickey et al., 1993). In the USA, the maximum dose of clomiphene citrate approved for use by the Food and Drug Administration is 100 mg/day for five days. Some authors, however, have found that higher doses are required, particularly in women who are overweight (Shepard, Balmaceda and Leija, 1979; Lobo et al., 1982; Dickey et al., 1997). Dickey et al., (1997) reported a series of 1681 pregnancies that occurred with a combination of clomiphene citrate and intrauterine insemination (in patients who did not necessarily have PCOS and may have had other subfertility factors). They used doses up to 250 mg for five days and found that overweight women required higher doses to achieve a pregnancy, with no apparent increase in the rate of miscarriage or multiple pregnancy.

Another approach for women who are unresponsive to five days of clomiphene citrate (>150 mg) is to increase the duration of therapy to ten days, which in one study enabled 14 previously unresponsive women to ovulate in 65% of 48 cycles, during which five conceived (Fluker, Wang and Rowe, 1996). Alternatively, adjunctive therapy with naltrexone, which, by its action as an opioid receptor blocker, can normalize gonadotrophin secretion in women with PCOS, has been found to increase the efficacy of clomiphene citrate in previously unresponsive patients (Roozenberg et al., 1997). Another attractive approach in clomiphene-resistant patients is the administration of progesterone prior to clomiphene citrate treatment (Homburg et al., 1988b), which, at an intramuscular dose of 50 mg over five days, caused a suppression of FSH and LH secretion. LH levels fell in seven out of ten women treated with progesterone, all became responsive to clomiphene (those whose LH levels were not suppressed remained unresponsive), and three conceived in the first cycle of treatment.

An ovulatory trigger in the form of human chorionic gonadotrophin (hCG) is very rarely required and should only be given if there has been repeated evidence of an unruptured follicle by ultrasound monitoring, as the majority (80%) of treatment cycles in which ovulation does not occur are characterized by failure of development of a dominant follicle (Polson et al., 1989).

Clomiphene is currently licensed for only six months' use in the UK because of the putative increased risk of ovarian cancer (there are no data on this association and tamoxifen). The paper on which this ruling was based found an association between clomiphene and ovarian cancer with more than 12 months' therapy, and in most cases of prolonged use the indication was unexplained infertility rather than anovulation (Rossing et al., 1994). It would seem reasonable that patients should be counselled about the possible risks if treatment is to continue beyond six months; for example, some patients might not respond to a dose of 50 mg that has been prescribed for three months and then ovulate in response to 100 mg. They can expect an increasing cumulative chance of conception over at least the next nine months, and so it is reasonable to suggest that they take clomiphene for a total of 12 months, provided that a full explanation is given (Balen and Jacobs, 1997; Kousta et al., 1997). If pregnancy has not occurred after 10–12 normal ovulatory cycles, it is then appropriate to offer the couple assisted conception.

If anti-oestrogens fail

The therapeutic options for patients with anovulatory infertility who are resistant to anti-oestrogens are either parenteral gonadotrophin therapy or laparoscopic ovarian diathermy. Here lies another problem with definition, as some (including the authors) consider clomiphene resistance to mean failure to ovulate (i.e. no response), whereas others take it to mean failure to conceive despite ovulation (which we would call clomiphene failure). Here, too, is a cause of considerable confusion when it comes to comparing pregnancy rates with either gonadotrophin therapy or laparoscopic ovarian diathermy.

Gonadotrophin therapy

Gonadotrophin therapy is indicated for women with anovulatory PCOS who have been treated with anti-oestrogens, either if they have failed to ovulate or if they have a response to clomiphene that is likely to reduce their chance of conception (e.g. persistent hypersecretion of LH, or negative post-coital tests due to the anti-oestrogenic effect on cervical mucus). Whether gonadotrophin therapy should be offered to women who have responded normally to clomiphene citrate but failed to conceive is another issue of some debate, with some (in particular manufacturers of gonadotrophin preparations) suggesting transfer to gonadotrophin therapy after six, or sometimes fewer, clomiphene-stimulated ovulatory cycles. In the authors' experience there is a greater consensus for the view argued above, that is, to provide careful monitoring of clomiphene therapy and assume that if conception has not occurred after 9–12 cycles of treatment, the next step is assisted conception and not alternative methods of ovulation induction.

It is essential to scrutinize carefully the criteria used to define patients who are selected for gonadotrophin therapy in published studies. It should be remembered that using the criteria suggested above, that is, the 20% or so that are resistant to clomiphene therapy, it will be the most 'resistant' of patients who require gonado-trophin therapy. Balen et al. (1994) have published the cumulative conception and livebirth rates in 103 women with PCOS who did not ovulate with anti-oestrogen therapy. Whilst the cumulative conception and livebirth rates after six months were 62% and 54%, respectively, and after 12 months 73% and 62%, respectively, the rate of multiple pregnancy was 19% and there were three cases of moderate to severe OHSS. The rate of multiple pregnancy fell to 4% after the introduction of real-time transvaginal ultrasound monitoring of follicular development. This emphasizes the central role of effective surveillance in programmes of ovulation induction, especially for women with PCOS who are at increased risk of OHSS and multiple pregnancy. If conception has failed to occur after six ovulatory cycles in a woman younger than 25 years, or after 12 ovulatory cycles in women older than 25, then it can be assumed that anovulation is unlikely to be the cause of the couple's infertility, and assisted conception – usually in-vitro fertilization (IVF) – is then indicated.

Gonadotrophins are available in the form of urinary derived human menopau-sal gonadotrophins (hMG) or follicle stimulating hormone (FSH). The gonado-trophins are glycoprotein hormones and it is the degree of glycosylation that affects the biological activity (half-life) (see Rose et al., 1999, for recent review). Biological activity can only be measured by bioassay and is not measurable by immunoassay. Pharmacopoeial monographs taking account of the inherent precision of the methods in bioassays allow 95% confidence limits of 80–125% of the stated dose on estimates of activity, in other words between 60 and 94 units of activity in a 75 unit ampoule (a potential variation of up to 57% between ampoules from differ-ent batches). The same pharmacopoeial requirements apply to the recombinantly derived FSH preparations. There is also evidence that there is heterogeneity between the different recombinantly derived preparations. The preparations of hMG are administered intramuscularly, whilst more highly purified preparations can now be given by subcutaneous injection, which can be self-administered and appear to be tolerated better by the patient.

The authors' current protocol is that treatment with gonadotrophins should be commenced within the first five days of a natural or induced menstrual bleed, when a pelvic ultrasound examination indicates that the endometrium is thin (less than 6 mm in depth) and that there are no ovarian cysts. The initial dose, until recently one ampoule per day of either hMG (75 IU FSH + 75 IU LH) or FSH (75 IU), is increased by one ampoule per day after 14 days in the first cycle of treatment (and seven days in subsequent cycles) if there is an inadequate response, as assessed by ultrasound scan. There is no value in increasing the initial dose before the fifth day (at the earliest) as recruitment of follicles takes between five and 15 days. Further increases are made at four–seven-day intervals. In subsequent cycles, the starting dose is determined by the patient's previous response and can be reduced in some cases to half an ampoule and increased in others to two ampoules per day (Balen and Jacobs, 1997).

In order to prevent the risks of overstimulation and multiple pregnancy, the traditional standard step-up regimens (when 75–150 IU are increased by 75 IU every three to five days: Thompson and Hansen, 1970; Lunenfeld and Insler, 1974; Wang and Gemzell, 1980) have been replaced by either low-dose step-up regimens (Brown et al., 1969; Hamilton-Fairley et al., 1991; Shoham, Patel and Jacobs, 1991a; Schoemaker et al., 1993; Balen et al., 1994) or step-down regimens (Fauser, Donderwinkel and Schoot, 1993). The low-dose step-up regimen employs a starting dose of 0.5–0.75 of an ampoule (37.5–50 IU), which is only increased after 14 days if there is no response, and then by only half an ampoule every seven days (Hamilton-Fairley et al., 1991). Treatment cycles using this approach can be quite long – up to 28–35 days – but the risk of multiple follicular growth appears to be small compared with conventional step-up regimens. With the 'step-down' protocol, follicular recruitment is achieved using two or three ampoules daily for three to four days before decreasing the dose to one ampoule to maintain follicular development (Fauser et al., 1993; van Santbrink et al., 1995a). Experimental studies have indicated that initiation of follicular growth requires a 10–30% increment in the dose of exogenous FSH and the threshold changes with follicular growth, due to an increased number of FSH receptors, so that the concentration of FSH required to maintain growth is less than that required to initiate it (Ben Rafael, Levy and Schoemaker, 1995). More recently, a 'sequential' step-up, step-down protocol has been employed, in which the FSH threshold dose is reduced by half when the leading follicle has reached 14 mm (Hugues et al., 1996). This approach also appears to reduce the number of lead follicles when compared with a classic step-up protocol (Hugues et al., 1996).

The rationale behind the development of low-dose stimulation regimens is to reduce the risks of both multiple pregnancy and OHSS, both of which are increased in women with PCO compared with normal ovaries. The reduction in these harmful side-effects has been further aided by the use of transvaginal ultrasound monitoring, whereas in the early days of the development of gonadotrophin therapy the only means of monitoring treatment was the measurement of urinary oestrogen metabolites – at best a semi-quantitative system.

Ovulation is triggered with a single intramuscular injection of hCG 10 000 units (occasionally 5000 units are given). The inclusion criterion for hCG administration should be the development of at least one follicle of at least 17 mm in its largest diameter, and there may be some benefit to waiting until the largest follcicle is > 20 mm (Silverberg et al., 1991). In order to reduce the risks of multiple pregnancy and OHSS, the exclusion criteria for hCG administration are the development of two or more follicles larger than 16 mm in diameter and/or more than four folli-cles larger than 14 mm in diameter. In overstimulated cycles hCG is withheld, the patient counselled about the risks and advised to refrain from sexual intercourse.

Multiple pregnancy and OHSS are avoidable and this should be a matter not of controversy but of responsible clinical practice. Multiple pregnancy is an undesir-able side-effect of fertility therapy because of the increased rates of perinatal mor-bidity and mortality. In the UK it is the unmonitored use of oral anti-oestrogens that accounts for more cases of triplets than gonadotrophin therapy or assisted con-ception (Levene, Wild and Steer, 1992). High-order multiple pregnancies (quadru-plets or more) result almost exclusively from ovulation induction therapies (Botting, Macfarlane and Price, 1990). Gonadotrophins should be given in low doses to women with anovulatory infertility and strict criteria should be employed before the administration of the ovulatory trigger. Hull (1992) reviewed the results of six studies of conventional dose gonadotrophin therapy (111 patients) and com-pared them with six studies of low-dose therapy (243 patients). The pregnancy rates per cycle (23%) and per ovulatory cycle (30%) were higher in the standard dose cycles than during low-dose therapy (11% and 15% respectively). The miscar-riage rate was also lower in the standard dose cycles (17% vs 37%), resulting in an ongoing pregnancy rate per cycle of 20% compared with 7% in the low-dose cycles. The multiple pregnancy rate, however, was 23% in the standard dose cycles com-pared with 9% in the low-dose cycles. Homburg, Levy and Ben-Rafael (1995) com-pared 25 women treated with a conventional protocol with 25 treated with a low-dose protocol and found a slightly higher pregnancy rate with the latter (40% vs 24% – not significant) and no multiple pregnancies or cases of OHSS, compared with 33% and 11% respectively in the conventional group.

It can be extremely difficult to predict the response to stimulation of a women with PCO – indeed this is the greatest therapeutic challenge in all ovulation induc-tion therapies. The PCO is characteristically quiescent – at least when viewed by ultrasound – before often exhibiting an exuberant and explosive response to stim-ulation. It can be very challenging to stimulate the development of a single domi-nant follicle, and whilst attempts have been made to predict a multifollicular response (Farhi and Jacobs, 1997) by looking at mid-follicular endocrine profiles and numbers of small follicles, it is harder to do so prior to commencing ovarian stimulation and hence determine the required starting dose of gonadotrophin. In order to prevent OHSS and multiple pregnancy, however, the strategy of cancelling cycles on day 8 of stimulation if there are more than seven follicles (≥ 8 mm) and an FSH:LH ratio of ≥ 1.6 (Farhi and Jacobs, 1997) would seem to be reasonable.

White and colleagues (1996) have recently reported their extensive experience of the low-dose regimen in 225 women, over 934 cycles of treatment and resulting in 109 pregnancies in 102 women (45%). Seventy-two per cent of the cycles were ovulatory (fewer than 5% of patients failed to ovulate) and 77% of these uniovulatory. The multiple pregnancy rate was 6%. Despite the low-dose protocol, 18% of cycles were abandoned because more than three large follicles developed – a further reminder of the sensitivity of the PCO even when attempts are made to reduce the response. At the start of their series, the starting dose was 75 IU, but this was reduced to 0.7 of an ampoule (i.e. 52.5 IU) for the last 429 cycles of treatment in order to reduce further the rate of multiple follicle development (84% of cycles with the lower starting dose were uniovulatory). Interestingly, their previously reported relatively high miscarriage rate of 35% when the higher starting dose was used fell to 20% with the 52.5 IU starting dose (White et al., 1996). Once again it was noted that the only factor that influenced the outcome significantly was the patient's BMI. Those with a BMI >25 kg/m^2 had a higher rate of abandoned cycles (31% vs 15% in those of normal weight), a lower cumulative conception rate over six cycles (46.8% vs 57% for the whole group) and a miscarriage rate of 31%. This confirms earlier findings of the adverse effects of obesity on outcome (Hamilton-Fairley et al., 1992).

The first observational study of the use of recombinantly derived FSH (follitropin beta, Puregon, Organ Labs Ltd, Cambridge) in the induction of ovulation in 11 patients with clomiphene-resistant PCOS using a low-dose step-up regimen has recently been published (Hayden, Rutherford and Balen, 1999). All of the patients exhibited a follicular response: six ovulated, of whom two conceived; treatment was cancelled in four cases because of overstimulation. One patient was anovulatory despite the development of a follicle. It has therefore been demonstrated that recombinantly derived FSH can be used successfully to stimulate follicular growth at a starting dose of 50 IU.

There are many published series in the literature that support the notion that carefully conducted ovulation induction therapy results in good cumulative conception rates in women with PCOS. It is beyond the scope of this chapter to provide details of each publication, and interested readers are referred to some relevant references: Schoot et al., 1992; Fauser, 1994; Schoot, 1995; van Santbrink et al., 1995b; Tadokoro et al., 1997.

Different gonadotrophin preparations

The 'purified' FSH preparations, or those with a reduced LH content, confer no therapeutic advantage over hMG as the LH content in hMG is trivial compared with the endogenous secretion of LH (Jacobs et al., 1987; Homburg et al., 1990a; Sagle et al., 1991; Fulghesu et al., 1992). Furthermore, pharmacokinetic studies do not indicate a significant difference when hMG and FSH are administered (Venturoli et al., 1986). It is also our experience that serum LH concentrations usually fall in response to normal ovarian–pituitary feedback as the dominant follicle grows, although some women with PCOS continue to oversecrete LH in the presence of follicular growth – a phenomenon that may be due to disordered production of non-steroidal ovarian factors in these patients (Balen and Rose, 1994).

A recent meta-analysis of eight randomized studies of patients undergoing IVF, however, suggested that treatment with FSH resulted in 50% higher pregnancy rates (Daya, 1995), with an overall odds ratio of 1.71 (95% confidence interval (CI) 1.12–2.62). The papers that made up the meta-analysis had small numbers and the result was skewed by small studies which needed to be combined in order to achieve significance – a well-known drawback of such reviews (Gardosi, 1998).

Adjuncts to gonadotrophin therapy

A number of prestimulation protocols have been used in order to suppress endogenous pituitary gonadotrophin secretion and ovarian activity before commencing gonadotrophin therapy. These include two to three months of the combined oral contraceptive pill or a GnRH agonist for six to eight weeks. It is our view that this approach simply prolongs the treatment cycle, resulting in fewer ovulations and hence fewer chances of conception in a given period of time without conferring a significant benefit on the pregnancy rates.

Hypersecretion of LH has a profound effect on conception and miscarriage (Homburg et al., 1988a; Balen et al., 1993a). Initial, non-randomized reports of GnRH agonist therapy in PCOS described encouraging rates of pregnancy (Fleming et al., 1985, 1988), but prospective randomized studies have indicated that GnRH agonists provide no benefit over hMG therapy alone and, in particular, do not reduce the tendency of the PCO to multifollicular development, cyst formation or OHSS (Homburg et al., 1990a; Buckler et al., 1993; Scheele et al., 1993). Miscarriage related to hypersecretion of LH is one condition that might benefit from pituitary desensitization, as suggested by preliminary studies of women with PCO undergoing ovulation induction for in-vivo and in-vitro fertilization (Balen et al., 1993b; Farhi et al., 1993; Homburg et al., 1993).

One potential advantage of the use of GnRH agonists is to enable accurate timing of ovulation and hence either intercourse or intrauterine insemination (the latter being used by some to further enhance the efficacy of treatment). Luteal support is, of course, required after a GnRH agonist is used either throughout the follicular phase (Donderwinkel et al., 1993), or simply instead of hCG to trigger ovulation (Fraser, 1994), the latter being an approach to prevent the development of OHSS (Emperaire and Ruffie, 1991).

Pulsatile GnRH has been used in an attempt to stimulate unifollicular growth in women with PCOS and thereby avoid the risks of exogenous gonadotrophins. Rates of ovulation, however, are disappointing (Eshel et al., 1988; Filicori et al., 1994) and miscarriage rates as high as 45% (Shoham, Homburg and Jacobs, 1990b;

Filicori et al., 1994). Pulsatile GnRH therapy is ideally suited to women with hypogonadotrophic hypogonadism, and it is interesting that some women with this condition also have PCO, responding in a typically 'polycystic' fashion to stimulation with respect to both ultrasound and endocrine findings (Shoham et al., 1992; Schachter et al., 1996). The effect of pulsatile GnRH may be improved when it is given together with gonadotrophins (Homburg et al., 1990b) or clomiphene citrate (Tan et al., 1996), or after pretreatment with a GnRH agonist (Filicori et al., 1994). Alternatively GnRH antagonists have been proposed as a possible therapy to permit normalization of LH secretion when exogenous pulsatile GnRH is superimposed (Dubourdieu et al., 1993). Whilst there is certainly an improvement in the endocrinopathy, an ovarian response was not obtained and so the theoretical promise of this approach has not been pursued (Dubourdieu et al., 1993). Thus, pulsatile GnRH therapy is rarely used nowadays for women with PCOS (Homburg, 1996).

Surgical ovulation induction

Laparoscopic ovarian surgery has replaced ovarian wedge resection as the surgical treatment for clomiphene resistance in women with PCOS. It is free of the risks of multiple pregnancy and ovarian hyperstimulation and does not require intensive ultrasound monitoring. Furthermore, ovarian diathermy appears to be as effective as routine gonadotrophin therapy in the treatment of clomiphene-insensitive PCOS (Abdel Gadir et al., 1990b; Kovacs et al., 1991; Donesky and Adashi, 1995; Cohen, 1996). In addition, laparoscopic ovarian surgery is a useful therapy for anovulatory women with PCOS who fail to respond to clomiphene and who persistently hypersecrete LH, need a laparoscopic assessment of their pelvis, or live too far away from the hospital to be able to attend for the intensive monitoring required for gonadotrophin therapy. Surgery does, of course, carry its own risks and should be performed only by properly trained laparoscopic surgeons. A systematic review of surgical versus medical treatment of PCOS has recently been carried out showing no difference in success rates.

Wedge resection of the ovaries was initially described by Stein and Leventhal (1935) at the time that PCO were diagnosed during a laparotomy. It was found that ovarian biopsies taken to make the diagnosis led to subsequent ovulation. The rationale was to 'normalize' ovarian size, and hence the endocrinopathy, by removing between 50% and 75% of each ovary. Until the introduction of clomiphene citrate therapy in 1961, wedge resection was the only treatment for anovulatory PCOS and it is interesting to note that, despite this, over a 30-year period such great care was taken in the selection of patients for treatment that Stein reported a personal experience of only 108 cases (Stein, 1966). Stein found that 95% of patients resumed normal menstrual cycles and 87% of those wishing to conceive did so on at least one occasion. Furthermore, he stated that surgery cured the condition such that the ovarian pathology did not recur (Stein, 1956, 1964).

A large review of 187 reports summarized data on 1079 ovarian wedge resections, with an overall rate of ovulation of 80% and pregnancy of 62.5% (range: 13.5–89.5%) (Goldzieher and Axelrod, 1963). Another 30 or so years later, Donesky and Adashi (1995) were able to increase the summated experience in the literature to 1766 treatments, with an average pregnancy rate of 58.8%. Wedge resection went out of favour in the 1970s because of the realization that significant postoperative adhesion formation occurred and that initial favourable reports of pregnancy rates were not sustained (Weinstein and Polishuk, 1975; Buttram and Vaquero, 1975; Adashi et al., 1981). In one series of seven patients, all were found to have extensive pelvic adhesions following wedge resection (Toaff, Toaff and Peyser, 1976). A microsurgical approach has been recommended (Eddy, Asch and Balmaceda, 1980) but this did not become popular. The operation is therefore rarely performed these days. Donesky and Adashi (1995) provide an excellent history of the surgical management of PCOS, which is recommended for a more comprehensive overview.

Whether patients respond to laparoscopic ovarian diathermy appears to depend on their pretreatment characteristics, with patients with high basal LH concentrations having better clinical and endocrine responses (Abdel Gadir et al. 1992a). In the study by Abdel Gadir et al., it was found that the pretreatment testosterone level, BMI and ovarian volume could not be used to predict outcome. A small prospective study was performed in which women were randomized to receiving either unilateral or bilateral laparoscopic ovarian diathermy (Balen and Jacobs, 1994). It was found that unilateral diathermy restored bilateral ovarian activity, with the contralateral, untreated ovary often being the first to ovulate after the diathermy treatment. It was also found that the only significant difference between the responders and non-responders was a post-diathermy fall in serum LH concentration.

Although the mechanism of ovulation induction by laparoscopic ovarian diathermy is uncertain, it appears that minimal damage to an unresponsive ovary either restores an ovulatory cycle or increases the sensitivity of the ovary to exogenous stimulation. Furthermore, the finding of an attenuated response of LH secretion to stimulation with GnRH (Rossmanith et al., 1991) suggests an effect on ovarian–pituitary feedback and hence pituitary sensitivity to GnRH. The authors' study goes one step further by demonstrating that unilateral diathermy leads to bilateral ovarian activity, suggesting that ovarian diathermy achieves its effect by correcting a perturbation of ovarian–pituitary feedback (Balen and Jacobs, 1994). The hypothesis is that the response of the ovary to injury leads to a local cascade of growth factors, and those such as insulin-like growth factor-1 (IGF-1), which interact with FSH, result in stimulation of follicular growth and the production of the hormone gonadotrophin surge attenuating/inhibitory factor (GnSAF/GnSIF), which leads to a fall in serum LH concentrations (Balen and Jacobs, 1994).

Laparoscopic ovarian surgery: methods and results

This topic is discussed in detail in Chapter 11 and is therefore only summarized here. Laparoscopic surgery has several obvious advantages over laparotomy and was first reported by Palmer and de Brux (1967) some years after the invention by Palmer of his ovarian biopsy forceps. The initial reports were of multiple biopsies with additional cautery only to stop bleeding. Commonly employed methods for laparoscopic surgery include monopolar electrocautery (diathermy: Gjonnaess, 1984) and laser (Daniell and Miller, 1989); multiple biopsy alone is less commonly used. In the first reported series, ovarian diathermy resulted in ovulation in 90% and conception in 70% of the 62 women treated (Gjonnaess, 1984). The outcome of 62 pregnancies was no different from that of the normal population (Gjonnaess, 1989) and the miscarriage rate was 15%.

A number of subsequent studies have produced similarly encouraging results, although the techniques used and degree of ovarian damage vary considerably. Gjonnaess (1984) cauterized each ovary at five to eight points, for five to six seconds at each point with 300–400 W. Using the same technique as Gjonnaess, Dabirashrafi et al. (1991) reported mild to moderate adhesion formation in 20% of patients. Naether et al. (1993) treated 5–20 points per ovary, with 400 W for approximately one second. They found that the rate of adhesions was 19.3% and that this was reduced to 16.6% by peritoneal lavage with saline (Naether and Fischer, 1993). In an earlier study, Naether, Weise and Fischer (1991) found that the post-diathermy fall in serum testosterone concentration was proportional to the degree of ovarian damage, with up to 40 cauterization sites being used in some patients. The greater the amount of damage to the surface of the ovary, the geater the risk of peri-ovarian adhesion formation. This led Armar to develop a strategy of minimizing the number of diathermy points (Armar et al., 1990). We have employed Armar's technique, in which the ovary is simply cauterized at four points. We have not performed routine follow-up laparoscopy on our patients, but the high pregnancy rate (86% of those with no other pelvic abnormality) reported by Armar and Lachelin (1993) indicates that the small number of diathermy points used in our method leads to a low rate of significant adhesion formation.

The risk of peri-ovarian adhesion formation may be reduced by abdominal lavage and early second-look laparoscopy, with adhesiolysis if necessary (Naether, 1995). Others have also used liberal peritoneal lavage to good effect (Armar et al., 1990; Balen and Jacobs, 1997). Greenblatt and Casper (1993) found no correlation between the degree of ovarian damage and subsequent adhesion formation, nor did they find benefit from the adhesion barrier Interceed (Ethicon Ltd), as assessed by second-look laparoscopy. In another interesting study, 40 women undergoing laser photocoagulation of the ovaries using an Nd-YAG laser set at 50 W at 20–25 points per ovary were randomized to second-look laparoscopy and adhesiolysis (Gurgan et al., 1992). Of those who underwent a second-look laparoscopy, adhesions that were described as minimal or mild were found in 68%, yet adhesiolysis did not appear to be necessary as the cumulative conception rate after six months was 47% compared with 55% in the expectantly managed group (not significant).

The difficulty when deciding how to perform laparoscopic ovarian diathermy is not knowing the 'dose response' for a particular patient. Whereas it has been shown that laparoscopic ovarian diathermy using 40 W for four seconds in four places on one ovary can lead to bilateral ovarian activity and ovulation (our usual protocol involves the same on each ovary: Balen and Jacobs, 1994), the ovulation rate was 50% and conception rate 40% (some patients were sensitized to exogenous stimulation). It has been proposed that the degree of ovarian destruction should be determined by the size of the ovary (Naether et al., 1994). Naether et al. have reported their method of laparoscopic electrocautery of the ovarian surface, which causes greater destruction of the ovary than the method we use as they apply 400 W at 5–20 sites on each ovary (Naether et al., 1994).

Despite such a large amount of ovarian destruction, in Naether et al.'s series of 206 patients, 45.2% of those who conceived required additional ovarian stimulation (with an 8% multiple pregnancy rate) and the overall miscarriage rate was 20% (Naether et al., 1994). We also believe that we are dealing with different patient populations, as we only recommend operation for women with irregular, anovulatory cycles who have not responded to anti-oestrogen therapy, whereas in Naether's series approximately 24% of the women operated on had regular cycles and 15% were ovulating before their operation.

Although it might be that unilateral ovarian diathermy is insufficient to induce spontaneous ovulations and pregnancies in all patients, the 'dose' of diathermy that is required needs to be better quantified and how it should be adjusted for individual patients should be evaluated. We therefore urge caution to those who practise any form of ovarian destruction, as we believe that we should be striving to cause as little damage as is necessary in order to induce ovulation. In general, the correct dose of any therapy is the lowest one that works. Furthermore, a combined approach may be suitable for some women whereby low-dose diathermy is followed by low-dose ovarian stimulation. Ostrzenski (1992), for example, commenced all his patients on either clomiphene or FSH therapy immediately after laser wedge resection, and Farhi, Soule and Jacobs (1995) also demonstrated an increased ovarian sensitivity to gonadotrophin therapy after laparoscopic ovarian diathermy.

An additional concern is the possibility of ovarian destruction leading to ovarian failure, an obvious disaster in a woman wishing to conceive. Cases of ovarian failure have been reported after both wedge resection and laparoscopic surgery (Toaff et al., 1976; Cohen, 1996). An unfortunate vogue has developed whereby women with PCO who have over-responded to superovulation for IVF are subjected to ovarian diathermy as a way of reducing the likelihood of subsequent OHSS (Rimmington, Walker and Shaw, 1997). If one accepts that appropriately performed ovarian diathermy works by sensitizing the ovary to FSH (and ovarian diathermy certainly makes the clomiphene-resistant PCO sensitive to clomiphene: Armar et al., 1990; Balen and Jacobs, 1994; Donesky and Adashi, 1995), then one could extrapolate that ovarian diathermy prior to superovulation for IVF should make the ovary more and not less likely to overstimulate. The amount of ovarian destruction that is required to reduce the chance of overstimulation is therefore likely to be considerable (as is, indeed, the case: Rimmington, personal communication). Great caution should therefore be taken before proceeding with such an approach because of concerns about permanent ovarian atrophy.

Laparoscopic ovarian diathermy appears to be as effective as routine gonadotrophin therapy in the treatment of clomiphene-insensitive PCOS (Abdel Gadir et al., 1990a). Abdel Gadir et al. (1990b) prospectively randomized 88 patients, who had failed to conceive after six clomiphene citrate cycles, to receiving hMG, FSH or laparoscopic ovarian diathermy. There were no differences in the rates of ovulation or pregnancy between the groups, although those treated with laparoscopic ovarian diathermy had fewer cycles with multiple follicular growth and a lower rate of miscarriage (Abdel Gadir et al., 1990b). This is the only prospective, randomized study to have attempted to compare the two therapies and really should be repeated with larger numbers.

Laser treatment seems to be as efficacious as diathermy and it has been suggested that it may result in less adhesion formation (Huber, Hosmann and Spona, 1988; Daniell and Miller, 1989; Keckstein et al., 1990), although the only study to compare the two techniques was non-randomized, reported similar ovulation and pregnancy rates, and did not examine adhesion formation (Heylen, Puttemans and Brosens, 1994). Various types of laser have been used from the CO_2 laser, to the Nd:YAG and KTP lasers. As with the use of laser in other spheres of laparoscopic surgery, whether laser or diathermy is employed appears to depend upon the preference of the surgeon and the availability of the equipment.

Conclusion

Unifollicular ovulation induction requires a subtle approach, particularly in women with PCOS. These days, with the high costs of gonadotrophin, even for unifollicular ovulation induction, there is little to choose between ovulation induction and laparoscopic ovarian diathermy. The potential financial costs of a multiple pregnancy, particularly if neonatal intensive care facilities are required, are of course immense. Other costs have to be counted in terms of the successful outcome of treatment, with a low rate of miscarriage and the birth of healthy, preferably singleton, babies, with no health risks to their mothers. It is here that laparoscopic ovarian surgery appears to provide a significant advantage: it is a single treatment that results in unifollicular ovulation, with correction of the endocrinopathy and an apparent low rate of miscarriage. Although there are risks associated with surgery and an anaesthetic, women require a test of tubal patency prior to gonadotrophin therapy and therefore many would be subjected to a laparoscopy in any case. The main concerns are the formation of adhesions and the potential for significant reduction in viable ovarian tissue, with the possibility of inducing premature ovarian failure. The evidence to date, however, is reassuring. The underlying principle of all methods of ovulation induction for women with PCOS must always be to use the lowest possible dose (of drug or surgery) to achieve unifollicular ovulation.

REFERENCES

Abdel Gadir, A., Alnaser, H.M.I., Mowafi, R.S. and Shaw R.W. (1992a). The response of patients with polycystic ovarian disease to human menopausal gonadotrophin therapy after ovarian electrocautery or a luteinizing hormone-releasing hormone agonist. *Fertility and Sterility* **57**, 309–13.

Abdel Gadir, A., Mowafi, R.S., Alnaser, H.M.I. et al. (1990b). Ovarian electrocautery versus human menopausal gonadotrophins and pure follicle stimulating hormone therapy in the treatment of patients with polycystic ovarian disease. *Clinical Endocrinology (Oxford)* **33**, 585–92.

Acbay, O. and Gundogdu, S. (1996). Can metformin reduce insulin resistance in polycystic ovary syndrome? *Fertility and Sterility* **65**, 946–9.

Adams, J., Franks, S., Polson, D.W. et al. (1985). Multifollicular ovaries: clinical and endocrine features and response to pulsatile gonadotrophin-releasing hormone. *Lancet* **ii**, 1375–8.

Adashi, E.Y., Rock, J.A., Guzick, D et al. (1981). Fertility following bilateral ovarian wedge resection: a critical analysis of 90 consecutive cases of the polycystic ovary syndrome. *Fertility and Sterility* **36**, 320–5.

Armar, N.A. and Lachelin, G.C.L. (1993). Laparoscopic ovarian diathermy: an effective treatment for anti-oestrogen resistant anovulatory infertility in women with polycystic ovaries. *British Journal of Obstetrics and Gynaecology* **100**, 161–4.

Armar, N.A., McGarrigle, H.H.G., Honour, J.W. et al. (1990). Laparoscopic ovarian diathermy in the management of anovulatory infertility in women with polycystic ovaries: endocrine changes and clinical outcome. *Fertility and Sterility* **53**, 45–9.

Balen, A.H. (1997). Anovulatory infertility and ovulation induction – recommendations for good clinical practice. *Journal of the British Fertility Society* 2, 83–7.

Balen, A.H. (1999). Pathogenesis of PCOS – the enigma unravels. *Lancet* 354, 966–70.

Balen, A.H., Braat, D.D.M., West, C., Patel, A. and Jacobs, H.S. (1994). Cumulative conception and live birth rates after the treatment of anovulatory infertility. An analysis of the safety and efficacy of ovulation induction in 200 patients. *Human Reproduction* 9, 1563–70.

Balen, A.H., Conway, G.S., Kaltsas, G. et al. (1995). Polycystic ovary syndrome: the spectrum of the disorder in 1741 patients. *Human Reproduction* 10, 2107–11.

Balen, A.H. and Jacobs, H.S. (1994). A prospective study comparing unilateral and bilateral laparoscopic ovarian diathermy in women with the polycystic ovary syndrome. *Fertility and Sterility* 62, 921–5.

Balen, A.H. and Jacobs, H.S. (1997). Ovulation induction. In *Infertility in Practice*, ed. A.H. Balen and H.S. Jacobs, pp. 131–80. Edinburgh: Churchill Livingstone.

Balen, A.H. and Rose, M. (1994). The control of luteinising hormone secretion in the polycystic ovary syndrome. *Contemporary Reviews in Obstetrics and Gynaecology* 6, 201–7.

Balen, A.H., Tan, S.L. and Jacobs, H.S. (1993a). Hypersecretion of luteinising hormone – a significant cause of subfertility and miscarriage. *British Journal of Obstetrics and Gynaecology* 100, 1082–9.

Balen, A.H., Tan, S.L., MacDougall, J. and Jacobs, H.S. (1993b). Miscarriage rates following in vitro fertilisation are increased in women with polycystic ovaries and reduced by pituitary desensitisation with buserelin. *Human Reproduction* 8, 959–64.

Ben Rafael, Z., Levy, T. and Schoemaker, J. (1995). Pharmacokinetics of follicle-stimulating hormone: clinical significance. *Fertility and Sterility* 63, 689–700.

Botting, B.J., Macfarlane, A.J. and Price, F.V. (ed.) (1990). *Three, Four and More. A Study of Triplet and Higher Order Births*. London: HMSO.

Brown, J.B., Evans, J.H., Adey, F.D., Taft, H.P. and Townsend, L. (1969). Factors involved in the induction of fertile ovulation with human gonadotrophins. *Journal of Obstetrics and Gynaecology of the British Commonwealth* 76, 289–307.

Buckler, H.M., Critchley, H.O., Cantrill, J.A. et al. (1993). Efficacy of low dose purified FSH in ovulation induction following pituitary desensitisation in polycystic ovary syndrome. *Clinical Endocrinology* 38, 209–17.

Burghen, G.A., Givens, J.R. and Kitabchi, A.E. (1980). Correlation of hyperandrogenism with hyperinsulinism in polycystic ovarian disease. *Journal of Clinical Endocrinology and Metabolism* 50, 113–16.

Buttram, V.C. and Vaquero, C. (1975). Post-ovarian wedge resection adhesive disease. *Fertility and Sterility* 26, 874–6.

Clark, A.M., Ledger, W., Galletly, C. et al. (1995). Weight loss results in significant improvement in pregnancy and ovulation rates in anovulatory obese women. *Human Reproduction* 10, 2705–12.

Cohen, J. (1996). Laparoscopy procedures for treatment of infertility related PCOS. *Human Reproduction Update* 2, 337–44.

Conway, G.S. (1990). Insulin resistance and the polycystic ovary syndrome. *Contemporary Reviews in Obstetrics and Gynaecology* 2, 34–9.

Dabirashrafi, H., Mohamad, K., Behjatnia, Y. et al (1991). Adhesion formation after ovarian electrocauterization on patients with PCO syndrome. *Fertility and Sterility* 55, 1200–1.

Daniell, J.F. and Miller, N. (1989). Polycystic ovaries treated by laparoscopic laser vaporization. *Fertility and Sterility* **51**, 232–6.

Daya, S. (1995). Follicle stimulating hormone versus human menopausal gonadotropin for in vitro fertilisation: results of a meta-analysis. *Hormone Research* **43**, 224–9.

DeFronzo, R.A., Barzilai, N. and Simonson, D.C. (1991). Mechanism of action of metformin in obese and lean noninsulin-dependent diabetic subjects. *Journal of Clinical Endocrinology and Metabolism* **73**, 1294–301.

Dickey, R.P., Olar, T.T., Taylor, S.N. et al. (1993). Relationship of biochemical pregnancy to pre-ovulatory endometrial thickness and pattern in ovulation induction patients. *Human Reproduction* **8**, 327–90.

Dickey, R.P., Taylor, S.N., Curole, D.N. et al. (1997). Relationship of clomiphene dose and patient weight to successful treatment. *Human Reproduction* **12**, 449–53.

Donderwinkel, P.F.J., Schoot, D.C., Pache, T.D., de Jong, F.H. and Fauser, B.C.J.M. (1993). Luteal function following ovulation induction in polycystic ovary syndrome patients using exogenous gonadotrophins in combination with a gonadotrophin-releasing hormone agonist. *Human Reproduction* **8**, 2027–32.

Donesky, B.W. and Adashi, E.Y. (1995). Surgically induced ovulation in the polycystic ovary syndrome: wedge resection revisited in the age of laparoscopy. *Fertility and Sterility* **63**, 439–63.

Dubourdieu, S., Nestour, E.L., Spitz, I.M., Charbonnel, B. and Bouchard, P. (1993). The combination of gonadotrophin-releasing hormone antagonist and pulsatile GnRH normalises LH secretion in polycystic ovarian disease but fails to induce follicular maturation. *Human Reproduction* **8**, 2056–60.

Dunaif, A., Scott, D., Finegood, D., Quintana, B. and Whitcomb, R. (1996). The insulin-sensitizing agent troglitazone improves metabolic and reproductive abnormalities in polycystic ovary syndrome. *Journal of Clinical Endocrinology and Metabolism* **81**, 3299–306.

Dunaif, A., Segal, K.R., Futterweit, W. and Dobrjansky, A. (1989). Profound peripheral insulin resistance, independent of obesity in polycystic ovary syndrome. *Diabetes* **38**, 1165–73.

Eddy, C.A., Asch, R.H. and Balmaceda, J.P. (1980). Pelvic adhesions following microsurgical and macrosurgical wedge resection of the ovaries. *Fertility and Sterility* **33**, 557–61.

Ehrmann, D.A., Cavaghan, M.K., Imperial, J. et al. (1997a). Effects of metformin on insulin secretion, insulin action and ovarian steroidogenesis in women with polycystic ovary syndrome. *Journal of Clinical Endocrinology and Metabolism* **82**, 1241–7.

Ehrmann, D.A., Schneider, D.J., Sobel, B.E. et al. (1997b). Troglitazone improves defects in insulin action, insulin secretion, ovarian steroidogenesis and fibrinolysis in women with polycystic ovary syndrome. *Journal of Clinical Endocrinology and Metabolism* **82**, 2108–16.

Emperaire, J.C. and Ruffie, A. (1991). Triggering of ovulation with endogenous LH may prevent ovarian hyperstimulation syndrome. *Human Reproduction* **6**, 506–10.

Eshel, A., Abdulwahid, N.A., Armar, N.A. and Jacobs, H.S. (1988). Pulsatile LHRH therapy in women with polycystic ovary syndrome. *Fertility and Sterility* **49**, 956–60.

ESHRE (1997). Female infertility: treatment options for complicated cases; *the ESHRE Capri Workshop. Human Reproduction* **12**, 1191–6.

Farhi, J., Homburg, R., Lerner, A. and Ben-Rafael, Z. (1993). The choice of treatment for anovulation associated with polycystic ovary syndrome following failure to conceive with clomiphene. *Human Reproduction* **8**, 1367–1371.

Farhi, J. and Jacobs, H.S. (1997). Early prediction of ovarian multifollicular response during ovulation induction in patients with polycystic ovary syndrome. *Fertility and Sterility* **67**, 459–62.

Farhi, J., Soule, S. and Jacobs, H. (1995). Effect of laparoscopic ovarian electrocautery on ovarian response and outcome of treatment with gonadotrophins in clomiphene citrate resistant patients with PCOS. *Fertility and Sterility* **64**, 930–5.

Fauser, B.C.J.M. (1994). Observations in favor of normal early follicle development and disturbed dominant follicle selection in polycystic ovary syndrome. *Gynecological Endocrinology* **8**, 75–82.

Fauser, B.C., Donderwinkel, P.F.J. and Schoot, D.C. (1993). The step-down principle in gonadotrophin treatment and the role of GnRH analogues. *Ballière's Clinical Obstetrics and Gynaecology* **7**, 309–30.

Filicori, M., Flamigni, C., Dellai, P. et al. (1994). Treatment of anovulation with pulsatile GnRH: prognostic factors and clinical results in 600 cycles. *Journal of Clinical Endocrinology and Metabolism* **79**, 1215–20.

Fleming, R., Haxton, M.J., Hamilton, M.P.R. et al. (1985). Successful treatment of infertile women with oligomenorrhoea using a combination of an LHRH agonist and exogenous gonadotrophins. *British Journal of Obstetrics and Gynaecology* **92**, 369–73.

Fleming, R., Jamieson, M.E., Hamilton, M.P.R. et al. (1988). The use of GnRH analogues in combination with exogenous gonadotropins in infertile women. *Acta Endocrinology* **119** (Suppl. 288), 77–84.

Fluker, M.R., Wang, I. and Rowe, T.C. (1996). An extended 10-day course of clomiphene citrate in women with CC-resistant ovulatory disorders. *Fertility and Sterility* **66**, 761–4.

Franks, S. (1992). Induction of ovulation. In *Infertility*, ed. A.A. Templeton and J.O. Drife, pp. 237–52. London: Springer Verlag.

Franks, S., Adams, J., Mason, H. and Polson, D. (1985). Ovulatory disorders in women with polycystic ovary syndrome. *Clinical Obstetrics and Gynecology* **12**, 605–32.

Franks, S., Gharani, N., Waterworth, D. et al. (1997). The genetic basis of polycystic ovary syndrome. *Human Reproduction* **12**, 2641–8.

Fraser, H.M. (1994). Risk of luteal phase inadequacy after GnRH agonist-induced ovulation. In *The Triggering of Ovulation in Stimualted Cycles: hCG or LH?*, ed. J.C. Emperaire, pp. 229–38. Carnforth, Lancashire: Parthenon Publishing Group.

Fulghesu, A.M., Lanzone, A., Gida, C. et al. (1992). Ovulation induction with human menopausal gonadotrophin versus follicle stimulating hormone after pituitary suppression by gonadotrophin-releasing hormone agonist in polycystic ovary disease: a cross over study. *Journal of Reproductive Medicine* **37**, 834–40.

Gardosi, J. (1998). Systematic reviews: insufficient evidence on which to base medicine. *British Journal of Obstetrics and Gynaecology* **105**, 1–4.

Gjonnaess, H. (1984). Polycystic ovarian syndrome treated by ovarian electrocautery through the laparoscope. *Fertility and Sterility* **41**, 20–5.

Gjonnaess, H. (1989). The course and outcome of pregnancy after ovarian electrocautery with PCOS: the influence of body weight. *British Journal of Obstetrics and Gynaecology* **96**, 714–19.

Goldzieher, J.W. and Axelrod, L.R. (1963). Clinical and biochemical features of polycystic ovarian disease. *Fertility and Sterility* 14, 631–53.

Greenblatt, E. and Casper, R.F. (1993). Adhesion formation after laparoscopic ovarian cautery for PCOS: lack of correlation with pregnancy rate. *Fertility and Sterility* 60, 766–9.

Grodstein, F., Goldman, M.B. and Cramer, D.W. (1994). Body mass index and ovulatory infertility. *Epidemiology* 5, 247–50.

Gurgan, T., Urman, B., Asku, T. et al. (1992). The effect of short internal laparoscopic lysis of adhesions in pregnancy rates following ND:YAG laser photocoagulation of PCO. *Obstetrics and Gynaecology* 80, 45–7.

Hamilton-Fairley, D., Kiddy, D., Watson, H., Paterson, C. and Franks, S. (1992). Association of moderate obesity with poor pregnancy outcome in women with polycystic ovary syndrome treated with low dose gonadotrophins. *British Journal of Obstetrics and Gynaecology* 99, 128–31.

Hamilton-Fairley, D., Kiddy, D.S., Watson, H., Sagle, M. and Franks, S. (1991). Low-dose gonadotrophin therapy for induction of ovulation in 100 women with polycystic ovary syndrome. *Human Reproduction* 6, 1095–9.

Hammond, M.G., Halme, J.K. and Talbert, L.M. (1983). Factors affecting the pregnancy rate in clomiphene citrate induction of ovulation. *Obstetrics and Gynaecology* 62, 196–202.

Hayden, C., Rutherford, A.J. and Balen, A.H. (1999). Induction of ovulation using a starting dose of 50 units of recombinant human follicle stimulating hormone (Puregon). *Fertility and Sterility* 71, 106–8.

Heylen, S.M., Puttemans, P.J. and Brosens, L.H. (1994). Polycystic ovarian disease treated by laparoscopic argon laser capsule drilling: comparison of vaporization versus perforation technique. *Human Reproduction* 9, 1038–42.

Homburg, R. (1996). Polycystic ovary syndrome – induction of ovulation. *Human Reproduction* 11, 29–39.

Homburg, R., Armar, N.A., Eshel, A., Adams, J. and Jacobs, H.S. (1988a). Influence of serum luteinising hormone concentrations on ovulation, conception and early pregnancy loss in polycystic ovary syndrome. *British Medical Journal* 297, 1024–6.

Homburg, R., Eshel, A., Kilborn, J., Adams, J. and Jacobs, H.S. (1990a). Combined luteinising hormone releasing hormone analogue and exogenous gonadotrophins for the treatment of infertility associated with polycystic ovaries. *Human Reproduction* 5, 32–5.

Homburg, R., Kilborn,. J., West, C. and Jacobs, H.S. (1990b). Treatment with pulsatile luteinising hormone-releasing hormone modulates folliculogenesis in response to ovarian stimulation with exogenous gonadotrophins in patients with polycystic ovaries. *Fertility and Sterility* 54, 737–40.

Homburg, R., Levy, T. and Ben-Rafael, Z. (1995). A comparative prospective study of conventional regimen with chronic low-dose administration of FSH for anovulation associated with polycystic ovary syndrome. *Fertility and Sterility* 59, 729–33.

Homburg, R., Levy, T., Berkovitz, D. et al. (1993). Gonadotropin-releasing hormone agonist reduces the miscarriage rate for pregnancies achieved in women with polycystic ovary syndrome. *Fertility and Sterility* 59, 527–31.

Homburg, R., Weissglass, L. and Goldman, J. (1988b). Improved treatment for anovulation in polycystic ovarian disease utilizing the effect of progesterone on the inappropriate gonado-trophin release and clomiphene citrate response. *Human Reproduction* **3**, 285–8.

Huber, J., Hosmann., J. and Spona, J. (1988). Polycystic ovarian syndrome treated by laser through the laparoscope. *Lancet* **ii**, 215.

Hugues, J.N., Cedrin-Durnerin, I., Avril, C. et al. (1996). Sequential step-up and step-down dose regimen: an alternative method for ovulation induction with FSH in polycystic ovary syndrome. *Human Reproduction* **11**, 2581–4.

Hull, M.G.R. (1992). Gonadotrophin therapy in anovulatory infertility. In *Gonadotrophins, GnRH Anologues and Growth Factors in Infertility: Future Perspectives*, ed. C.M. Howles, pp. 56–70. Sussex: Medifax International.

Jacobs, H.S., Porter, R., Eshel, A. and Craft, I. (1987). Profertility uses of luteinising hormone releasing hormone agonist anologues. In *LHRH and its Analogs*, ed. B.H. Vickery, and J.J. Nestor, pp. 303–22. Lancaster: MTP Press Ltd.

Keckstein, G., Rossmanith, W., Spatzier, K. et al. (1990). The effect of laparoscopic treatment of polycystic ovarian disease by CO-laser or Nd:YAG laser. *Surgical Endoscopy* **4**, 103–7.

Kiddy, D.S., Hamilton-Fairley, D., Bush, A. et al. (1992) Improvement in endocrine and ovarian function during dietary treatment of obese women with polycystic ovary syndrome. *Clinical Endocrinology* **36**, 105–11.

Kiddy, D.S., Hamilton Fairley, D., Seppala, M. et al. (1989). Diet-induced changes in sex hormone binding globulin and free testosterone in women with normal or polycystic ovaries: correlation with serum insulin and insulin-like growth factor-1. *Clinical Endocrinology (Oxford)* **31**, 757–63.

Kiddy, D.S., Sharp, P.S., White, D.M. et al. (1990). Differences in clinical and endocrine features between obese and non-obese subjects with polycystic ovary syndrome: an analysis of 263 consecutive cases. *Clinical Endocrinology (Oxford)* **32**, 213–20.

Kousta, E., White, D.M. and Franks, S. (1997). Modern use of clomiphene citrate in induction of ovulation. *Human Reproduction Update* **3**, 359–65.

Kovacs, G., Buckler, H., Bangah, M. et al. (1991). Treatment of anovulation due to PCOS by laparoscopic ovarian electrocautery. *British Journal of Obstetrics and Gynaecology* **98**, 30–5.

Levene, M.I., Wild, J. and Steer, P. (1992). Higher multiple births and the modern management of infertility in Britain. *British Journal of Obstetrics and Gynaecology* **99**, 607–13.

Lobo, R.A., Gysler, M., March, C.M. et al. (1982). Clinical and laboratory predictors of clomiphene response. *Fertility and Sterility* **37**, 168–74.

Lunenfeld, B. and Insler, V. (1974). Classification of amenorrhoeic states and their treatment by ovulation induction. *Clinical Endocrinology* **3**, 223–7.

Michelmore, K., Balen, A.H., Dunger, D. and Vessey, M. (1999). Polycystic ovaries and associated clinical and biochemical features in young women in the normal population. *Clinical Endocrinology* **51**, 779–86.

Naether, O.G.J. (1995). Significant reduction of adnexal adhesions following laparoscopic electrocautery of the ovarian surface by lavage and artificial ascites. *Gynaecological Endoscopy* **4**, 17–19.

Naether, O.G.J., Baukloh, V., Fischer, R. and Kowalczyk, T. (1994). Long-term follow-up in 206 infertility patients with polycystic ovarian syndrome after laparoscopic electrocautery of the ovarian surface. *Human Reproduction* 9, 2342–9.

Naether, O.G.J. and Fischer, R. (1993). Adhesion formation after laparoscopic electrocoagulation of the ovarian surface in polycystic ovary patients. *Fertility and Sterility* 60, 95–9.

Naether, O.G.J., Fischer, R., Weise, H.C. et al. (1993). Laparoscopic electrocoagulation of the ovarian surface in infertile patients with polycystic ovarian disease. *Fertility and Sterility* 60, 88–94.

Naether, O., Weise, H.C. and Fischer, R. (1991). Treatment with electrocautery in sterility patients with polycystic ovarian disease. *Geburtsh Frauenheilk* 51, 920–4.

Nestler, J.E., Clore, J.N. and Blackard, W.G. (1989). The central role of obesity (hyperinsulinemia) in the pathogenesis of polycystic ovary syndrome. *American Journal of Obstetrics and Gynecology* 5, 1095–7.

Nestler, J.E. and Jakubowicz, D.J. (1996). Decreases in ovarian cytochrome P450c17alpha activity and serum free testosterone after reduction of insulin secretion in polycystic ovary syndrome. *New England Journal of Medicine* 335, 617–23.

Nestler, J.E., Jakubowicz, D.J., Evans, W.S. and Pasquali, R. (1998). Effects of metformin on spontaneous and clomiphene-induced ovulation in the polycystic ovary syndrome. *New England Journal of Medicine* 338, 1876–80.

Nugent, D., Salha, O., Balen, A.H. and Rutherford, A.J. (1998). Ovarian neoplasia and subfertility treatments. *British Journal of Obstetrics and Gynaecology* 105, 584–91.

Ostrzenski, A. (1992) Endoscopic carbon dioxide laser ovarian wedge resection in resistant polycystic ovarian disease. *International Journal of Fertility* 37, 295–9.

Palmer, R. and de Brux, J. (1967). Resultants histologiques, biochemiques et therapeutiques obtenus chez les femmes dont les ovaires avaient ete diagnostiques Stein–Leventhal a la coelioscopie. Bulletin Federation. *Societes Gynaecology Obstetris Languages Francais* 19 405–12.

Polson, D.W., Kiddy, D.S., Mason, H.D. and Franks, S. (1989). Induction of ovulation with clomiphene citrate in women with polycystic ovary syndrome: the difference between responders and nonresponders. *Fertility and Sterility* 51, 30–4.

Prelevic, G.M. (1997). Insulin resistance and polycystic ovary syndrome. *Current Opinion in Obstetrics and Gynecology* 9, 193–201.

Rajkhowa, M., Bicknell, J., Jones, M. and Clayton, R.N. (1994). Insulin sensitivity in women with polycystic ovary syndrome: relationship to hyperandrogenaemia. *Fertility and Sterility* 61, 605–12.

Rajkhowa, M. and Clayton, R.N. (1995). Polycystic ovary syndrome. *Current Opinion in Obstetrics and Gynecology* 5, 191–200.

Rimmington, M.R., Walker, S.M. and Shaw, R.W. (1997). The use of laparoscopic ovarian electrocautery in preventing cancellation of in-vitro fertilization treatment cycles due to risk of ovarian hyperstimulation syndrome in women with polycystic ovaries. *Human Reproduction* 7, 1443–1447.

Roozenberg, B.J., van Dessel, H.J.H.M., Evers, J.L.H. and Bots, R.S.G.M. (1997). Successful induction of ovulation in normogonadotrophic clomiphene resistant anovulatory women by combined naltrexone and clomiphene citrate treatment. *Human Reproduction* 12, 1720–2.

Rose, M.P., Gaines Das, R.E. and Balen, A.H. (1999). Definition and measurement of FSH. *Endocrine Reviews.*

Rossing, M.A., Dalling, J.R., Weiss, N.S. et al. (1994). Ovarian tumors in a cohort of infertile women. *New England Journal of Medicine* 331, 335–9.

Rossmanith, W.G., Keckstein, J., Spatzier, K. and Lauritzen, C. (1991). The impact of ovarian laser surgery on the gonadotrophin secretion in women with polycystic ovarian disease. *Clinical Endocrinology (Oxford)* 34, 223–30.

Sagle, M.A., Hamilton-Fairley, D., Kiddy, D. and Franks, S. (1991). A comparative, randomised study of low-dose human menopausal gonadotrophin and FSH in women with polycystic ovary syndrome. *Fertility and Sterility* 55, 56–60.

Schachter, M., Balen, A.H., Patel, A. and Jacobs, H.S. (1996). Hypogonadotrophic patients with ultrasonographically diagnosed polycystic ovaries have aberrant gonadotropin secretion when treated with pulsatile gonadotropin releasing hormone – a new insight into the pathophysiology of polycystic ovary syndrome. *Gynecological Endocrinology* 10, 327–35.

Scheele, F., Hompes, P.G.A., van der Meer, M., Schoute, E. and Schoemaker, J. (1993). The effects of a gonadotrophin-releasing hormone agonist on treatment with low dose FSH in polycystic ovary syndrome. *Human Reproduction* 8, 699–704.

Schoemaker, J., van Weissenbruch, M.M., Scheele, F. and van der Meer, M. (1993). The FSH threshold concept in clinical ovulation induction. *Baillière's Clinical Obstetrics and Gynaecology.* 7, 297–308.

Schoot, D.C. (1995). *Exogenous Follicle Stimulating Hormone and Development of Human Ovarian Follicles.* Carnforth, Lancashire: Parthenon Publishing Group.

Schoot, D.C., Pache, T.D., Hop, W.C., de Jong, F.H. and Fauser, B.C.J.M. (1992). Growth patterns of ovarian follicles during induction of ovulation with decreasing doses of human menopausal gonadotrophin following presumed selection in polycystic ovary syndrome. *Fertility and Sterility* 57, 1117–20.

Shepard, M.K., Balmaceda, J.P. and Leija, C.G. (1979). Relationship of weight to successful induction of ovulation with clomiphene citrate. *Fertility and Sterility* 32, 641–5.

Shoham, Z., Borenstein, R., Lunenfeld, B.and Pariente, C. (1990a). Hormonal profiles following clomiphene citrate therapy in conception and nonconception cycles. *Clinical Endocrinology* 33, 271–8.

Shoham, Z., Conway, G.S., Patel, A. and Jacobs, H.S. (1992). Polycystic ovaries in patients with hypogonadotrophic hypogonadism: similarity of ovarian response to gonadotrophin stimulation in patients with polycystic ovary syndrome. *Fertility and Sterility* 58, 37–45.

Shoham, Z., Homburg, R. and Jacobs, H.S. (1990b). Induction of ovulation with pulsatile GnRH. *Baillière's Clinical Obstetrics and Gynaecology* 4, 589–608.

Shoham, Z., Patel, A. and Jacobs, H.S. (1991a). Polycystic ovary syndrome: safety and effectiveness of stepwise and low-dose administration of purified follicle stimulating hormone. *Fertility and Sterility* 55, 1051–6.

Shoham, Z., Zosmer, A. and Insler, V. (1991b). Early miscarriage and fetal malformations after induction of ovulation (by clomiphene citrate and/or human menopausal gonadotrophins), in vitro fertilisation and gamete intrafallopian transfer. *Fertility and Sterility* 55, 1–11.

Silverberg, K.M., Olive, D.L., Burns, W.N. et al. (1991). Follicular size at the time of human chorionic gonadotrophin administration predicts ovulation outcome in human menopausal gonadotrophin-stimulated cycles. *Fertility and Sterility* **56**, 296–300.

Stein, I.F. (1956). Ultimate results of bilateral ovarian wedge resection: twenty five years follow-up. *International Journal of Fertility* **1**, 333–44.

Stein, I.F. (1964). Duration of fertility following ovarian wedge resection – Stein–Leventhal syndrome. *Western Journal of Surgery* **78**, 124–7.

Stein, I.F. (1966). Wedge resection of the ovaries: the Stein Leventhal syndrome. In *Ovulation: Stimulation, Suppression, Detection*, ed. R.B. Greenblatt, pp. 150–7. Philidelphia: JB Lippincot.

Stein, I.F. and Leventhal, M.L. (1935). Amenorrhoea associated with bilateral polycystic ovaries. *American Journal of Obstetrics and Gynecology* **29**, 181–91.

Tadokoro, N., Vollenhoven, B., Clark, S. et al. (1997). Cumulative pregnancy rates in couples with anovulatory infertility compared with unexplained infertility in an ovulation induction programme. *Human Reproduction* **12**, 1939–44.

Tan, S.L., Farhi, J., Homburg, R. and Jacobs, H.S. (1996). Induction of ovulation in clomiphene-resistant polycystic ovary syndrome with pulsatile GnRH. *Obstetrics and Gynecology* **88**, 221–6.

Thompson, C.R. and Hansen, L.M. (1970). Pergonal (menotropins): a summary of clinical experience in the induction of ovulation and pregnancy. *Fertility and Sterility* **21**, 844–53.

Toaff, R., Toaff, M.E. and Peyser, M.R. (1976) Infertility following wedge resection of the ovaries. *American Journal of Obstetrics and Gynecology* **124**, 92–6.

van Santbrink, E.J.P., Donderwinkel, P.F.J., van Dessel, T.J.H.M. and Fauser, B.C.J.M. (1995a). Gonadotrophin induction of ovulation using a step-down dose regimen: single centre clinical experience in 82 patients. *Human Reproduction* **10**, 1048–53.

van Santbrink, E.J.P., Hop, W.C., van Dessel, T.J.H.M., de Jong, F.H. and Fauser, B.C.J.M. (1995b). Decremental FSH and dominant follicle development during the normal menstrual cycle. *Fertility and Sterility* **64**, 37–43.

Velasquez, E.M., Acosta, A. and Mendoza, S.G. (1997a). Menstrual cyclicity after metformin therapy in PCOS. *Obstetrics and Gynecology* **90**, 392–5.

Velasquez, E.M., Mendoza, S., Hamer, T., Sosa, F. and Glueck, C.J. (1994). Metformin therapy in polycystic ovary syndrome reduces hyperinsulinaemia, insulin resistance, hyperandrogenaemia and systolic blood pressure, while facilitating normal menses and pregnancy. *Metabolism* **43**, 647–54.

Velasquez, E.M., Mendoza, S.G., Wang, P. and Glueck, C.J. (1997b). Metformin therapy is associated with a decrease in plasminogen activator inhibitor-1, lipoprotein(a) and immunoreactive insulin levels in patients with PCOS. *Journal of Clinical Endocrinology and Metabolism* **82**, 524–30.

Venn, A. and Lumley, J. (1994). Clomiphene citrate and pregnancy outcome. *Australian and New Zealand Journal of Obstetrics and Gynaecology* **34**, 56–66.

Venturoli, S., Orsini, L.F., Paradisi, R., Fabbri, R. et al. (1986). Human urinary FSH and hMG in induction of multiple follicle growth and ovulation. *Fertility and Sterility* **45**, 30–5.

Wang, C.F. and Gemzell, C. (1980). The use of human gonadotrophins for induction of ovulation in women with polycystic ovarian disease. *Fertility and Sterility* **33**, 479–86.

Weinstein, D. and Polishuk, W. (1975). The role of wedge resection of the ovary as a cause of mechanical sterility. *Surgery, Obstetrics and Gynecology* **141**, 417–18.

White, D.M. and Polson, D.W., Kiddy, D. et al. (1996). Induction of ovulation with low-dose gonadotrophins in polycystic ovary syndrome: an analysis of 109 pregnancies in 225 women. *Journal of Clinical Endocrinology Metabolism* **81**, 3821–4.

Zaadstra, B.M., Seidell, J.C., Van Noord, P.A. et al. (1993). Fat and female fecundity: prospective study of effect of body fat distribution on conception rates. *British Medical Journal* **306**, 484–7.

11

Laparoscopic surgical treatment of infertility related to polycystic ovary syndrome

Jean Cohen

Introduction

Polycystic ovary syndrome (PCOS) characterized by chronic anovulation, and/or androgen excess, hypersecretion of luteinizing hormone (LH), obesity and infertility is a relatively common condition in women during the reproductive years. The consistent morphological feature is a peripheral ring of small follicles in association with increased ovarian stroma. It remains an incompletely understood entity, with varying degress of severity and partial symptomatologies.

Wedge resection of ovaries was proposed by Stein in 1935 (Stein and Leventhal, 1935), and for many years it was the only treatment for polycystic ovaries (PCO). However, when treatments with anti-oestrogens (clomiphene citrate) became available (Greenblatt, 1961), and the good results obtained with these treatments became known, this surgical technique, with its associated problems of peri-ovarian adhesion formation, almost disappeared. Subsequently, numerous publications have indicated the advantages of laparoscopic techniques (biopsy, cauterization, multi-electrocoagulation, laser etc.) in cases of non-response to medical treatment. The first attempts at laparoscopy were made in France following the development of Raoul Palmer's ovarian biopsy forceps (Palmer and Cohen, 1965; Cohen et al. 1972a, 1972b).

Techniques

Electrocautery

Biopsy

The first publication concerning pregnancies obtained after laparoscopic ovarian biopsy with cauterization with Palmer forceps dates back to 1972. At this time, Cohen and colleagues (1972a) reported 21 pregnancies after 51 successive ovarian biopsies. They came to the conclusion that this procedure has a therapeutic effect on some types of ovarian infertility (Cohen et al., 1972b).

In 1989, Cohen reported on 778 ovarian biopsies performed between 1971 and 1987 with a pregnancy rate (PR) of 31.8% distributed as 36.6% in less than three months, 32.2% between three and eight months and 31% after this time (Cohen, 1989).

As early as 1972, numerous French authors confirmed spontaneous pregnancies after laparoscopic ovarian biopsy. Among those publications, Sykes (63% PR for 70 cases: Sykes and Ginsburg, 1972), Mintz (44% PR for 157 cases: Mintz and de Brux, 1971), Tescher (23% PR for 85 cases: Tescher, Chassagnard and Boury-Heyler, 1972), Cohen and Chassagnard (1974: 23% PR for 92 cases), Devaut (1977: 33% PR for 32 cases), Scarpa (55% PR for 29 cases: Scarpa and Malaponte, 1978), Fouquet (1978: 50% PR for 100 biopsies). Diquelou, Boyer and Cicquel (1988) performed 68 ovarian biopsies and obtained 13 pregnancies within three months (19%) and 24 pregnancies within 12 months (35%). The rate of success was 34% in women with PCO and 40% in those with unexplained infertility. As early as 1972, Cohen and colleagues indicated that there was no association between pathological examination of the biopsied ovary and the occurrence of pregnancy.

In the 778 cases of Cohen (Cohen and Audebert, 1989), the authors observed three complications due to the ovarian biopsy:

two cases of ovarian haemorrhage linked to trauma of ovarian blood vessels which were impossible to coagulate: one case was treated by immediate laparotomy, and the second one by delayed laparotomy for haematocele;

one bowel perforation due to an electric spark, leading to a perforation on the ninth day post-laparoscopy; it was treated by a simple suture.

In all other cases where ovarian bleeding occurred during the biopsy, haemostasis could be obtained either by cauterization or by pressure on the two sides of the biopsy with the forceps.

In some cases, the authors reviewed the biopsied ovary a few years later (on the occasion of caesarean section, ectopic pregnancy or laparoscopy). The aspect usually observed was that of a simple depression on the surface of the ovary. In no case have adhesions been observed on the biopsied capsule.

Multipunctures

Gjonnaess (1984) proposed the use of laparoscopic multi-electrocauterization in PCOS. The ovulation rate in this study was 92% and the pregnancy rate 69%. In a publication in 1989 (Gjonnaess, 1989), with a follow-up of ten years, the same author reported the outcome of pregnancy for 89 women who became pregnant after electrocauterization. The abortion rate was 15%, which is less than that following clomiphene or wedge resection.

In a recent publication, Gjonnaess (1994) reported the results concerning 252 women with PCOS treated with ovarian electrocauterization during the years 1979–91: ovulation was obtained in 92% of the total series, and pregnancy in 84%. The response was influenced by body weight, with an ovulation range of 96–97% for the slim and moderately obese women, decreasing to 70% in the very obese ones.

When ovulation was established, the pregnancy rate per se was independent of body weight, being 92% for slim and 95% for overweight women. In the responders (who ovulated following ovarian electrocautery), the annual rate of cessation of ovulation was 3–4% only. Even after a period of contraceptive use following the ovarian electrocautery, ovulation was resumed and pregnancy obtained within a few months. Therefore, the author proposes electrocautery as the primary treatment for women with PCOS undergoing laparoscopy for any reason, infertility being a present or only a potential problem.

Greenblatt and Casper (1987) looked at cauterization with small scissors. Eight to ten punctures were made on each ovary with a current of 4 amp, until penetration of the cortex. Six cases of PCOS were studied and compared to six controls with regular cycles. Three to four days after laparoscopy, a decrease of androtestosterone, testosterone, oestradiol and LH was observed in the PCOS group. An increase in FSH was also seen. These modifications are independent of anaesthesia and laparoscopy as they did not occur in the control group. Four of the six women with PCOS became pregnant during the same month.

Sumioki and Utsunomiya (1998) reported on multiple punch resection cautery of ovaries with monopolar forceps done on six to ten surface follicles. The authors estimated that this technique reduces the ovarian volume by one-tenth. Seven cases were observed. Four days after laparoscopy, a decrease in LH, a diminution of LH pulse amplitude and a decrease of androgens were observed. Follicle stimulating hormone (FSH) and prolactin were not modified. The observed modifications were still apparent at the sixth week post-laparoscopy. Four of the six women became pregnant between 12 and 44 weeks after their operation.

Pellicer and Remohi (1992) treated 76 patients with PCOS; 58 had electrocautery, six had laser vaporization, and the remainder had both treatments. All patients failed to respond to clomiphene or human menopausal gonadotrophin (hMG) treatment. Thirty-three patients had anovulatory cycles. The pregnancy rate after laparoscopic treatment was 52.6% and the ovulation rate 67.1%.

Armar and Lachelin (1993) made a study of 50 women with PCO treated over a period of three years and three months. Diathermy was applied to each ovary for four seconds at a time in four separate places. Forty-three women (86%) ovulated within an average time of 23 days. Thirty-three women became pregnant (50 pregnancies with eight spontaneous abortions). The abortion rate of 14% is very low;

of the 22 women who had no pelvic abnormality other than PCO, 19 (86%) had one or more successful pregnancies.

Campo et al. (1993) treated 23 women with PCO who failed to become pregnant following ovulation induction. Treatment was by either multiple laparoscopic biopsy or a longitudinal incision on the surface of the ovary. Fifty-six per cent of patients ovulated and 13 pregnancies occurred, with an abortion rate of 8%.

Kovacs and colleagues (1991) treated ten patients with PCO with ovarian electrocautery on ten different points on each ovary. Seven women ovulated. The authors observed a significant and persistent fall in serum testosterone levels and a transient fall with subsequent rise in inhibin levels.

Gadir and colleagues (1990) consider laparoscopic electrocautery of the ovaries to be 'the' treatment of PCO. Eighty-eight patients who failed to respond to clomiphene were divided into three groups:

A   electrocautery

B   hMG

C   pure FSH.

After treatment, the ovulation rates (as seen by hormones and ultrasound) were, A = 71.4%, B = 70.6%, C = 66.7%. The pregnancy rates per cycle were 9.5%, 12.6% and 8.8%, respectively. The spontaneous abortion rates were 21.4%, 53.3% and 40%. The birth rates were 37.9%, 23.3% and 20.7%. The authors concluded that ovarian electrocautery is the best treatment for PCOS.

Balen and Jacobs (1994) carried out a prospective study on ten patients with resistant PCOS, comparing unilateral and bilateral laparoscopic diathermy. Diathermy was applied three or four times for four seconds. The results were evaluated within six weeks. Unilateral ovarian diathermy resulted in ovulation from both ovaries. Fifty per cent of the patients responded to diathermy, and those who responded had a significantly greater fall in serum LH concentrations than those who failed to respond.

Farhi, Soule and Jacobs (1995) reported a retrospective study of 22 women to evaluate the effect of ovarian electrocautery on the ovarian response to gonadotrophic stimulation and on pregnancy rate in clomiphene citrate-resistant women with PCOS and high basal serum LH levels. Markedly reduced basal serum LH concentrations and normal menstrual cyclicity were recorded in 41% of patients after laparoscopic ovarian electrocautery. Comparison of gonadotrophin-stimulated cycles before and after electrocautery revealed significantly higher rates of ovulation and pregnancy after electrocautery as well as a significant reduction in the number of ampoules, daily effective dose, and duration of the induction phase with hMG and in daily effective dose with FSH. The results indicate an increased ovarian sensitivity to gonadotrophins after laparoscopic ovarian electrocautery. The authors recommend a preference for laparoscopic ovarian electrocautery over medical treatment in all or selected groups of clomiphene citrate-resistant PCOS patients.

Almeida and Risk (1998) reported a case of ovarian drilling by microlaparoscopy under local anaesthesia.

Laparoscopic laser

Laparoscopic laser drilling has been used in the treatment of PCO for the last 15 years. According to its proponents, the laser provides controllable power density, sufficient depth of penetration and predictable thermodamage of surrounding tissues. It may also diminish the risk of adhesions.

Few series have been published. All types of laser have been used: CO_2 laser, argon, YAG. With the YAG laser, Huber et al. (1988) perform three to five drills on each ovary (5–10 mm long and 4 mm deep). They obtained five spontaneous ovulations in eight patients treated. For the three other patients, clomiphene induced ovulation, contrary to the results obtained before laparoscopy.

Daniell and Miller (1989) treated 85 women with PCO with different laser models. The women were poor responders to clomiphene. During laparoscopy, ovarian vaporization was performed by argon, CO_2 or potassium titanyl phosphate (KTP). A two-puncture technique was used to drain all the visible small subcapsular follicles of each ovary and drill randomly placed craters in the ovarian stroma. Ovulation occurred spontaneously in 71%. Postoperatively, 56% conceived within six months of laparoscopy. The KTP laser at 20 W is used to vaporize multiple sites over each ovary. Small wells up to 2 cm deep are developed. The technique is straightforward, even in patients who are obese. The effect is transient. Kurtz and Daniell (1993) encountered no complications in more than 120 cases.

Ostrzenski (1992) used translaparoscopic CO_2 laser ovarian wedge resection. The free ovarian surface was vaporized to a width of 1 cm. There was a 92% pregnancy rate and a 8% postsurgical adhesion rate among 12 cases that were incorporated in the study.

Heylen, Puttemans and Brosens (1994) treated 44 anovulatory patients with laparoscopic argon laser. Spontaneous ovulation occurred in 80% of the women, and spontaneous conception in 55%.

Donesky and Adashi (1995) reviewed 29 relevant studies identified in the English-language articles. Pregnancies after laparoscopic ovulation induction procedures have been reported in an average of 55% of treated subjects (range 20–65%).

Although lasers provide greater control over the type of damage induced in the ovary, this does not appear to translate into a clinical advantage. The impact of the different techniques on reducing adhesion formation remains theoretical.

Table 11.1. Results of percoelioscopics treatments in polycystic ovary syndrome

Authors	Years	Techniques	Number of cases	Spontaneous ovulation(%)	Pregnancies (%)
Cohen et al.	1972b	Biopsy	51		41
Gjonnaess	1984	Cauterization	62	92.0	84
Greenblatt and Casper	1987	Cauterization	6	71.0	56
Cohen	1989	Cauterization	778		31.8
Huber et al.	1988	Laser	8	41.7	
Daniell and Miller	1989	Laser	85	83.8	66.7
Utsunomiya et al.	1990	Biopsy	16	93.8	50.0
Gadir et al.	1990	Cauterization	29	26.5	43.8
Tasaka et al.	1990	Cauterization	11	91	36
Gurgan et al.	1991	Cauterization	40	71	57
Kovacs et al.	1991	Cauterization	10	70	20
Gurgan et al.	1992	Laser	40	70	50
Pellicer and Remohi	1992	Cauterization/laser	131	67.1	52.6
Ostrzenski	1992	Laser	12	92	92
Armar and Lachelin	1993	Cauterization	50	86	66
Campo et al.	1993	Resection coelio	23	56	56
Gjoannes	1994	Cauterization	252	92	84

Results

The results of laparoscopic treatments of PCO are presented in Table 11.1. They are homogeneous whatever the technique: more than 50% spontaneous ovulation and a mean percentage of 50% of pregnancies are obtained.

Lower spontaneous abortion rates were reported in several studies with laparoscopic series compared to medical treatment. Cohen and Leal de Meirelles (1983) reported early pregnancy loss in 22 of 179 patients (12%); Gjonnaess (1989) reported early pregnancy loss in only 13 of 89 patients (15%) who conceived after laparoscopic electrocautery. Gadir et al. (1990) reported early pregnancy loss in 3 of 14 (21%) patients randomized to undergo laparoscopic cautery. In contrast, 8 of 14 (57%) in the hMG group and 4 of 10 (40%) in the pure FSH group of the same study aborted.

Naether and colleagues (1994) evaluated 206 patients up to 72 months after laparoscopic surgery: 145 patients achieved a total of 211 conceptions, giving a pregnancy rate of 70%. They showed that the effects are not temporary. There were 18% miscarriages and three ectopic implantations.

Complications

The risk of laparoscopy could be postoperative adhesions. In a review of 18 studies, El Helw, Ghorab and Elattar (1996) reported adhesion formation ranging between 0 and 100%. The wide variation can be explained by patient selection bias. Gjonnaess (1984) found no adhesion during caesarean sections of pregnant patients. Dabirashrati and colleagues (1991) published a complete study: 17 women were electrocauterized; eight second-look laparoscopies were performed, with no adhesions. In a second group of 21 patients who all had a second-look laparoscopy, four minimal adhesions and one moderate (according to American Fertility Society classification) were observed.

Naether and Fischer (1993) evaluated the incidence and extent of previous adhesion formations subsequent to laparoscopic electrocoagulation from a total of 199 PCOS patients. Fifty cases of laparoscopy and 12 caesarean sections served as second-look investigations. A subgroup of 30 patients had abdominal lavage and artificial ascites after surgery, and underwent 'early' second look two to 14 days after laparoscopy. Adhesion formation was detected in 19.3%. The incidence was reduced to 16.5% with the use of abdominal lavage. The adhesions found were due to bleeding of the ovarian capsule. Adhesiolysis was possible during 'early' second look.

Greenblatt and Casper (1993) observed peri-ovarian adhesions of varying severity in eight women after laparoscopic cautery. Intercede adhesion barrier (Ethicon) showed no protective effect. Despite this finding, seven of the eight women spontaneously conceived without any further therapy.

Gurgan, Yarali and Urman (1994) reported a review of 12 publications concerning adhesion formation as a complication of laparoscopic treatment of PCOS. Adhesion formation rates as assessed by second-look laparoscopy ranged from 0 to 100%. The mean adhesion score of the group treated with CO_2 laser was significantly higher than that of the electrocautery group (Table 11.2).

The rate of adhesions seems to be very different from one author or one technique to the other. The adhesions may be due to some bleeding on the ovarian surface or to premature contact between the ovary and the bowel after cauterization. In this author's experience, the risk is very low, and less than the risk observed after laparotomy. All authors agree that adhesions do not exclude the possibility of pregnancy.

Ruiz Velasco (1996) considers that gonadal atrophy and/or premature ovarian failure caused by an excess of ovarian destruction is more common than is believed (the cases are mostly unpublished).

Table 11.2. Peri-adnexal adhesion formation rates as assessed by second-look laparoscopy following surgical treatment of polycystic ovary syndrome

References	n	Technique	Adhesions (%)
Portuondo et al. (1984)	24	Ovarian biopsy	0
Grochmal (1988)	30	Nd: YAG laser	3
Lyles et al. (1989)	6	Cautery/ND:YAG laser	100
Daniell and Miller (1989)	8	CO_2KTP laser	0
Keckstein (1989)	7	CO_2 laser	43
	4	Nd:YAG laser	0
Gurgan et al. (1991)	7	Cautery	86
	10	Nd:YAG laser	80
Armar and Lachelin (1993)	50	Cautery	24
Gurgan et al. (1992)	20	Nd:YAG laser	68
Naether and Fischer (1993)	26	Cautery	35
Naether et al. (1994)	62	Cautery	19
Dabirashrati et al. (1991)	8	Cautery	0

Mode of action of laparoscopic procedures

The first postoperative endocrine alterations were described by Greenblatt and Casper (1987) and Sumioki and colleagues (1988). These authors have observed a significant decrease of LH and androgen levels during the days immediately after surgery, which is still persistent at six weeks. It is enough to explain how the endocrinological disorders of PCOS are corrected and how pregnancies occur. Both sets of authors agree that the trauma of the ovary is enough to induce a decrease in the production of local androgens, followed by a fall in oestradiol, and a decrease of the positive feedback on LH.

Recently, Sumioki and Utsunomiya (1998) proposed a mechanism of mono-folliculogenesis by ovarian drilling in PCOS:
• vicious cycle of high androgen and high LH pulsation;
• pituitary hyper-response and positive feedback from high androgen;
• high inhibition in atretic PCO follicle;
• high androgen and cytochrome P450c 17α enzyme activity.

Greenblatt and Casper (1987) ascribe an important role to inhibin. Sakata and colleagues (1990) studied nine anovulatory patients with PCO submitted to laparoscopic cauterization of their ovaries. The rates of bioactive LH, immunoreactive LH, FSH, androstenedione and testosterone were studied before and after cauterization and in five controls. Eight women ovulated spontaneously and three became pregnant. The authors noticed a decrease of androgens as well as of immuno-reactive LH, and they are the first to point out a decrease of bioactive LH.

Pellicer and Remohi (1992) studied 13 anovulatory patients after cauterization and confirmed the decrease in the levels of LH, testosterone and androstenedione ($p<0.05$); the level of insulin (IGF1) remained unchanged.

Campo and colleagues (1993) confirmed the rapid decrease in the levels of androstenedione and plasma testosterone in all cases after cauterization of the ovaries. However, the variations of these levels are not linked to the clinical successes; these authors found no variation in the levels of LH. On the contrary, the mean values of FSH and its pulsatility increased significantly in the patients who became pregnant.

It seems that all the authors agree that the ovarian traumas are associated with:
• a significant and immediate decrease of androgens;
• a secondary increase of FSH which could be related to a decrease of intra-ovarian inhibin

However, the most difficult aspect of the problem is how to explain how a physical trauma induces endocrine modifications. As all the authors do not perform the same technique (multiperforation, single or multi biopsy, laser), it seems unlikely that it is the volume of the injured tissues that is responsible. The only common factor is heat damage of the ovary.

However, Mio and colleagues (1991) have shown in 18 patients with PCO that with transvaginal ultrasound-guided follicular aspiration they could obtain an 87–100% ovulation rate per patient and 50% pregnancy. Most of the persistent follicles were punctured and their contents aspirated during the mid-luteal phase. The same ovarian stimulation regimen as used in the previous cycles was administered in the cycles after the aspiration. A significant decrease of basal LH was observed. This method, simpler and less invasive than laparoscopy, may be revolutionary if further experiments confirm its efficacy.

Szilagyi and colleagues (1993) questioned whether restitution of menstrual cyclicity and ovulation was associated with changes in opioidergic and dopaminergic activity, known to be aberrant in these women. Opioidergic and dopaminergic tone was assessed in patients with PCO before and after laser vaporization ($n=4$) or classical ovarian wedge resection ($n=4$). Blood samples for the determination of LH, FSH and prolactin were frequently obtained following opioidergic and/or dopaminergic antagonism affected by nalaxone (4 mg IU) or metoclopramide (10 mg IU). In response to either surgical approach, circulating LH levels decreased ($p<0.01$), while FSH concentrations remained unaltered. Further, LH and FSH concentrations did not change following challenges with naloxone or metoclopramide. This applied to conditions before and after surgery. Prolactin release in response to metoclopramide was markedly higher ($p<0.01$) following ovarian surgery. Thus, both ovarian laser and classical wedge resection can restore normal menstrual cyclicity in patients with PCO, although they failed to alter opioidergic and dopaminergic activity. This suggests that ovarian surgery is effective in influencing gonadal control, but that the central opioidergic and dopaminergic control of gonadotrophin secretion remains unaffected.

Graf and colleagues (1994) studied two patients after ovarian wedge resection. They found that testosterone decreased immediately and LH amplitudes were reduced in one of the PCO patients.

One may consider again the two hypotheses formulated in 1983 (Cohen and Leal de Meirelles, 1983):

- the burning of the ovary provokes a secondary hyperhaemia, inducing an increase in the concentration of gonadotrophins by surface unity;
- electrocoagulation stimulates the ovarian nerves, which transmit the excitation to the superior centres.

Zaidi and colleagues (1995) studied the stromal blood flow in three groups of patients on day 2 or 3 of ovarian stimulation:

- 63 women with regular cycles,
- 13 women with PCO on ultrasound scan,
- 12 women with anovulatory cycles and PCO.

A subjective assessment of the intensity and quantity of coloured areas in the ovarian stroma suggested that they were to be greater in the last two groups compared with the first group.

Mean (SEM) ovarian stromal peak systolic blood flow velocity (Vmax) was 16.88 (1.79) and 16.89 (2.36) cm/s in groups two and three respectively. These velocities were significantly greater than the mean (SEM) ovarian stromal Vmax of group one: 8.74 (0.68) cm/s ($p < 0.001$). Mean (SEM) ovarian stromal time averaged maximum velocity (TAMX) was 10.55 (0.91) and 10.89 (1.80) cm/s in groups two and three respectively, both significantly greater than mean ovarian stromal TAMX of group one ($p < 0.001$). There was no significant difference in pulsatility index (PI) between the three groups. There thus appears to be significantly greater ovarian stromal blood flow velocity in women with polycystic ovaries as detected by colour and pulsed Doppler ultrasound. However, at present there is no study into the possible changes of velocity after laparoscopic ovarian treatment of PCO, which would permit verification of our first hypothesis.

Shawki and colleagues (1998) studied the effect of ovarian drilling on ovarian blood flow in 35 patients. Assessment of P1 of the ovarian artery before and after drilling showed it to decrease in 62% of cases by 30%. Spontaneous ovulation occurred in 58% of cases.

Brian Cohen (1989) hypothesized that drainage of androgens and inhibin from surface follicles could reverse the excessive collagenization of overlaying ovarian cortex and facilitate a softening of the ovaria tunica. Neighbouring follicles that are not undergoing astresia may then mature and gain access to the ovarian surface, facilitating normal ovulation.

It remains a mystery as to how the laparoscopic techniques bring about the resumption of endocrinological function. What is certain, though, is that laparoscopic techniques suppress less ovarian tissue than wedge resection but have the same effect.

Conclusions

Considerable data have been collected on the impact of laparoscopic treatment for PCOS on the resumption of ovulation and the rate of pregnancy in infertile patients, which is greater than 50%. A significant difficulty encountered in the evaluation of the studies is their lack of uniformity. There was great variation in the diagnostic criteria used to define PCOS; none of the studies includes a treatment-independent control group; and some of the patients became pregnant with medical treatment after laparoscopy (the same treatment having been inefficient before).

Nevertheless, the large number of reports of clinical experience allow us to highlight the *advantages* of the laparoscopic surgical method:
- elimination of the risk of ovarian hyperstimulation syndrome and multiple gestations;
- multiple ovulatory cycles from a single treatment;
- high pregnancy rate;
- its usefulness for the diagnosis of unexplained infertility;
- a lower rate of spontaneous abortion;
- elimination of intensive monitoring and high-cost treatment with gonadotrophin.

The laparoscopic techniques have the advantage over surgical wedge resection in terms of:
- cost savings,
- fewer postoperative adhesions.

They have the advantage over gonadotrophin therapy in terms of:
- serial repetitive ovulatory events resulting from a single treatment;
- no increased risk of ovarian hyperstimulation or multiple pregnancies;
- a lower incidence of spontaneous abortion;
- appreciation of the ovarian reserve by the count of the number of early follicles.
  The *disadvantages* of the laparoscopic techniques are:
- the need for anaesthesia;
- the non-permanent ovulatory effect;
- possible postoperative adhesions.

The possible adverse effects (postoperative adhesions, bowel lesions) indicate that the technique must be performed by a well-trained gynaecologist.

Laparoscopy must not be considered as first-line treatment. Clomiphene citrate remains the first-line therapy for the anovulatory patient with PCOS. For resistant patients, the laparoscopic techniques have many advantages over gonadotrophin therapy, and must be offered. On the other hand, when a gynaecologist diagnoses PCOS (by ultrasound imaging or hormonal results) and performs laparoscopy for infertility, cauterization of the ovaries may be done at the same time in order to avoid a secondary surgical laparoscopy.

This treatment option deserves further study by means of randomized, controlled trials.

REFERENCES

Almeida, O.D. and Risk, B. (1998). Microlaparoscopic ovarian drilling under local anaesthesia. *Middle East Fertility Society Journal* 3, 189–91.

Armar, N.A. and Lachelin, G. (1993). Laparoscopic ovarian diathermy: an effective treatment for anti-oestrogen resistant anovulatory infertility in women with PCOS. *British Journal of Obstetrics and Gynaecology* 100, 161–4.

Balen, A. and Jacobs, H. (1994). A prospective study comparing unilateral laparoscopic ovarian diathermy in patients with PCO. *Fertility and Sterility* 62, 921–5.

Campo, S., Felli, A., Lamanna, M.A. et al. (1993). Endocrine changes and clinical outcome after laparoscopic ovarian resection in women with PCO. *Human Reproduction* 8, 359–63.

Cohen, B.M. (1989). Laser laparoscopy for polycystic ovaries. *Fertility and Sterility* 52, 167–8.

Cohen, B.M. and Chassagnard, N. (1974). Analyse de 92 biopsies d'ovaire per-coelioscopique. Thesis, Doctor of Medicine, University of Paris.

Cohen, J. and Audebert, A.J.M. (1989). De la 'mecanique' au fonctionnel: place des traitements chirurgicaux en endoscopiques dans les dystrophies ovariennes. In *Dystrophies Ovairennes*, pp. 183–92. Paris: Masson Editeur.

Cohen, J., Audebert A., De Brux, J. and Giorgi, H. (1972a). Biopsie ovarienne et survenue d'une grossesse. *Nouvelle Presse Medicale* 1, 1294.

Cohen, J., Audebert A., De Brux, J. and Giorgi, H. (1972b). Les sterilites pour dysovulation: role pronotisque et therapeutique de la biopsie ovairienne percoelioscopique. *Journal of Gynaecology, Obstetrics and Reproduction* 1 657–71.

Cohen, J. and Leal de Meirelles, H. (1983). Fertilité apres biopsie ovarienne percoelioscopique. A propos de 477 cas en sterilité. *Journal of Gynaecology, Obstetrics and Reproduction* 12, 73–9.

Dabirashrati, H., Mohamad, K., Behjatnia, Y. et al. (1991). Adhesion formation after ovarian electrocauterization on patients with PCO syndrome. *Fertility and Sterility* 55, 1200–1.

Daniell, J.F. and Miller, R. (1989). Polycystic ovaries treated by laparoscopic laser vaporization. *Fertility and Sterility* 51, 232–6.

Devaut, F. (1977). Interet de la biopsie d'ovaire per-coelioscopique à propos de 69 cas. Thesis, Doctor of Medicine, University of Paris.

Diquelou, J.Y., Boyer, S. and Cicquel, J.M. (1988). Therapeutic role of ovarian biopsy done by laparoscopy in polycystic ovarian and unexplained infertility. *Human Reproduction* 3, (Suppl.) 80.

Donesky, B. and and Adashi, E. (1995). Surgically induced ovulation in the PCO syndrome: wedge resection revisited. *Fertility and Sterility* 63, 439–63.

El Helw, B., Ghorab, M.N. and Elattar, E. (1996). Surgical induction of ovulation in women with polycystic ovary syndrome: a critical analysis of published data. *Middle East Fertility Society Journal* 1, 101–15.

Farhi, J., Soule, S. and Jacobs, H. (1995). Effect of laparoscopic ovarian electrocautery on ovarian response and outcome of treatment with gonadotrophins in clomiphene citrate resistant patients with PCOS. *Fertility and Sterility* 64, 930–5.

Fouquet, A. (1978). Interet diagnostique et therapeutique de lap biopsie d'ovaire. Thesis, Doctor of Medicine, University of Paris.

Gadir, A., Mowafie, R., Huda, M.I. et al. (1990). Ovarian electrocautery versus pure FSH therapy in the treatment of PCOS. *Clinical Endocrinology* 33, 585–92.

Gjonnaess, H. (1984). Polycystic ovarian syndrome treated by ovarian electrocautery through the laparascope. *Fertility and Sterility* 41, 20–5.

Gjonnaess, H. (1989). The course and outcome of pregnancy after ovarian electrocautery with PCOS: the influence of body weight. *British Journal of Obstetrics and Gynaecology* 96, 714–19.

Gjonnaess, H. (1994). Ovarian electrocautery in the treatment of women with PCOS. *Acta Obstetricia et and Gynaecologica Scandinavica* 73, 407–12.

Graf, M.A., Bielfed, P., Graf, C. and Distler, W. (1994). Pattern of gonadotrophin secretion in patients with hyperandrogenaemic amenorrhea before and after ovarian wedge resection. *Human Reproduction* 9, 1022–6.

Greenblatt, E. and Casper, R.F. (1987). Endocrine changes after laparoscopic ovarian cautery in polycystic ovarian syndrome. *American Journal of Obstetrics and Gynecology* 42, 517–18.

Greenblatt, E. and Casper, R.F. (1993). Adhesion formation after laparoscopic ovarian cautery for PCOS: lack of correlation with pregnancy rate. *Fertility and Sterility* 60, 766–9.

Greenblatt, R.B. (1961). Chemical induction of ovulation. *Fertility and Sterility* 12, 402–4.

Grochmal, S. (1988). Contact Nd:YAG laser superior to CO_2 for the treatment of ovarian disease. *Laser Practice Reports* 3 IS.

Gurgan, T., Kisnisci, H., Yarali, H. et al. (1991). Evaluation of adhesion formation after laparoscopic treatment of PCOD. *Fertility and Sterility* 56, 1176–8.

Gurgan, T., Urman, B., Aksu, T. et al. (1992). The effect of short internal laparoscopic lysis of adhesions on pregnancy rates following ND:YAG laser photocoagulation of PCO. *Obstetrics and Gynaecology* 80, 45–7.

Gurgan, T., Yarali, H. and Urman, B. (1994). Laparoscopic treatment of PCO decrease. *Human Reproduction* 9, 573–7.

Heylen, S.M., Puttemans, P.J. and Brosens, I.A. (1994). Polycystic ovarian disease treated by laparoscopic argon laser capsule drilling: comparison of vaporization versus perforation technique. *Human Reproduction* 9, 1038–42.

Huber, J., Hosmann, J. and Spona, J. (1988). Polycystic ovarian syndrome treated by laser through the laparoscope. *Lancet* **ii**, 215.

Keckstein, J. (1989). Laparoscopic treatment of PCOS. *Baillère's Clinical Obstetrics and Gynaecology* **3**, 563–81.

Kovacs, G.T., Buckler, H., Bangah, M. et al. (1991). Treatment of anovulation due to PCOS by laparoscopic ovarian cautery. *British Journal of Obstetrics and Gynaecology* **98**, 30–5.

Kurtz, B.R. and Daniell, J.F. (1993). The role of lasers in the laparoscopic treatment of infertility and endometriosis. *Reproductive Medicine Review* **2**, 85–94.

Lyles, R., Goldzieher, J.W. et al. (1989). Early second look laparoscopy after the treatment of PCO. Presented at the 45th annual meeting of the American Fertility Society, San Francisco, 13–16 November 1989. Program supplement published by *Fertility and Sterility*, p. 526.

Mintz, M. and de Brux, J. (1971) La biopsie per-coelioscopique de l'ovaire dans les amenorrhees, spaniomenorrhees et troubles ovulatoires. (Etude critique de ses indications en fonction des suites proches et lointaines de 157 cas.) *Comptes Rendus de la Societe Francaise de Gynecologie*, **8**, 609–29.

Mio, Y., Toda, T., Tanikawa, M. et al. (1991). Transvaginal ultrasound guided follicular aspiration in the management of anovulatory infertility associated with polycystic ovaries. *Fertility and Sterility* **56**, 1060–5.

Naether, O.G.J., Baukloh, V., Fischer, R. and Kowalczyk, T. (1994). Long-term follow-up in 206 infertility patients with polycystic ovarian syndrome after laparoscopic electrocautery of the ovarian surface. *Human Reproduction* **9**, 2342–9.

Naether, O.G.J. and Fischer, R. (1993). Adhesion formation after laparoscopic electrocoagulation of the ovarian surface in polycystic ovary patients. *Fertility and Sterility* **60**, 95–9.

Ostrzenski, A. (1992). Endoscopic carbon dioxide laser wedge resection in resistant PCO. *International Journal of Fertility* **37**, 295–9.

Palmer, R. and Cohen, J. (1965). Biopsies percoelioscopiques. *Minerva Gynaecologica* **17**, 238–9.

Pellicer, A. and Remohi, J. (1992). *Management of the PCOS by Laparoscopy*. Basel: Karger.

Portuondo, J., Melshor, J., Neyro, J. et al. (1984). Periovarian adhesions following ovarian wedge resections or laparoscopic biopsy. *Endoscopy* **16**, 143–5.

Ruiz Velasco, V. (1996). Laparoscopic management of the polycystic ovary. World Congress on Human Reproduction, May 1996, Philadelphia.

Sakata, M., Tasaka, K., Kurachi, H. et al. (1990). Changes of bio-active LH laser laparoscopic ovarian cautery in patients with PCOS. *Fertility and Sterility* **53**, 610–13.

Scarpa, F. and Malaponte, E. (1978). La laparoscopoia e la biopsia ovarica come studio dela funzione ovarica nelle amenorree primarie e secondarie. *Minerva Gynaecologica* **30**, 871–80.

Shawki, H., Shawki,O., Zaki, S. et al. (1998). Effect of laparoscopic ovarian drilling in PCO disease on ovarian blood flow. *Egyptian Journal of Fertility and Sterility* **2**, 5–58.

Stein, I.F. and Leventhal, M.L. (1935). Amenorrhea associated with bilateral polycystic ovaries. *American Journal of Obstetrics and Gynecology* **29**, 181–91.

Sumioki, H., Korencaga, M., Utsunomyiya, T., Kadota, T. and Matsuoka, K. (1988). Wedge resection revisited in the age of laparoscopy. *Fertility and Sterility* **50**, 567–72.

Sumioki, H. and Utsunomiya, T. (1998). Ovarian drilling. In *Fertility and Reproduction Medicine*, ed. R. Kempers, J. Cohen, A.F. Haney and J.B. Youngers, pp. 537–9. New York: Elsevier Science.

Sykes, O.W. and Ginsburg, J. (1972). The use of laparoscopic biopsy to assess gonadal function. *American Journal of Obstetrics and Gynecology* **112**, 211–18.

Szilagyi, A., Hole, R., Keckstein, J. and Rossmanith, W. (1993). Effect of ovarian surgery on the dopaminergic and opioidergic control of gonadotrophin and prolactin secretion in women with PCO disease. *Gynecological Endocrinology* **7**, 159–66.

Tasaka, K., Sakata, M., Kurachi, H. et al. (1990). Electrocautery in PCOS. *Hormone Results* **33**, 40–2.

Tescher, M., Chassagnard, N. and Boury-Heyler, C. (1972). Interet therapeutique des biopsies ovariennes dans les sterilites par anovulation. *Comptes Rendus de la Sociétè Francaise de Gynecologie* **5**, 327–35.

Utsunomiya, T., Sumioki, T. and Taniguchi, I. (1990). Hormonal and clinical effects of multi-follicular puncture and resection of PCOS. *Hormone Research* **33** (Suppl. 2), 35.

Zaidi, J., Campbell, S., Pittrof, R. et al. (1995). Ovarian stromal blood flow in women with PCO – a possible marker for diagnosis? *Human Reproduction* **10**, 1992–6.

12

In-vitro fertilization and the patient with polycystic ovaries

Adam Balen

Introduction

Many patients with polycystic ovaries (PCO) may be referred for in-vitro fertilization (IVF) either because there is another reason for their infertility or because they fail to conceive despite ovulating for more than six months (i.e. their infertility remains unexplained). An understanding of the management of such patients is therefore important to specialists involved in IVF.

The association of enlarged, sclerocystic ovaries with amenorrohoea, infertility and hirsutism, as described by Stein and Leventhal in 1935, is now described as the polycystic ovary syndrome (PCOS). In recent years, it has become apparent that PCO may be present in women who are non-hirsute and who have a regular menstrual cycle. Thus, a clinical spectrum exists between the typical Stein–Leventhal picture (PCOS), on the one hand, and the symptomless women with PCO, on the other. Even the clinical picture of patients with the PCOS exhibits considerable heterogeneity (Balen et al., 1995). This heterogeneous disorder may present, at one end of the spectrum, with the single finding on pelvic ultrasound of polycystic ovarian morphology. At the other end of the spectrum, symptoms such as obesity, hyperandrogenism, menstrual cycle disturbance and infertility may occur, either singly or in combination (Table 12.1). Metabolic disturbances (elevated serum concentrations of luteinizing hormone (LH), testosterone, insulin and prolactin) are common and may have profound implications on the long-term health of women with PCOS. The PCOS is a familial condition, and a number of canditate genes have been implicated. It appears to have its origins during adolescence and is thought to be associated with significant weight gain during puberty (Balen and Dunger, 1995).

Table 12.1. The spectrum of clinical manifestations of the heterogenous polycystic ovary syndrome

Symptoms (% patients affected)	Associated endocrine manifestations	Possible late sequelae
Obesity (38)	↑Androgens (testosterone and androstenedione)	Diabetes mellitus (11%)
Menstrual disturbance (66)		Cardiovascular disease
Hyperandrogenism (48)	↑Luteinizing hormone	Hyperinsulinaemia
Infertility (73% of anovulatory infertility)	↑LH:FSH ratio	Low low-density lipoprotein
	↑Free oestradiol	Endometrial carcinoma
Asymptomatic (20)	↑Fasting insulin	Hypertension
	↑Prolactin	
	↓Sex hormone binding globulin	

Diagnosis

The diagnosis of PCO is best made not on the clinical presentation, but rather on the ovarian morphology. With the advent of high-resolution ultrasound, identification of PCO is simple, and ovarian biopsy, which is invasive and possibly damaging to future fertility because it can cause adhesions, is unnecessary. Ovaries are described as polycystic if there are ten or more cysts, 2–8 mm in diameter, arranged around a dense stroma or scattered throughout an increased amount of stroma (Adams et al., 1985). This is discussed in greater detail in Chapter 6.

High-resolution ultrasound scanning has made possible an accurate estimate of the prevalence of PCO in the general population. Several studies have estimated the prevalence of PCO in 'normal adult' women and have found rates of approximately 20% (Polson et al., 1988; Tayob et al., 1990; Clayton et al., 1992; Farquhar et al., 1994). It is important to differentiate between PCO and PCOS. The former describes the morphological appearance of the ovary, whereas the latter term is only appropriate when PCO are found in association with a menstrual disturbance, most commonly oligomenorrhoea, the complications of hyperandrogenization (seborrhoea, acne and hirsutism) and obesity.

The PCOS is often associated with endocrinological abnormalities, and in particular with alterations in the serum concentrations of LH, prolactin, oestrogens and androgens (in particular, testosterone and androstenedione). In about 40% of cases, plasma concentrations of LH are raised (Balen et al., 1995). In a proportion of patients with PCOS, moderate hyperprolactinaemia (usually between 600 and 2000 mU/l) is present. Futterweit (1984) reported a 27% prevalence of raised prolactin levels in 394 women. Hyperprolactinaemia may be caused by stimulation of pituitary lactotrophs by acyclical oestrogen production (Franks et al., 1985), rather than by a primary pituitary defect. Oestrogen levels may be altered in patients with PCOS who are anovulatory. Oestradiol levels are similar to those found in normal women during the early follicular phase of the cycle. Oestrone levels are raised, mostly because of extra-ovarian conversion of androstenedione (Baird, Corker and Davidson, 1977; Yen, 1980), which largely takes place in adipose tissue. Finally, the PCO tends to produce an excess of androgens. As with the clinical picture, these endocrine changes are variable, and patients with PCOS may have normal hormone concentrations. Thus, their measurement is not as helpful as ultrasound in making the diagnosis.

Even today, a universally agreed definition of either the polycystic ovary or the polycystic ovary syndrome is not available. The PCO is usually detected by ultrasound, the images of which correlate well with histopathological studies. The original ultrasound definition was provided by transabdominal ultrasonography (Adams et al., 1985), which is still used in present-day publications (Obrhai et al., 1990; Balen et al., 1995). Whereas Swanson et al. (1981) described a characteristic appearance without the need for a particular number of cysts, Adams et al. (1985) proposed a quantifiable definition, with a prerequisite number of at least ten cysts in a single plane. It is now accepted that transvaginal sonography provides greater resolution and the need to redefine the ultrasound criteria for the PCO (Fox et al., 1991). Indeed, Fox et al., (1991) suggested the requirement of at least 15 cysts per ovary in their study.

Apart from the number of cysts, it is necessary to consider the stromal thickness or density – the latter usually being a subjective assessment – and the ovarian volume, neither of which is clearly defined. Van Santbrink, Hop and Fauser (1997) recently characterizsed PCOS by taking values for the diagnostic criteria of the syndrome (increased follicle number and ovarian volume, elevated serum concentrations of testosterone, androstenedione and LH) as the 95th percentile of a control population. They found considerable overlap between the sonographic and endocrine criteria for the diagnosis of PCOS in women with normogonadotrophic oligomenorrhoea or infertile women with amenorrhoea. The predictive value of PCO detected by ultrasound for endocrine parameters, however, was limited (van Santbrink et al., 1997) – a finding supported by others.

Recent studies with computerized, three-dimensional reconstructions of ultrasound images of the polycystic ovary have shown that the major factor responsible for the increase in ovarian volume is an increase in the stroma, with little contribution from the cysts themselves (Kyei-Mensah et al., 1998). Zaidi et al. (1995), using colour and pulsed Doppler ultrasound, have shown that the stroma of the PCO has a very high rate of blood flow, consistent with histological studies showing increased stromal vascularity and the recent finding of large amounts of vascular endothelial growth factor (VEGF) in the theca cells of the PCO (Kamat et al., 1995).

There have been many reviews over the years which have attempted to piece together the complexities of the syndrome, but that is beyond the scope of this chapter (Goldzieher and Axelrod, 1963; Yen, 1980; Vaitukaitis, 1983; Franks, 1989). It is fascinating to follow the evolving ideas on the spectrum and pathogenesis of PCOS, yet at the same time frustrating that a consensual definition cannot be accepted – and this has meant that when we turn to the literature on the treatment of the condition it proves impossible to compare studies from different centres which use differing starting points.

Hypersecretion of LH is particularly associated with menstrual disturbances and infertility. Indeed, it is this endocrine feature that appears to result in reduced conception rates and increased rates of miscarriage in both natural and assisted conception (Balen et al., 1993b). The finding of a persistently elevated early to mid-follicular phase LH concentration in a woman who is trying to conceive suggests the need to suppress LH levels by either pituitary desensitization, with a gonadotrophin-releasing hormone (GnRH) agonist, or laparoscopic ovarian diathermy prior to IVF. There are, however, no large prospectively randomized trials that demonstrate a therapeutic benefit from a reduction in serum LH concentrations during ovulation induction protocols.

The author, and others, have found that the patient's body mass index (BMI) correlates with an increased rate of hirsutism, cycle disturbance and infertility (Kiddy et al., 1992; Balen et al., 1995). Obese women with PCOS hypersecrete insulin, which stimulates ovarian secretion of androgens, and is associated with hirsutism, menstrual disturbance and infertility. It is seldom necessary to measure the serum insulin concentration, as this will not overtly affect the management of the patient, but the prevalence of diabetes in obese women with PCOS is 11% and so a measurement of impaired glucose tolerance is important in these women. Obese women (BMI >30 kg/m2) should therefore be encouraged to lose weight prior to IVF. Weight loss improves the symptoms of PCOS and improves the patient's endocrine profile (Kiddy et al., 1992; Clark et al., 1995).

Heterogeneity of the polycystic ovary syndrome

Balen et al. (1995) have carefully characterized a large population of women with PCOS who have presented with both the ultrasound finding of PCO and at least one sign or symptom of the syndrome (oligo/amenorrhoea, obesity, hyperandrogenism and/or elevated serum LH and testosterone concentrations). As might have been expected, with increasing severity of signs (obesity) or endocrine status (elevated serum LH or testosterone concentrations), there was an increased risk of infertility. In this large series of 1871 women, there was great heterogeneity of signs and symptoms, and ovarian morphology, as assessed by ultrasound scan, was found to be the unifying diagnostic criterion.

Prevalence

The prevalence of PCO in patients referred for IVF is not well known. Three studies suggest that many patients will have PCO. The first involved a review of ultrasound scans performed in the early follicular phase of an IVF treatment cycle and noted that 50% of 42 patients had PCO (Jacobs et al., 1987). A more recent study of patients attending the Hallam Medical Centre identified 58 (33%) with PCO compared with 117 (67%) with normal ovaries (Balen, Tan and Jacobs, 1993b). In patients referred for natural cycle IVF (all had regular ovulatory menstrual cycles), 43.5% had PCO (MacDougall et al., 1994).

Polycystic ovaries with or without clinical symptoms are therefore a common finding in patients referred for IVF. It must be stressed that the first-line treatment for PCOS is *not* IVF. Occasionally, the IVF specialist will be presented with a patient with PCOS, referred for IVF, who either has never had induction of ovulation or has been inadequately stimulated. Provided there is no other cause for her infertility, for example tubal damage, it then behoves the clinician to try induction of ovulation.

Infertility in patients with PCO is caused either by PCOS (i.e. failure to ovulate at a normal rate, and/or hypersecretion of LH) or any of the other causes of infertility, or a combination of the two. Ovulation induction is appropriate for the first group (PCOS). In-vitro fertilization may be necessary in the second group (other causes) and in patients with PCOS who have failed to conceive despite at least six ovulatory cycles (i.e. who have coexisting 'unexplained' infertility).

The response of the polycystic ovary to stimulation for IVF

The response of the PCO to stimulation in the context of ovulation induction aimed at the development of unifollicular ovulation is well documented and differs significantly from that of normal ovaries (Buyalos and Lee, 1996). The response tends to be slow, with a significant risk of ovarian hyperstimulation and/or cyst formation (Balen et al., 1994, 1995). Conventional IVF nowadays depends on inducing multifollicular recruitment (Balen and Jacobs, 1997). It is thus to be expected that the response of the PCO within the context of an IVF programme should also differ from that of the normal ovary, but this has previously been assumed rather than documented. Jacobs et al. (1987) described an increase in follicle production in patients with PCO, and others (Smitz et al., 1991) refer to the 'explosive' nature of the ovarian response. Dor et al. (1990) compared 16 patients with PCOS with a control group with normal ovaries, who were all udergoing in-vitro fertilization, and noted an increase in follicle numbers, oocytes and oestrogen levels, associated with a decrease in fertilization rates.

There are several possible explanations for this 'explosive' response. There are many partially developed follicles present in the PCO and these are readily stimulated to give rise to the typical multifollicular response. Thecal hyperplasia (with, in some cases, raised levels of LH and/or insulin) provides large amounts of androstenedione and testosterone, which act as substrates for oestrogen production. Granulosa cell aromatase, although deficient in the 'resting' PCO, is readily stimulated by follicle-stimulation hormone (FSH). Therefore, normal quantities of FSH act on large amounts of substrate (testosterone and androstenedione) to produce large amounts of intra-ovarian oestrogen. Ovarian follicles, of which there are too many in the PCO, are increasingly sensitive to FSH (receptors for which are stimulated by high local concentrations of oestrogen) and as a result there is multiple follicular development associated with very high levels of circulating oestrogen. In some cases, this may result in the ovarian hyperstimulation syndrome (OHSS), to which patients with PCO are particularly prone.

There are two additional factors to be considered. The first is that many women with PCOS, particularly those who are obese, have compensatory hypersecretion of insulin in response to the insulin resistance specifically related to PCOS and that caused by obesity. Because the ovary is spared the insulin resistance, it is stimulated by insulin, acting, as it were, as a co-gonadotrophin. Insulin augments theca cell production of androgens in response to stimulation by LH (Franks, 1995) and granulosa cell production of oestrogen in response to stimulation by FSH (Adashi et al., 1985).

The second factor to be considered relates to the already mentioned widespread expression of VEGF in the PCO. VEGF is an endothelial cell mitogen which stimulates vascular permeability, hence its involvement in the pathophysiology of OHSS (see Chapter 10). It is normally confined in the ovary to the blood vessels and is responsible there for invasion of the relatively avascular graafian follicle by blood vessels after ovulation. The increase of LH at mid-cycle leads to expression of VEGF, which has recently been shown to be an obligatory intermediatry in the formation of the corpus luteum (Ferrara et al., 1998). In PCO, however, Kamat et al. (1995) have shown widespread expression of VEGF in theca cells in the increased stroma. Recent studies (Agrawal et al., 1998) have shown that, compared with women with normal ovaries, women with PCO and PCOS have increased serum VEGF, both before and during LHRH analogue therapy and gonadotrophin treatment.

The above data serve to remind us of the close relationship of PCO and OHSS and also provide a possible explanation for the multifollicular response of the PCO to gonadotrophin stimulation. Thus, one of the mechanisms which underpins the unifollicular response of the normal ovary is diversion of blood flow within the ovaries, first from the non-dominant to the dominant ovary and, second, from cohort follicles to the dominant follicle. This results in diversion of FSH away from the cohort follicles and permits them to undergo atresia. We postulate that the widespread distribution of VEGF in the PCO prevents this diversion of blood flow, leaving a substantial number of small and intermediate-sized follicles in 'suspended animation' and ready to respond to gonadotrophin stimulation. The distribution of VEGF in the PCO therefore helps to explain one of the fundamental features of the PCO, namely, the loss of the intra-ovarian auto-regulatory mechanism which permits unifollicular ovulation to occur.

The outcome of IVF in 76 patients diagnosed as having PCO on pretreatment ultrasound scan was examined and compared with that of 76 control patients who had normal ovaries. The subjects were matched for age, cause of infertility and stimulation regimen (MacDougall et al., 1993). Despite receiving significantly less human menopausal gonadotrophin (hMG), patients with ultrasound-diagnosed PCO had significantly higher serum oestradiol concentrations on the day of human chorionic gonadotrophin (hCG) administration (5940 ± 255 versus 4370 ± 240 pmol/l; $p < 0.001$), developed more follicles (14.9 ± 0.7 vs 9.8 ± 0.6; $p < 0.001$) and produced more oocytes (9.3 ± 0.6 vs 6.8 ± 0.5; $p = 0.003$). Fertilization rates were, however, reduced in PCO patients ($52.8 \pm 3.4\%$ vs $66.1 \pm 3.4\%$; $p = 0.007$). There was no significant difference in cleavage rates. The pregnancy rate per embryo transfer was 25.4% in the PCO group and 23.0% in the group with normal ovaries. There were three high-order multiple pregnancies in the PCO group, but none in the group with normal ovaries. Of the PCO patients, 10.5% developed moderate/severe OHSS, compared with none in the controls ($p = 0.006$). Patients with and without PCO undergoing IVF had similar pregnancy and livebirth rates as each had similar numbers of good-quality embryos for transfer. The study indicated the importance of the diagnosis of polycystic ovarian morphology prior to 'controlled' ovarian stimulation, because it is less likely to be controlled in women with PCO and these patients are more likely to develop OHSS and multiple pregnancy. Similar observations in women with PCO undergoing IVF have been reported by others (Homburg et al., 1993a).

It should be noted that there are a small number of PCO patients who are poor responders rather than over-responders. Such patients are often very resistant to gonadotrophin stimulation and may benefit from the addition of growth hormone (Owen et al., 1991).

Preconception counselling

Women with PCO encounter specific problems during assisted conception treatment cycles. By our diagnostic criteria, many women are unaware that their ovaries are polycystic and may have presented with another cause of subfertility. When

PCO have been diagnosed by ultrasound, it is helpful to discuss this finding with the patient, as a preliminary knowledge of the behaviour of the PCO in response to superovulation regimens allows both an explanation of the drugs chosen and advice about potential problems – specifically OHSS and multiple pregnancy (Balen and Jacobs, 1997).

Some women will have already been diagnosed as having either PCO or PCOS and may be aware of the sequelae. The latter group will usually have had endocrinological and metabolic problems, and for them preconception counselling should involve more than an outline of the consequences of treatment. There are additional problems that may occur during pregnancy, and there may be a chance to reduce their risk by appropriate measures such as weight loss, even before embarking upon assisted conception regimens.

There are thus two aspects to the counselling and subsequent management of women with PCO: firstly, the general behaviour of the PCO itself and, secondly, additional features of PCOS. Ovaries that are morphologically polycystic contain multiple antral follicles and are extremely sensitive to stimulation. It is the woman with PCOS who will benefit most from preconception counselling. Not only does she have an endocrine disorder, but also a metabolic one. She may therefore have hyperandrogenism and insulin resistance – it is the consequences of the latter which have a particular bearing on pregnancy. Hyperinsulinaemia may lead to obesity, which in turn is associated with hypertension, pre-eclampsia and gestational diabetes (MacGillivray, 1983; Treharne, 1984). Although hypertension and pre-eclampsia have been directly associated with PCOS (Diamant, Rimon and Evron, 1982), it appears that it is the resultant obesity that is the prime factor (Gjonnaess, 1989). Dietary restriction and reduction of weight gain during pregnancy do not reduce the incidence of pre-eclampsia (MacGillivray, 1983), yet, if an ideal weight can be attained before conception, pre-eclampsia may be avoided (Treharne, 1984).

It is established that women with PCO exhibit insulin resistance, particularly if they are obese (Conway, 1990), and it has been postulated that hyperinsulinaemia may have an aetiological role in PCOS, possibly through effects on ovarian insulin-like growth factor 1 (IGF-1) receptors (Dunaif and Graf, 1989). Even if not aetiological, exposure to high insulin or IGF-1 levels is thought to result in increased ovarian androgen secretion (Conway, 1990). Fasting insulin levels are raised in two-thirds of obese and in one-third of lean women with PCOS; those women with hyperinsulinaemia are more likely to present with menstrual disturbances and hyperandrogenism than those with normal insulin levels (Conway, 1990). The most effective management is dietary advice and weight loss. One should also be aware that type 2 diabetes mellitus may be precipitated by some treatments, such as synthetic sex steroids (Fox and Wardle, 1990). Screening women with PCOS for glucose intolerance is now becoming part of normal practice in the Endocrine Unit at The Middlesex Hospital. Gestational diabetes is also more prevalent amongst women with PCOS, our study quoting a prevalence of 8.1%, as compared with a population prevalence of 0.25% (Gjonnaess, 1989). Of the 89 pregnancies studied, the rate was greatest (19%) in the obese women; none of those with a normal weight became diabetic in pregnancy. Although dietary restriction is employed in the management of obesity, active steps towards weight loss during pregnancy itself are not advised (Treharne, 1984).

Obesity in pregnancy also leads to an increased incidence of urinary tract infections, fetal malpresentations and dystocia, post-partum haemorrhage and thromboembolism. The perinatal mortality rate in the infants of obese women (greater than the 110th centile, Metropolitan Life Insurance tables) is also double that of the normal population (Treharne, 1984). Current research suggests that, in later life, women with PCOS may be at risk from hypertension, type 2 diabetes mellitus and cardiovascular disease, because insulin resistance is also associated with a reduction of the cardioprotective high-density lipoprotein 2. Women with endometrial hyperplasia and carcinoma are traditionally obese, with hypertension and diabetes, and they are likely to have PCO. Thus, preconception counselling is important not only to advise short-term weight loss, in order to reduce maternal and neonatal morbidity, but also to prevent later morbidity by encouraging obese women to become slim, and non-obese women to stay slim (Balen and Jacobs, 1997).

There has been disagreement in the past about the association of PCOS with congenital abnormalities, especially as treatment regimens may have an influence (Ahlgren, Kallen and Rannevik, 1976). The miscarriage rate is increased in women with PCO (Sagle et al., 1988). This is thought to be secondary to an abnormal endocrine environment, specifically hypersecretion of LH, affecting either oocyte maturation or endometrial receptivity (Sagle et al., 1988; Regan, Owen and Jacobs, 1990). There is, however, no evidence of an increased incidence of congenital abnormalities either in women with PCOS (Gjonnaess, 1989) or in women undergoing ovulation induction (Harlap, 1976; Kurachi et al., 1983) and IVF (Medical Research Council, 1990; Beral et al., 1990). That PCOS does not cause congenital anomalies is also supported by the high prevalence of the syndrome in the author's clinic, whose statistics are included in the reports of the Medical Research Council (1990) and Beral et al. (1990). Couples can thus be given appropriate reassurance at the time of their first consultation.

Implications of polycystic ovary syndrome in relation to fertility

Anovulation is the main cause of infertility in women with PCOS. Many regimens have been evolved to induce ovulation, and the interested reader is referred to

Chapter 10 of this book. In recent years, there has been increasing evidence that hypersecretion of LH is deleterious both to fertility and pregnancy outcome (Stanger and Yovich, 1985; Abdulwahid et al., 1985; Howles et al., 1986; Homburg et al., 1988; Balen et al., 1993a). LH has several functions in the control of the developing follicle. In the early follicular phase, low levels of LH induce a change in function of the theca interstitial cells from progesterone to androgen production (Erickson et al., 1985). FSH then promotes the conversion of androgen to oestradiol by the granulosa cells. Not only does LH initiate theca cell androgen production, it is also involved in the reversal to progesterone secretion at the time of the pre-ovulatory surge. LH is also involved in suppression of the oocyte maturation inhibitor (OMI). The action of OMI is to maintain the meiotic arrest of the oocyte at the diplotene stage of prophase 1. The precise nature of OMI is uncertain; it is known that cyclic adenosine monophosphate (cAMP) activates OMI or is itself OMI (Downs, 1990). By reducing cAMP in the oocyte, LH enables the reactivation of meiosis and hence the attainment of oocyte maturity prior to ovulation (Dekel, Galiani and Aberdam, 1990). Inappropriate release of LH may profoundly affect this process such that the released egg is either unable to be fertilized (Homburg et al., 1988) or, if fertilized, miscarries (Regan et al., 1990).

Recently, there has been debate about the predictive value of an elevated follicular phase LH for either conception or pregnancy outcome. It was first demonstrated in 1985 that oocytes obtained from women undergoing IVF who had a serum LH value greater than one standard deviation above the mean on the day of hCG administration had a significantly reduced rate of fertilization and cleavage (Stanger and Yovich, 1985). This relationship has subsequently been confirmed with urinary LH measurements in the Bourn Hall IVF programme (Howles et al., 1986) and in our ovulation induction clinic (Homburg et al., 1988). It has also been shown that not only are ovulation and fertilization affected by high tonic LH levels, but also miscarriage is more likely (Homburg et al., 1988). A study of women attending a recurrent miscarriage clinic demonstrated that 82% had PCO (Sagle et al., 1988), and women attending this clinic were also found to have abnormalities in follicular phase LH secretion (Watson et al., 1989). A field study of 193 women planning to become pregnant showed that mid-follicular phase LH levels of greater than 10 IU/l were associated with both a significant drop in conception rate (67%) and a major increase in miscarriage rate (65%), compared with those women with normal LH levels (88% and 12% respectively) (Regan et al., 1990). There has been some disagreement over the significance of an elevated LH, with the Monash group suggesting no deleterious affect in IVF cycles (Thomas et al., 1989; Kovacs et al., 1990). In this study, it was considered that only cycles that result in a pregnancy should be used to provide the normal range of LH concentrations, and that by taking LH levels above the 75th centile, no adverse effect on fertilization or cleavage was detected. An effect on miscarriage was not addressed.

The occurrence of a 'premature' endogenous LH surge in exogenously stimulated cycles is not related to basal hypersecretion of LH, but is a reflection of endocrine feedback from the leading follicle(s). The 'prematurity' is not an indication of abnormality, but rather of a surge that has occurred before the planned intervention by egg collection. If an LH surge is identified at its initiation, the treatment cycle is sometimes abandoned, but it may instead be augmented with hCG (as the LH surge is usually markedly attenuated: Messinis, Templeton and Baird, 1986a) and therapy continued. If, however, the surge is established – also demonstrated by a rising serum progesterone – the patient may have ovulated by the time that oocyte retrieval is attempted (Van Uem et al., 1986). Others have had similar experiences, with women who do not conceive having significantly higher LH values in the 24–48 hours prior to hCG administration (Lejeune, et al., 1986; Howles, Macnamee and Edwards, 1987; Punnonen, et al., 1988). This has led to the practice of cancelling cycles in which a spontaneous surge is observed, unless it is 'caught' within 12 hours of its onset. This approach requires intense endocrine monitoring, with serum or urine LH measurements at least four-hourly.

Basal hypersecretion of LH is a defect found only in PCOS. There is increasing evidence that both high follicular phase LH levels and an endogenous LH surge are deleterious to conception and pregnancy outcome (Balen et al., 1993a). While the precise mechanism resulting in hypersecretion of LH in PCOS is unclear (Balen and Rose, 1994), the therapeutic approach to ovulation induction in women with PCO should be aimed at preventing inappropriate gonadotrophin levels.

To assess the risk of miscarriage after IVF with respect to age, cause of infertility, ovarian morphology and treatment regimen, an analysis was performed of the first 1060 pregnancies conceived between July 1984 and July 1990 as a result of 7623 IVF cycles (Balen et al., 1993b). Superovulation was achieved with hMG and/or purified FSH together with either clomiphene citrate or GnRH agonist buserelin – the latter either as a short 'flare' regimen or as a 'long' regimen to induce pituitary desensitization. The miscarriage rate was 23.6% in women with normal ovaries, compared with 35.8% in those with PCO ($p = 0.0038$; 95% confidence interval (CI) 4.68–23.10). There was no difference in the miscarriage rate between treatment with hMG or FSH. Women whose ovaries were normal on ultrasound were just as likely to miscarry if they were treated with clomiphene or with the 'long' buserelin protocol. Those with PCO, however, had a significant reduction in the rate of miscarriage when treated with 'long' buserelin 20.3% (15/74) compared with clomiphene citrate 47.2% (51/108) ($p = 0.0003$; 95% CI 13.82–40.09) (Table 12.2).

In this series of 1060 consecutive IVF pregnancies, the rate of miscarriage was 26.6%, which is similar to the miscarriage rates of other large IVF series (reviewed

Table 12.2. Miscarriage rate by ovarian morphology and treatment with either clomiphene citrate (CC) or long buserelin (LTB)

	Successful	Miscarriage	Total
(a) Normal ovaries + CC	122	31 (20.3%)	153
(b) Normal ovaries + LTB	70	24 (25.5%)	94
(c) Polycystic ovaries + CC	57	51 (47.2%)	108
(d) Polycystic ovaries + LTB	59	15 (20.3%)	74

Notes:
(a) vs (b) N.S., (a) vs (c) $p < 0.00005$, (b) vs (d) N.S., (c) vs (d) $p = 0.0003$.

in Balen and Yovich, 1992). It is difficult to compare figures obtained after assisted conception procedures with miscarriage rates after spontaneous conceptions because of the more intensive early pregnancy monitoring and earlier diagnosis of pregnancy after IVF treatment. If one takes the timing of the miscarriage into account, the abortion rates that follow natural and assisted conception are similar (Steer et al., 1989).

The outcome of pregnancy from 25 units in Australia and New Zealand following IVF and gamete intrafallopian transfer (GIFT) in 1988–89 has been reported (Saunders, Lancaster and Pedisich, 1992). In 2646 pregnancies following stimulation with a clomiphene citrate regimen, the spontaneous miscarriage rate was 23.8%, compared with a 19.5% miscarriage rate in 731 pregnancies which resulted after a buserelin regimen ($p < 0.05$). The type of buserelin regimen was not known to the authors. There was no correlation with the cause of infertility, and ovarian morphology was not studied.

The high rate of miscarriage in those who received clomiphene may be related to the deleterious effects of elevated serum LH levels. Clomiphene citrate causes an exaggerated early follicular phase release of both gonadotrophins, and the resultant elevated LH may reduce the chance of conception and increase the risk of miscarriage (Shoham et al., 1990). The protective effect of GnRH agonists, such as buserelin, is presumably mediated by the functional hypogonadotrophic hypogonadism and suppressed LH levels that they induce. This notion is consistent with the observation that it was the 'long' protocol of treatment with buserelin, but not the 'short' or 'ultrashort' protocols, that was associated with the reduction in miscarriage rates. It is well documented that the use of the 'short' or 'ultrashort' protocols of GnRH agonists is associated with a rise of LH concentrations to pre-ovulatory surge levels (Tan et al., 1992) so that the developing ovarian follicle may be exposed to inappropriately high LH levels, especially in patients with PCO, in whom return to baseline levels of LH takes longer than average. In this respect, the use of the 'short' or 'ultrashort' protocols of GnRH agonists exposes the patient to the same adverse effects as when clomiphene citrate is used.

Our study cannot distinguish between the proposed beneficial effect of pituitary desensitization and the detrimental effect of clomiphene citrate. This issue, however, has been clarified by Homburg et al. (1993b), who studied the outcome of 97 pregnancies in women with PCOS. The patients were treated by either ovulation induction or IVF with either hMG alone or hMG after pituitary desensitization with the GnRH agonist decapeptyl. The miscarriage rate in the agonist-treated patients (17.6%) was significantly lower than the miscarriage rate in the women treated with hMG alone (39.1%; $p = 0.03$). The study demonstrates that pituitary desensitization is the important factor in reducing miscarriage rates in women with PCO, rather than clomiphene citrate being the adverse factor, as clomiphene was not given to the patients in that study.

The use of a GnRH agonist to achieve pituitary desensitization has become popular in IVF clinics because of the flexibility in programming oocyte recovery. There is debate as to whether the improved pregnancy rates observed by some clinics (Rutherford et al., 1988; Frydman et al., 1988a) is seen consistently (Polson et al., 1991). We have found, however, that in women with an ultrasound diagnosis of PCO, the use of the GnRH agonist buserelin is associated with a significant reduction in the rate of miscarriage in the particular group of women at greatest risk. However, there appears to be no beneficial effect on the rate of miscarriage for women with normal ovaries. Pretreatment pelvic ultrasonography is therefore important in order to select the treatment regimen that will optimize outcome.

Superovulation strategies for women with polycystic ovaries and/or polycystic ovary syndrome

When ovarian stimulation is required for IVF, a different approach to therapy is necessary because the objective is to achieve multifollicular development, resulting in the collection of several appropriately mature eggs, but without causing OHSS. The latter is a particular problem in women with PCOS, as they usually exhibit greater sensitivity than women with normal ovaries to exogenous stimulation (Salat-Baroux and Antoine, 1990). Women with PCOS may require IVF for reasons other than their ovarian dysfunction (for example, tubal damage, male factors etc.). In addition, there is a group of women who do not conceive with either oral anti-oestrogens or gonadotrophin therapy (Wang and Gemzell, 1980), and for these women assisted conception is a reasonable option (Ashkenazi et al., 1989, Dor et al., 1990). Such a patient, who is still not pregnant following at least six ovulatory cycles, becomes a case of 'unexplained' infertility. There have been no specific studies examining whether IVF confers any advantages over other treatments, such as GIFT, for women with PCO, and therefore treatment should be individualized to the other needs of the patient. It is important to be able to assess fertilization and this can be examined either by IVF or with spare oocytes collected during GIFT. We will consider the various regimens used with specific reference to PCOS.

The initial experience in ovulation induction for IVF was with a combination of clomiphene citrate either with both hMG and FSH, or sometimes with a high-dose gonadotrophin alone (Fleming and Coutts, 1990). Irrespective of ovarian morphology, these treatment regimens do not suppress pituitary responsiveness to the secretory products of the developing follicle. Premature luteinization and a premature LH surge may both occur, with deleterious effects on the developing oocytes (Gemzell, Kemman and Jones, 1978; Stanger and Yovich, 1985) or ovulation prior to oocyte recovery. These problems are more often encountered in women with PCOS (Gemzell et al., 1978; Fleming and Coutts, 1988). As already mentioned, the mechanism resulting in inappropriate LH release in PCOS is not yet understood.

Many strategies have evolved to achieve superovulation for IVF, and several were evaluated at the Hallam Medical Centre (Riddle et al., 1987; Sharma et al., 1989). It is interesting to note that, contrary to earlier beliefs, ovarian stimulation resulting in the collection of large numbers of oocytes (more than ten) results in a poor outcome, the optimum number being between seven and nine (Sharma et al., 1988). This is of particular relevance to women with PCO, in whom there are often a high number of oocytes, yet poor rates of fertilization and implantation (Dor et al., 1990) – the overall effect being to achieve an equivalent pregnancy rate to a control group (Dor et al., 1990) but a higher miscarriage rate.

The above experience relates to the use of clomiphene with exogenous gonadotrophins. The move towards pituitary desensitization with a GnRH agonist (Porter et al., 1984) has become almost universal in assisted conception clinics. The reversible hypogonadotrophic hypogonadism so produced permits unimpeded control over follicular development (Fleming et al., 1985) and improved pregnancy rates in IVF programmes (Rutherford et al., 1988; Frydman et al., 1988b). As already mentioned, the suppression of endogenous LH by GnRH agonists is of particular relevance and advantage to the woman with PCOS (Jacobs et al., 1987; Fleming and Coutts, 1988). Thus, many oocyte-containing follicles may develop in the sensitive PCO free from the adverse environment of high tonic LH levels. These oocytes appear to fertilize better than those obtained in cycles without pituitary desensitization (Abdalla et al., 1990), suggesting that it is indeed the abnormal hormonal milieu, rather than the PCO itself, that is the problem for women with PCOS.

Short and long protocols

There are few studies that specifically compare different treatment regimens for women with and without PCOS, and those that do vary in their definition and diagnosis of the syndrome (Jacobs et al., 1987; Salat-Baroux et al., 1988a; Tanbo et al., 1990). The two particular aims of therapy in this group of women are the correction of the abnormal hormone milieu, by suppressing elevated LH and androgens, and the avoidance of ovarian hyperstimulation. Pituitary desensitization avoids the initial surge of gonadotrophins, with the resultant ovarian steroid release that occurs in the short GnRH protocol. While the long protocol theoretically provides controlled stimulation, the polycystic ovary is still more likely than the normal ovary to become hyperstimulated (Salat-Baroux and Antoine, 1990). With both long and short protocols, significantly more eggs are collected from women with PCO than from those with normal ovaries (Jacobs et al., 1987) and, interestingly, the total dose of exogenous gonadotrophins is the same for either regimen. It has also been proposed that a longer period of desensitization (30 instead of 15 days) is of benefit by reducing androgen levels (Salat-Baroux et al., 1988a); in this study, the longer duration of treatment did not improve pregnancy rates but did, apparently, decrease the incidence of hyperstimulation.

The other debate in ovulation induction for women with PCOS is whether the use of FSH alone has any benefit over hMG: is the hypersecretion of LH responsible for the exaggerated response to stimulation of the PCO? Does minimizing circulating LH levels by giving FSH alone improve outcome? Preparations of purified urinary FSH contain some LH activity, usually less than 1%, and preliminary work suggested that ovulation induction can be achieved without exogenous LH (Jones, Garcia and Rosenwaks, 1984). In patients with hypogonadotrophic hypogonadism, follicular maturation is, however, often incomplete and inconsistent (Couzinet et al., 1988; Shoham et al., 1991) as LH, by its action on the thecal cells, is required for full ovarian steroidogenesis. Thus, the presence of some LH is facilitatory to normal follicular development. Most studies have found no benefit from the use of FSH alone in the ovulation induction for either in-vivo (Jacobs et al., 1987; Homburg et al., 1990; Sagle et al., 1991) or in-vitro fertilization (Messinis et al., 1986b; Jacobs et al., 1987; Salat-Baroux et al., 1988b; Bentick et al., 1988; Larsen, 1990; Tanbo et al., 1990). The most probable reason is that there are only 75 units of LH activity in each ampoule and, when hMG is given in standard doses to patients who are receiving treatment with buserelin, the serum LH levels barely rise to above 5 IU/l. In patients with PCOS, the serum LH concentration is usually two to four times that level – that is, the serum level represents a higher 'secretion rate' than that mimicked by injections of hMG.

A recent meta-analysis of eight randomized studies of patients undergoing IVF, however, suggested that treatment with FSH resulted in 50% higher pregnancy rates than treatment with hMG (Daya, 1995), with an overall odds ratio of 1.71 (95% CI 1.12–2.62). The papers that contributed to the meta-analysis had small numbers and the result was skewed by small studies, which needed to be combined in order to achieve significance – a potential drawback of meta-analyses. It should also be mentioned that the studies cited by Daya were of patients with both normal ovaries and PCO. To settle this matter, it will be necessary to perform a large prospective, randomized study, either in one centre or in multiple centres. We have calculated that to show a 5% improvement in outcome there would have to be 900 patients in each arm of the study. For the time being, we and others (Buyalos and Lee, 1996) conclude that there is little to choose between the different gonadotrophin preparations in patients with PCO with respect to pregnancy rates or other clinical parameters. Furthermore, regarding the propensity of the PCO to overrespond, we consider that it is the dose of FSH rather than whether it is given with or without LH that is important.

We recommend the long protocol of pituitary desensitization for women identified as having PCO, and a dose of 75–150 units of FSH or hMG for women under the age of 35, and 150 units for older women. This is intentionally lower than our usual starting dose of 225 units for women under the age of 35 years. The dose may, of course, be modified if the patient has exhibited either an exuberant or poor response in a previous cycle. Follicular development is then monitored principally by daily ultrasonography from day eight of stimulation, with additional measurements of serum oestradiol being helpful in some cases.

Luteal support and ovarian hyperstimulation syndrome

The OHSS is a well-recognized complication of ovulation induction. In its severe form, it is characterized by ascites, ovarian enlargement with cyst formation, pleural effusion and electrolyte disturbances (Schenker and Weinstein, 1978). Oliguria and vascular complications may ensue, and there have been fatalities. It is believed to be relatively rare in patients undergoing ovarian stimulation for IVF, despite the multiple follicular development and high oestrogen levels that commonly occur, and it has been suggested that the protective mechanism is mediated through aspiration of ovarian follicular fluid at the time of oocyte collection (Friedman et al., 1984). However, it does occur in IVF (Golan et al., 1989; Smitz et al., 1991; MacDougall, Tan and Jacobs, 1992) and, when severe, is the only lifethreatening condition associated with ovarian stimulation in IVF.

It has been apparent for some time that patients with PCO undergoing straightforward ovulation induction are particularly at risk of developing OHSS (Lunenfeld and Insler, 1974; Schenker and Weinstein, 1978). Recently this has been confirmed in IVF as well (Smitz et al., 1991; MacDougall et al., 1992). In a total population of 1302 patients, we recently identified 15 patients who underwent ovarian stimulation for IVF or other assisted conception techniques at the Hallam Medical Centre, between July 1989 and July 1990, and developed OHSS of sufficient severity to merit hospital admission (prevalence of 1.2% with 0.6% having severe OHSS). Fifty-three per cent of these patients had ultrasonically diagnosed PCO and 87% were undergoing their first attempt at IVF. All had received luteal support in the form of hCG. Although the pregnancy rate in this group was very high (93.3%), the multiple pregnancy rate was 57%, with a miscarriage rate of 14.3% (MacDougall et al., 1992). As a result of this analysis, we recommend that all patients undergoing IVF have a pelvic ultrasound scan performed either prior to or early in the treatment cycle. If PCO are identified, the dose of gonadotrophins should be minimized (see above).

It has been observed that OHSS is rare in patients with hypopituitary hypo-gonadism (Lunenfeld and Insler, 1974). The use of LHRH agonists has been rec-ommended in patients with PCO (Salat-Baroux et al., 1988b), in the hope that, by converting the patient to a hypogonadal state, OHSS could be prevented. Unfortunately, this does not seem to be the case (Smitz et al., 1991) and, in fact, a number of recent reports suggest that OHSS is actually more common when LHRH agonists are used, especially if patients have PCO (Charbonnel et al., 1987). Incidentally, this observation provides further evidence to suggest that the primary lesion in the PCOS is in the ovary itself, since its response to gonadotrophin stim-ulation is abnormal even after suppression of abnormal gonadotrophin secretion.

Recent studies have suggested that the increased propensity of PCO to become overstimulated is due to increased expression of VEGF in the stroma of the PCO, which itself has increased blood flow, as assessed by colour Doppler (Zaidi et al., 1995). A recent study explored this association further by performing pulsed and colour Doppler studies together with measurements of serum VEGF concentra-tions in 36 women with normal ovaries and 24 women with PCO (ten of whom had the syndrome) undergoing IVF. Serum VEGF concentrations and blood flow were significantly higher in the women with PCO/PCOS than in those with normal ovaries, and this might explain the greater risk of OHSS in these patients (Agrawal et al., 1998; MacDougall et al., 1992).

Careful monitoring of oestrogen levels and numbers of follicles by ultrasound scan during stimulation for IVF can also help to identify those at risk. In patients thought to be at risk of OHSS (age less than 30 years, and/or PCO $+/-$ oestrogen levels greater than 8000 pmol/l and/or more than 20 follicles at oocyte collection), luteal support in the form of hCG should be withheld. It is now our practice to use progesterone pessaries instead of hCG as luteal support in all patients.

Transfer of a maximum of two embryos in this group reduces the multiple preg-nancy rate, with its attendant obstetric and neonatal problems. Alternatively, embryos may be frozen for transfer at a later date, and, in the case of patients on LHRH analogues, the analogue continued until the onset of menstruation (by giving a long-acting depot) and hormone replacement therapy for the frozen embryo replacement cycle commenced at that stage.

Conclusion

Women with PCOS may have presented with symptoms of endocrine or metabolic disturbance prior to seeking assisted conception, or they may be diagnosed at their first attendance to the infertility clinic, a proportion of them having PCO on ultrasound scan but no symptoms. Women with PCO require careful management to achieve follicular maturation in an environment free from elevated LH levels in order to enhance fertilization and pregnancy outcome. The sensitivity of the PCO to exogenous stimulation and the risk of OHSS have been emphasized.

REFERENCES

Abdalla, H.I., Ahuja, K.K., Leonard, T. et al. (1990). Comparative trial of luteinising hormone releasing hormone analogue/HMG and clomiphene citrate/HMG in an assisted conception programme. *Fertility and Sterility* 53, 473–8.

Abdulwahid, N.A., Adams, J., Van der Spuy, Z.M. and Jacobs, HS. (1985). Gonadotrophin control of follicular development. *Clinical Endocrinology* 23, 613–26.

Adams, J., Polson, D.W., Abdulwahid, N. et al. (1985). Multifollicular ovaries: clinical and endocrine features and response to pulsatile gonadotrophin releasing hormone. *Lancet* ii, 1375–8.

Adashi, E.Y., Resnick, C.E., D'Ercole, A.J., Svoboda, M.E. and Van Wyk, J.J. (1985). Insulin-like growth factors as intraovarian regulators of granulosa cell growth and function *Endocrinology Review* 6, 400–20.

Agrawal, R., Sladkevicius, P., Engman, L. et al. (1998). Serum vascular endothelial growth factor concentrations and ovarian stromal blood flow are increased in women with polycystic ovaries. *Human Reproduction* 13, 651–5.

Ahlgren, M., Kallen, B. and Rannevik, G. (1976). Outcome of pregnancy after clomiphene therapy. *Acta Obstetricia et Gynecologica Scandinavica* 55, 371–5.

Ashkenazi, J., Feldberg, D., Dicker, D. et al. (1989). In-vitro fertilisation – embryo transfer in women with refractory polycystic ovary disease. *European Journal of Obstetrics, Gynecology and Reproductive Biology* 30, 157–61.

Baird, D.T., Corker, C.S. and Davidson, D.W. (1977). Pituitary–ovarian relationships in polycystic ovary syndrome. *Journal of Clinical Endocrinology and Metabolism* 45, 798–809.

Balen, A.H. (1995). Effects of ovulation induction with gonadotrophins on the ovary and uterus and implications for assisted reproduction. *Human Reproduction* 10, 2233–7.

Balen, A.H., Tan, S.L.and Jacobs, H.S. (1993a) Hypersecretion of luteinising hormone – a significant cause of infertility and miscarriage. *British Journal of Obstetrics and Gynaecology* 100, 1082–9.

Balen, A.H., Tan, S.L., MacDougall, J. and Jacobs, H.S. (1993b). Miscarriage rates following in-vitro fertilisation are increased in women with polycystic ovaries and reduced by pituitary desensitisation with buserelin. *Human Reproduction* 8, 959–64.

Balen, A.H. and Yovich, J.L. (1992). Miscarriage following assisted conception. In *Spontaneous*

Abortion, Diagnosis and Treatment, ed. I. Stabile, J.G. Grudzinskas and T. Chard, pp. 133–48. London: Springer-Verlag.

Balen, A.H., Braat, D.D.M., West, C., Patel, A. and Jacobs, H.S. (1994). Cumulative conception and live birth rates after the treatment of anovulatory infertility. An analysis of the safety and efficacy of ovulation induction in 200 patients. *Human Reproduction* **9**, 1563–70.

Balen, A.H., Conway, G.S., Kaltsas, G. et al. (1995). Polycystic ovary syndrome: the spectrum of the disorder in 1741 patients. *Human Reproduction* **8**, 2107–11.

Balen, A.H. and Dunger, D. (1995). Pubertal maturation of the internal genitalia (Commentary). *Ultrasound in Obstetrics and Gynaecology* **6**, 164–5.

Balen, A.H. and Jacobs, H.S. (1997). Ovulation induction. In *Infertility in Practice*, ed. A.H. Balen and H.S. Jacobs, pp. 131–80. Edinburgh: Churchill Livingstone.

Balen, A.H. and Rose, M. (1994). The control of luteinising hormone secretion in the polycystic ovary syndrome. *Contemporary Reviews in Obstetrics and Gynaecology* **6**, 201–7.

Bentick, B., Shaw, R.W., Iffland, C.A., Burford, G. and Bernard, A. (1988). A randomised comparative study of purified follicle stimulating hormone and human menopausal gonadotrophin after pituitary desensitisation with buserelin for superovulation and in-vitro fertilisation. *Fertility and Sterility* **50**, 79–84.

Beral, V., Doyle, P., Tan, S.L., Mason, B.A. and Campbell, S. (1990). Outcome of pregnancies resulting from assisted conception. *British Medical Bulletin* **46**(3), 753–68.

Buyalos, R.P. and Lee, C.T. (1996). Polycystic ovary syndrome: pathophysiology and outcome with IVF. *Fertility and Sterility* **65**, 1–10.

Charbonnel, B., Krempf, M., Blanchard. P., Dano, F. and Delage, C. (1987). Induction of ovulation in polycystic ovary syndrome with a combination of a luteinising hormone-releasing hormone analog and exogenous gonadotrophins. *Fertility and Sterility* **47**, 920–4.

Clark, A.M., Ledger, W., Galletly, C. et al. (1995). Weight loss results in significant improvement in pregnancy and ovulation rates in anovulatory obese women. *Human Reproduction* **10**, 2705–12.

Clayton, R.N., Ogden, V., Hodgekinson, J. et al. (1992). How common are polycystic ovaries in normal women and what is their significance for the fertility of the population? *Clinical Endocrinology* **37**, 127–34.

Conway, G.S. (1990). Insulin resistance and the polycystic ovary syndrome. *Contemporary Review of Obstetrics and Gynaecology* **2**, 34–9.

Couzinet, B., Lestrat, N., Brailly, S., Forest, M. and Schaison, G. (1988). Stimulation of ovarian follicular maturation with pure follicle stimulating hormone in women with gonadotrophin deficiency. *Journal of Clinical Endocrinology and Metabolism* **66**, 552–6.

Daya, S. (1995). Follicle stimulating hormone versus human menopausal gonadotropin for in vitro fertilisation: results of a meta-analysis. *Hormone Research* **43**, 224–9.

Dekel, N., Galiani, D. and Aberdam, E. (1990). Regulation of rat oocyte maturation: involvement of protein kinases. In *Fertilisation in Mammals*, ed. B.D. Bavister, J. Cummins and E.R.S. Roldan, pp. 17–24. Norwell, USA: Serono Symposia.

Diamant, Y.Z., Rimon, E. and Evron, S. (1982). High incidence of pre-eclamptic toxaemia in patients with polycystic disease. *European Journal of Obstetrics, Gynecology and Reproductive Biology* **14**, 199–204.

Dor, J., Shulman, A., Levran, D. et al. (1990). The treatment of patients with polycystic ovary syndrome by in-vitro fertilisation: a comparison of results with those patients with tubal infertility. *Human Reproduction* 5, 816–18.

Downs, S.M. (1990). Maintenance of meiotic arrest in mammalian oocytes. In *Fertilisation in Mammals*, ed. B.D. Bavister, J. Cummins and E.R.S. Roldan, pp. 5–16. Norwell, USA: Serono Symposia.

Dunaif, A. and Graf, M. (1989). Insulin administration alters gonadal steroid metabolism independent of changes in gonadotropin secretion in insulin-resistant women with the polycystic ovary syndrome. *Journal of Clinical Investigation* 83, 23–9.

Erickson, G.F., Magoffin, D.A., Dyer, C.A. and Hofeditz, C. (1985). The ovarian androgen producing cells: a review of structure/function relationships. *Endocrinology Review* 6, 371–99.

Farquhar, C.M., Birdsall, M., Manning, P. and Mitchell, J.M. (1994). Transabdominal versus transvaginal ultrasound in the diagnosis of polycystic ovaries on ultrasound scanning in a population of randomly selected women. *Ultrasound Obstetrics and Gynaecology* 4, 54–9

Ferrara, N. Chen, H., Davis-Smyth, T. et al. (1998). Vascular endothelial growth factor is essential for corpus luteum angiogenesis. *Nature Medicine* 4, 336–40.

Fleming, R. and Coutts, J.R.T. (1988). Luteinising hormone releasing hormone analogues for ovulation induction, with particular reference to polycystic ovary syndrome. In *Anti-Hormones in Clinical Gynaecology*, ed. D. Healy, *Baillière's Clinical Obstetrics and Gynaecology* 2, 677–88.

Fleming, R. and Coutts, J.R.T. (1990). Induction of multiple follicular development for in-vitro fertilisation. In *Assisted Human Conception*, ed. R.G. Edwards. *British Medical Bulletin* 46, 596–615.

Fleming, R., Haxton, M.J., Hamilton, M.P.R. et al. (1985). Successful treatment of infertile women with oligomenorrhoea using a combination of a luteinising hormone releasing hormone agonist and exogenous gonadotrophins. *British Journal of Obstetrics and Gynaecology* 92, 369–74.

Fox, R., Corrigan, E., Thomas, P.A. and Hull, M.G.R. (1991). The diagnosis of polycystic ovaries in women with oligo-amenorrhoea: predictive power of endocrine tests. *Clinical Endocrinology* 34, 127–31.

Fox, R. and Wardle, P.G. (1990). Maturity onset diabetes mellitus in association with polycystic ovarian disease. *Journal of Obstetrics and Gynaecology* 10, 555–6.

Franks, S. (1989). Polycystic ovary syndrome: a changing perspective. *Clinical Endocrinology* 31, 87–120.

Franks, S. (1995). Medical progress article: polycystic ovary syndrome. *New England Journal of Medicine* 333, 853–61

Franks, S., Adams, J., Mason, H. and Polson, D. (1985). Ovulatory disorders in women with polycystic ovary syndrome. In *Reproductive Endocrinology*, ed. H.S. Jacobs. *Clinical Obstetrics and Gynaecology* 12, 605–32.

Franks, S., Mason, S., Polson, D.W. et al. (1988). Mechanism and management of ovulatory failure in women with polycystic ovary syndrome. *Human Reproduction* 3, 531–4.

Friedman, C.L., Schmidt, G.E., Chang, F.E. and Kim, M.H. (1984). Severe ovarian hyperstimulation following follicular aspiration. *American Journal Obstetrics and Gynecology* 150, 436–7.

Frydman, R., Belaisch-Allart, J., Parneix, I. et al. (1988a). Comparison between flare up and down regulation of luteinising hormone releasing hormone agonists in an in-vitro fertilisation programme. *Fertility and Sterility* **50**, 471–5.

Frydman, R., Fries, N., Testart, J. et al. (1988b). Luteinising hormone releasing hormone agonists in in-vitro fertilisation: different methods of utilization and comparison with previous ovulation stimulation treatments. *Human Reproduction* **3**, 559–61.

Futterweit, W. (1984). Pathologic anatomy of polycystic ovarian disease. In *Polycystic Ovarian Disease*, ed. W. Futterweit, pp. 41–6. New York: Springer-Verlag.

Gemzell, C.A., Kemman, E. and Jones, J.R. (1978). Premature ovulation during administration of human menopausal gonadotrophins in non-ovulatory women. *Infertility* **1**, 1–10.

Gjonnaess, H. (1989). The course and outcome of pregnancy after ovarian electrocautery in women with polycystic ovarian syndrome: the influence of body weight. *British Journal of Obstetrics and Gynaecology* **96**, 714–19.

Golan, A., Ron-el, R., Herman, A. et al. (1989). Ovarian hyperstimulation syndrome: an update review. *Obstetrics and Gynaecology Survey* **44**, 430–40.

Goldzieher, J.W. and Axelrod, L.R. (1963). Clinical and biochemical features of polycystic ovarian disease. *Fertility and Sterility* **14**, 631–53.

Harlap, S. (1976). Ovulation induction and congenital malformation. *Lancet* **ii**, 961.

Homburg, R., Armar, N.A., Eshel, A., Adams, J. and Jacobs, H.S. (1988). Influence of serum luteinising hormone concentrations on ovulation, conception and early pregnancy loss in polycystic ovary syndrome. *British Medical Journal* **297**, 1024–6.

Homburg, R., Berkowitz, D., Levy, T. et al. (1993a). In-vitro fertilisation and embryo transfer for the treatment of infertility associated with polycystic ovary syndrome. *Fertility and Sterility* **60**, 858–63.

Homburg, R., Eshel, A., Kilborn, J., Adams, J. and Jacobs, H.S. (1990). Combined luteinising hormone releasing hormone analogue and exogenous gonadotrophins for the treatment of infertility associated with polycystic ovaries. *Human Reproduction* **5**, 32–5.

Homburg, R., Levy, T., Berkovitz, D. et al. (1993b). Gonadotropin releasing hormone agonist reduces the miscarriage rate for pregnancies achieved in women with polycystic ovaries. *Fertility and Sterility* **59**, 527–31.

Howles, C.M., Macnamee, M.C. and Edwards, R.G. (1987). Follicular development and early luteal function of conception and non-conception cycles after human in-vitro fertilisation: endocrine correlates. *Human Reproduction* **2**, 17–21.

Howles, C.M., Macnamee, M.C., Edwards, R.G., Goswamy, R. and Steptoe, P.C. (1986). Effect of high tonic levels of luteinising hormone on outcome of in-vitro fertilisation. *Lancet* **i**, 521–2.

Jacobs, H.S., Porter, R., Eshel, A. and Craft, I. (1987). Profertility uses of luteinising hormone releasing hormone agonist anologues. In *LHRH and its Analogs*, ed. B.H. Vickery and J.J. Nestor, pp. 303–22. Lancaster: MTP Press Ltd.

Jones, G.S., Garcia, J.E. and Rosenwaks, Z. (1984). The role of pituitary gonadotropins in follicular stimulation and oocyte maturation in the human. *Journal of Clinical Endocrinology and Metabolism* **59**, 178–83.

Kamat, B.R., Brown, L.F. and Manseau, E.J. (1995). Expression of vascular endothelial growth factor permeability factor by human granulosa and theca lutein cells. Role in corpus luteum development. *American Journal of Pathology* **146**, 157–65.

Kiddy, D.S., Hamilton-Fairley, D., Bush, A. et al. (1992). Improvement in endocrine and ovarian function during dietary treatment of obese women with polycystic ovary syndrome. *Clinical Endocrinology* **36**, 105–11.

Kovacs, G.T., Baker, H.W.G., Burger, H.G., Lee, J. and Summerbell, D. (1990). Prognosis of pregnancies conceived by donor insemination with respect to the late follicular phase luteinising hormone levels. *British Journal of Obstetrics and Gynaecology* **97**, 654–6.

Kurachi, K., Aono, T., Minagawa, J. and Miyake, A. (1983). Congenital malformations of newborn infants after clomiphene-induced ovulation. *Fertility and Sterility* **40**, 187–9.

Kyei-Mensah, A.A., Tan, S.L., Zaidi, J. and Jacobs, H.S. (1998). Relationship of ovarian stromal volume and androgen concentrations in women with PCOS. *Human Reproduction* **13**, 1437–41.

Larsen, T. (1990). Comparison of urinary human follicle stimulating hormone and HMG for ovarian stimulation in polycystic ovary syndrome. *Fertility and Sterility* **53**, 426.

Lejeune, B., Degueldre, M., Camus, M. et al. (1986). In vitro fertilisation and embryo transfer as related to endogenous luteinising hormone rise or human chorionic gonadotrophin administration. *Fertility and Sterility* **45**, 377–83.

Lunenfeld, B. and Insler, V. (1974). Classification of amenorrhoeic states and their treatment by ovulation induction. *Clinical Endocrinology* **3**, 223–37.

MacDougall, J.M., Tan, S.L., Balen, A.H. and Jacobs, H.S. (1993). A controlled study comparing patients with and without polycystic ovaries undergoing in-vitro fertilisation and the ovarian hyperstimulation syndrome. *Human Reproduction* **8**, 233–7.

MacDougall, J.M., Tan, S.L., Hall, V. et al. (1994). Comparison of natural with clomiphene citrate-stimulated cycles in IVF: a prospective randomised trial. *Fertility and Sterility* **61**, 1052–7.

MacDougall, J..M., Tan, S.L. and Jacobs, H.S. (1992). In-vitro fertilisation and the ovarian hyperstimulation syndrome. *Human Reproduction* **7**, 597–600.

MacGillivray, I. (1983). *Pre-eclampsia – the Hypertensive Disease of Pregnancy*, pp. 44–5 and 227–8. London: W.B. Saunders Co.

Medical Research Council (1990). Births in Great Britain resulting from assisted conception, 1978–87. *British Medical Journal* **330**, 1229–33.

Messinis, I.E., Templeton, A. and Baird, D.T. (1986a). Relationships between the characteristics of endogenous luteinising hormone surge and the degree of ovarian hyperstimulation during superovulation induction in women. *Clinical Endocrinology* **25**, 393–400.

Messinis, I.E., Templeton, A.A. and Baird, D.T. (1986b). Comparison between clomiphene plus human menopausal gonadotrophin and clomiphene plus pulsatile follicle stimulating hormone in induction of multiple follicular development in women. *Human Reproduction* **4**, 223–6.

Obrhai, M., Lynch, S.S., Holder, G. et al. (1990). Hormonal studies on women with polycystic ovaries diagnosed by ultrasound. *Clinical Endocrinology (Oxford)*, **32**, 467–74.

Owen, E.J., West, C.A., Mason, B.A. and Jacobs, H.S., (1991). Cotreatment with growth hormone for poor responders in IVF–ET. *Fertility and Sterility* **56**, 1104–10.

Polson, D.W., MacLachlan, V., Krapez, J.A., Wood, C.A. and Healy, D.L. (1991). A controlled study of gonadotrophin releasing hormone agonist (buserelin acetate) before folliculogenesis in routine IVF patients. *Fertility and Sterility* **56**, 509–14.

Polson, D.W., Wadsworth, J., Adams, J. and Franks, S. (1988). Polycystic ovaries: a common finding in normal women. *Lancet* **ii**, 870–2.

Porter, R.N., Smith, W., Craft, I.L., Abdulwahid, N.A. and Jacobs, H.S. (1984). Induction of ovulation for in-vitro fertilisation using buserelin and gonadotrophins. *Lancet* **ii**, 1284–5.

Punnonen, R., Ashorn, R., Vilja, P. et al. (1988). Spontaneous luteinising hormone surge and cleavage of in vitro fertilised embryos. *Fertility and Sterility* **49**, 479–82.

Regan, L., Owen, E.J. and Jacobs, H.S. (1990). Hypersecretion of luteinising hormone, infertility and miscarriage. *Lancet* **336**, 1141–4.

Riddle A, Sharma V, Mason, B. et al. (1987). Two years experience of ultrasound directed oocyte recovery. *Fertility and Sterility* **48**, 454.

Rutherford, A.J., Subak-Sharpe, R.J., Dawson, K.J. et al. (1988). Improvement of in-vitro fertilisation after treatment with buserelin, an agonist of luteinising hormone releasing hormone. *British Medical Journal* **296**, 1765–8.

Sagle, M., Bishop, K., Alexander, F.M. et al. (1988). Recurrent early miscarriage and polycystic ovaries. *British Medical Journal* **297**, 1027–8.

Sagle, M.A., Hamilton-Fairley, D., Kiddy, D.S. and Franks, S. (1991). A comparative, randomised study of low dose human menopausal gonadotrophin and follicle stimulating hormone in women with polycystic ovary syndrome. *Fertility and Sterility* **55**, 56–60.

Salat-Baroux, J., Alvarez, S., Antoine, J.M. et al. (1988a). Comparison between long and short protocols of luteinising hormone releasing hormone agonist in the treatment of PCOD by in-vitro fertilisation. *Human Reproduction* **3**, 535–9.

Salat-Baroux, J., Alvarez, S., Antoine, J.M. et al. (1988b). Results of in-vitro fertilisation in the treatment of polycystic ovary disease. *Human Reproduction* **3**, 331–5.

Salat-Baroux, J. and Antoine, J.M. (1990). Accidental hyperstimulation during ovulation induction. In *Ovulation Induction*, ed. P.G. Crosignani. *Ballière's Clinical Obstetrics and Gynaecology* **4**, 627–37.

Schenker, J.G. and Weinstein, D. (1978). Ovarian hyperstimulation syndrome: a current survey. *Fertility and Sterility* **30**, 255.

Sharma, V., Riddle, A., Mason, B.A., Pampiglione, J. and Campbell, S. (1988). An analysis of factors influencing the establishment of a clinical pregnancy in an ultrasound-based ambulatory in-vitro fertilisation program. *Fertility and Sterility* **49**, 468–78.

Sharma, V., Riddle, A., Mason, B., Whitehead, M. and Collins, W. (1989). Studies on folliculogenesis and in-vitro fertilisation outcome after the administration of follicle stimulating hormone at different times during the menstrual cycle. *Fertility and Sterility* **51**, 298–303.

Saunders, D.M., Lancaster, P.A.L. and Pedisich, E.L. (1992). Increased pregnancy failure rates after clomiphene following assisted reproductive technology. *Human Reproduction* **7**, 1154–8.

Shoham, Z., Borenstein, R., Lunenfeld, B. and Pariente, C. (1990). Hormonal profiles following clomiphene citrate therapy in conception and nonconception cycles. *Clinical Endocrinology* **33**, 271–8.

Shoham, Z., Balen, A.H., Patel, A. and Jacobs, H. (1991). Results of ovulation induction using hMG or purified FSH in hypogonatrophic hypogonadism patients. *Fertility and Sterility* **56**, 1048–53.

Smitz, J., Camus, M., Devroey, P., Evard, P. et al. (1991). Incidence of severe ovarian hyperstimulation syndrome after gonadotrophin releasing hormone agonist/HMG superovulation for in-vitro fertilisation. *Human Reproduction* 6, 933–7.

Stanger, J.D. and Yovich, J.L. (1985). Reduced in-vitro fertilisation of human oocyte from patients with raised basal luteinising hormone levels during the follicular phase. *British Journal of Obstetrics and Gynaecology* 92, 385–93.

Steer, C., Campbell, S, Davies, M., Mason, B. and Collins, W. (1989). Spontaneous abortion rates after natural and assisted conception. *British Medical Journal* 299, 1317–18.

Stein, I.F. and Leventhal, M.L. (1935). Amenorrhoea associated with bilateral polycystic ovaries. *American Journal of Obstetrics and Gynecology* 29, 181–91.

Swanson, M., Sauerbrei, E.E. and Cooperberg, P.L. (1981). Medical implications of ultrasonically detected polycystic ovaries. *Journal of Clinical Ultrasound* 9, 219–22.

Tan, S.L., Kingsland, C., Campbell, S. et al. (1992). The long protocol of administration of gonadotrophin releasing hormone agonist is superior to the short protocol for ovarian stimulation for in vitro fertilisation. *Fertility and Sterility* 57, 810–14.

Tanbo, T., Dale, P.O., Kjekshus, E., Haug, E. and Abyholm, T. (1990). Stimulation with HMG versus follicle stimulating hormone after pituitary suppression in polycystic ovary syndrome. *Fertility and Sterility* 53, 798–803.

Tayob, Y., Robinson, G., Adams, J. et al. (1990). Ultrasound appearance of the ovaries during the pill-free interval. *British Journal of Family Planning* 16, 94–6.

Thomas, A., Okamoto, S., O'Shea, F. et al. (1989). Do raised serum luteinising hormone levels during stimulation for in-vitro fertilisation predict outcome? *British Journal of Obstetrics and Gynaecology* 96, 1328–32.

Treharne, I. (1984). Obesity in pregnancy. In *Progress in Obstetrics and Gynaecology*, vol. 4, ed. J. Studd, pp. 127–38. Edinburgh: Churchill Livingstone.

Vaitukaitis, J.L. (1983). Polycystic ovary syndrome – what is it? *New England Journal of Medicine* 309, 1245–6.

van Santbrink, E.J.P., Hop, W.C. and Fauser, B.C.J.M. (1997). Classification of normogonadotrophic infertility: polycystic ovaries diagnosed by ultrasound versus endocrine characteristics of polycystic ovary syndrome. *Fertility and Sterility* 67, 452–8.

Van Uem, J.F.H.M., Garcia, J.E., Liu, H.C. and Rosenwaks, Z. (1986). Clinical aspects with regard to the occurrence of an endogenous luteinising hormone surge in gonadotrophin-induced normal menstrual cycles. *Journal of In-Vitro Fertilisation and Embryo Transfer* 3, 345–9.

Wang, C.F. and Gemzell, C. (1980). The use of human gonadotrophins for the induction of ovulation in women with polycystic ovary syndrome. *Clinical Endocrinology* 12, 479–86.

Watson, H., Hamilton-Fairley, D., Kiddy, D. et al. (1989). Abnormalities of follicular phase luteinising hormone secretion in women with recurrent early miscarriage. *Journal of Endocrinology* 123 (suppl.), Abstract 25.

Yen, S.S.C. (1980). The polycystic ovary. *Clinical Endocrinology* 12, 177–207.

Zaidi, J., Campbell, S., Pittrof, R. et al. (1995). Ovarian stromal blood flow in women with polycystic ovaries: a possible new marker for diagnosis. *Human Reproduction* 10, 1992–6

13

Possible future treatment of polycystic ovary syndrome: immature oocyte collection and in-vitro maturation

Carl Wood and Alan Trounson

Introduction

The treatment of anovulation associated with polycystic ovary syndrome (PCOS) has gone the 'full circle'. The syndrome was first recognized by Stein and Leventhal (1935), who treated it by wedge resection. Due to the complication of adhesion formation (Toaff, Toaff and Peyser, 1976), surgical treatment was abandoned when clomiphene citrate became available. Clomiphene citrate is the first line of treatment because it is simple to use, an oral medication, cheap, and not associated with high-order multiple pregnancies or serious hyperstimulation. Only 20–40% of anovulatory women with PCOS do not conceive with clomiphene citrate. Subsequently, the use of gonadotrophins for resistant cases also became widely used. It has the disadvantage that it is relatively expensive, complicated to administer, and has to be intensively monitored. Even with careful monitoring, it has a 13% multiple pregnancy rate and 3% triplet or higher rate, with its associated complications (Healy, 1992). The use of ovulation induction for PCOS is discussed in detail in Chapter 10. However, with the report from Gjonnaess (1984) of the laparoscopic approach to ovarian cautery, the use of a surgical approach to the treatment of clomiphene-resistant anovulation in women with PCOS has been revisited. A recent meta-analysis of success rates of surgical treatment indicates that they resemble those obtained by medical treatment (Farquhar et al., 1999). Nevertheless, there are still concerns about the theoretical complications of surgical treatment, including operative trauma or heat damage, postoperative adhesions, and the risk of premature menopause due to damage to primordial follicles within the ovarian cortex. The surgical treatment of PCOS is discussed in detail in Chapter 11.

In conclusion, there are still some concerns about all the methods currently available, and new techniques need to be developed for the twenty-first century. A possibility is the collection of immature oocytes and their subsequent maturation.

Immature oocyte collection and in-vitro maturation

Pregnancies and births have resulted in women from oocytes recovered from ovari-
ectomy specimens (Cha et al., 1991). By modifying the collection needle, using
lower pressures (Trounson, Wood and Kausche, 1994), immature oocytes can regularly be collected by transvaginal ultrasound controlled aspiration, their subsequent in-vitro maturation resulting in pregnancy (Cha et al., 1996). This was
particularly easy in women with multiple peri-ovarian follicles such as occur with
polycystic ovaries (PCO). Normal births have also been reported by Trounson et al.
(1994), Barnes et al. (1996) and Russell et al. (1996) from in-vitro matured oocytes.

Primary oocytes recovered from small and growing follicles of ≥ 3 mm in the
ovaries of untreated women can be matured in vitro, will fertilize and develop in
vitro, and, when transferred to the patient, develop to term. However, the implantation rate of cleaved embryos has been disappointingly low, and when embryos are
allowed to develop beyond the four-cell stage in vitro, retardation of development
and blockage are frequently observed, with relatively few embryos developing to
blastocysts.

It is possible that follicles of <10 mm diameter in the human contain develop-
mentally incompetent oocytes. However, the development to term and birth of
normal babies from germinal vesicle stage oocytes recovered from small follicles
and matured in vitro suggest that further research will identify the factors necessary to improve embryo developmental competence. The application of immature
oocyte collection and in-vitro maturation as an alternative to ovulation stimulation with high doses of gonadotrophins for in-vitro fertilization (IVF) remains a
priority for research in human medicine (Trounson et al., 1998).

In order to determine whether developmental competence could be improved, a
number of factors have been examined. Treatment of patients with pure follicle stimulating hormone (FSH) early in the follicular phase, or treatment with oestrogen
prior to oocyte recovery, had no apparent effect on any parameters of oocyte developmental competence. There was no indication that a medium made specifically for
human oocyte maturation improved oocyte developmental competence.

Fertilization rates using in-vitro matured oocytes can be significantly increased
from around 30% for insemination in vitro to around 50% using intracytoplasmic
sperm injection (ICSI) (Trounson et al., 1996). However, the improvement in the
development of oocytes with two pronuclei is only significant in PCOS patients and
not in naturally cycling, non-PCOS patients (Trounson et al., 1996). ICSI can be
justified for in-vitro matured oocytes in couples where the female partner has
PCOS.

Cha et al. have recently reported encouraging results from immature oocytes in
women with PCOS (Cha et al., 1996). Immature follicular oocytes collected from
38 PCOS patients resulted in a mean number of 12.0 ± 6.3 oocytes collected per

patient. Of 545 immature follicular oocytes, 320 (58.7%) matured after 48 hours of culture. ICSI was used and the fertilization rate was 78.8% (252/320). A co-culture system using Vero cells was used for in-vitro culture of fertilized oocytes: 124 embryos developed through the in-vitro culture were transferred to 39 cycles (mean: 4.3 embryos/patient). Ten patients became pregnant (25.6%). These findings suggest in-vitro culture of immature follicular oocytes from PCOS patients could be a valuable alternative treatment.

Oocyte cryopreservation

The use of immature oocyte collection to assist women with PCOS may be enhanced by freezing the oocytes. This allows flexibility of the future planning of a pregnancy, avoiding the increased risk of chromosomal abnormalities with increasing age and the performance of surgical procedures before clinical complications of PCOS, such as diabetes, cardiovascular disease and obesity, become severe. Oocytes can be collected at any stage of the menstrual cycle by transvaginal ultrasound needling of the ovaries, or as an additional procedure at the time of laparoscopic ovarian drilling for infertility.

The success rate of oocyte freezing has been limited by technical difficulties resulting from the reduced competence of embryos formed after successful oocyte thawing, fertilization, and early embryo development. The problems associated with oocyte freezing arise from their large size and variable membrane permeability, making it difficult to achieve sufficient dehydration to prevent ice formation and maybe also increasing chromosomal abnormalities by increasing spindle abnormalities.

A new procedure of vitrification – a non-freezing method that stores oocytes in a physical form comparable to glass – may overcome the problem with freezing. Two pregnancies have been obtained in a small number of patients using this technique, and laboratory studies of oocytes of other species appear promising.

Conclusion

It is likely that further research will result in the improvements in embryo developmental competence that will make this technique an attractive alternative.

REFERENCES

Barnes, F.L., Kausche, A., Tiglias, J. et al. (1996). Production of embryos from *in vitro*-matured primary human oocytes. *Fertility and Sterility* 55, 109–13.

Cha, K.Y., Chung, H.M., Han, S.Y. et al. (1996). Successful *in vitro* maturation, fertilization and pregnancy by using immature follicular oocytes collected from unstimulated polycystic ovarian syndrome patients [Abstract 0–044]. In *Proceedings of the American Society of Reproductive Medicine, Boston, November 2–6, 1996*, p. S23. Boston: American Society of Reproductive Medicine.

Cha, K.Y., Koo, J.J., Ko, J.J. et al. (1991). Pregnancy after in vitro fertilization of human follicular oocytes collected from non-stimulated cycles, their culture in vitro and their transfer in a donor oocyte program. *Fertility and Sterility* 55, 109–13.

Farquhar, C., Vanderkerckhove, P., Arnot, M. and Lilford, R. (1999). Laparoscopic 'drilling' by diathermy or laser for ovulation induction in anovulatory polycystic syndrome (Cochrane Review). In *The Cochrane Library*, Issue 1. Oxford: Update Software.

Gjonnaess, H. (1984). Polycystic ovarian syndrome treated by ovarian electrocautery through the laparoscope. *Fertility and Sterility* 41, 20–5.

Healy, D.L. (1992). Aetiology, investigation and management of ovulatory problems. *Current Opinion in Obstetrics and Gynecology* 2, 8–11.

Russell, J.B., Knezevich, K.M., Fabian, K. et al. (1996). *In vitro* oocyte maturation: clinical applicability [Abstract 0–042]. In *Proceedings of the American Society of Reproductive Medicine, Boston, November 2–6, 1996*, p. S22. Boston: American Society of Reproductive Medicine.

Stein, F.I. and Leventhal, M.L. (1935). Amenorrhoea associated with bilateral polycystic ovaries. *American Journal of Obstetrics and Gynecology* 29, 181–91.

Toaff, R., Toaff, M.E. and Peyser, M.R. (1976). Infertility following wedge resection of the ovaries. *American Journal of Obstetrics and Gynecology* 124, 92–6.

Trounson, A.O., Anderiesz, C., Jones, G.M. et al. (1998). Oocyte maturation. *Human Reproduction* 13 (Suppl. 1). 101–11.

Trounson, A.O., Bongso, A., Szell, A. et al. (1996). Maturation of human and bovine primary oocytes in vitro for fertilization and embryo production. *Singapore Journal of Obstetrics and Gynaecology* 27, 78–84.

Trounson, A., Wood, C., and Kausche, A. (1994). *In vitro* maturation and the fertilization and developmental competence of oocytes recovered from untreated polycystic ovarian patients. *Fertility and Sterility* 62, 353–62.

14

Pregnancy outcome for women with polycystic ovary syndrome

William M. Buckett, Alice Benjamin and Seang Lin Tan

Introduction

Polycystic ovary syndrome (PCOS) was first described by Stein and Leventhal (1935), although the overweight, hirsuit, amenorrhoeic phenotype they originally described, we now realize, probably reflects the severe end of the spectrum of the syndrome. Diagnosis is made primarily by ultrasound and endocrine changes, although there remains some controversy about the significance of ultrasound-only diagnosed PCOS when the clinical phenotype and endocrine pattern are normal (Polson et al., 1988; Abdel Gadir et al., 1992). The ultrasound features of PCOS are enlarged ovaries, thickened ovarian stroma, multiple peripheral cysts (2–10 mm diameter) and an increased intra-ovarian stromal blood flow (Adams, Polson and Franks, 1986; Zaidi et al., 1995). The endocrine pattern is characterized by raised serum luteinizing hormone (LH) levels in the early follicular phase or raised LH:FSH (follicle stimulating hormone) ratio and raised levels of testosterone and androstenedione, often associated with reduced levels of sex hormone binding globulin (SHBG) (DeVane et al., 1975; Hull, 1987). However, not all these features are present in every case of PCOS, and it is clear that the syndrome, primarily anovulation associated with hyperandrogenaemia, is an end-point of multiple causes, and this is reflected in the unknown aetiology of the syndrome.

Pregnancies following all treatments for infertility have been associated with higher risks of adverse outcomes when compared to spontaneously conceived pregnancies in fertile women. Early complications include first and second trimester miscarriage and also ectopic pregnancy, probably because of an underlying susceptibility to these complications in the women undergoing treatment. Later complications include pregnancy-induced hypertension, haemorrhagic complications, preterm birth, low birth weight babies, and increased perinatal morbidity and mortality (Tanbo and Åbyholm, 1996). However, these complications generally reflect the increased number of multiple pregnancies, the higher maternal age and the lower parity in women who conceive after infertility treatment when compared to the general population (from national registries) following spontaneous conception. Studies matching for age and parity have shown conflicting results. There still appears to be an increased incidence of preterm delivery, caesarean section, low birth weight babies, and small for gestational age babies (Tan et al., 1992; Petersen et al., 1995; Tanbo et al., 1995; FIVNAT, 1995). However, some studies have shown an increased risk of pregnancy-induced hypertension, pre-eclampsia and placenta praevia (Tanbo et al., 1995), while others report a reduced risk of pre-eclampsia and a similar incidence of placenta praevia (FIVNAT, 1995). These differences presumably reflect differences in the population undergoing treatment, as the various diagnoses have not been controlled for.

Early pregnancy loss, multiple pregnancy, and later complications of pregnancy have all been reported in women with PCOS, following spontaneous conception as well as following treatment for anovulation. This chapter reviews the current evidence for an association between PCOS and early pregnancy loss, multiple pregnancy, ovarian hyperstimulation syndrome (OHSS) and ectopic pregnancy and the later complications of pregnancy, as well as any benefits of current infertility or early pregnancy therapy, including the surgical treatment of PCOS.

Early pregnancy loss

Of all clinical pregnancies, about 15% end in a first trimester loss or miscarriage, usually as a result of genetic errors, but about 1% women have recurrent miscarriage (Stirrat, 1990). While the cause for recurrent miscarriage is impossible to identify in most cases, the incidence of PCOS amongst women with recurrent miscarriage is high (Regan, Owen and Jacobs, 1990), with one study suggesting the ultrasound incidence of polycystic ovaries (PCO) was as high as 82% (Watson et al., 1993). Several studies have shown a clear relationship between the raised serum LH often found in association with PCOS and early pregnancy loss (Regan et al., 1990; Balen, Tan and Jacobs, 1993b).

Hypersecretion of luteinizing hormone

The tonic hypersecretion of LH from the pituitary occurs during the follicular phase of the menstrual cycle and is one of the pathognomonic features of PCOS. Early studies comparing women with PCOS and hypogonadotrophic hypogonadism undergoing ovulation induction showed higher miscarriage rates amongst women with PCOS, and this was more marked in those with higher early follicular phase LH levels (Homburg et al., 1988). The aetiology of the hypersecretion of LH remains poorly understood.

Several hypotheses exist to explain the adverse effect of LH. Some workers believe that the persistently raised LH levels cause premature ageing of the oocyte so that the fertilization rate is decreased and the quality of any resulting embryo is reduced (Balen et al., 1993b). Other studies have suggested that embryo quality is similar in women with PCOS compared with those undergoing in-vitro fertilization (IVF) for other indications (Hardy et al., 1995). Other suggested mechanisms by which LH may exert a deleterious effect include the raised LH causing increased secretion of androgens, which then leads to suppressed granulosa cell function, or an endometrial abnormality from disordered prostaglandin synthesis (Bonney and Franks, 1990).

The use of gonadotrophin-releasing hormone (GnRH) agonists to achieve pituitary suppression of FSH and, more importantly, LH has been incorporated in protocols for assisted conception treatments, primarily with the intention of eliminating a spontaneous LH surge leading to premature ovulation and thereby simplifying treatment (Tan, 1994). Although some studies of women with PCOS who underwent IVF or gamete intrafallopian transfer (GIFT) and became pregnant showed that those who had pituitary desensitization appeared to have lower miscarriage rates (Abdalla et al., 1990; Balen et al., 1993c), other studies have not shown this (Dor et al., 1992). Similarly, there is controversy when pituitary desensitization is used in conjunction with ovulation induction (Dor et al., 1992). A prospective, placebo-controlled, double-blind study assessed the use of GnRH agonist to achieve pituitary suppression in the treatment of recurrent miscarriage and found no significant decrease in the miscarriage rate, despite lower LH levels in the treatment group (Clifford et al., 1996).

Obesity

Despite the association between the hypersecretion of LH in women with PCOS and miscarriage, and the observation that it is often the lean PCOS women who have an increased probability of miscarriage (Conway, Honour and Jacobs, 1989), increased miscarriage rates have also been reported in women with PCOS who are obese and who have normal early follicular LH levels (Hamilton-Fairley et al., 1992). Programmes directed at weight loss in these women have been shown to increase the response to ovulation induction treatment and also to reduce the chance of miscarriage (Clark et al., 1998).

These findings would suggest that the altered insulin sensitivity and associated hyperinsulinaemia may have a role in the early pregnancy loss associated with PCOS, either independently or synergistically.

Hyperandrogenaemia

Raised serum levels of free testosterone and androstenedione and reduced levels of SHBG are found in association with PCOS (DeVane et al., 1975; Hull, 1987). These changes have also been reported in women with recurrent miscarriage without the other features of PCOS (including raised LH or PCO by ultrasound) (Tulppala et al., 1993; Okon et al., 1998). The measurement of androgens with and without progesterone has also been reported to predict miscarriage in early pregnancy (Takeuchi et al., 1993; Aksoy et al., 1996).

Conclusions

It is clear that there is an association between PCOS and early pregnancy loss, and that this is most marked in women with hypersecretion of LH. However, the picture is complicated by the heterogeneity of the syndrome and the differences in diagnostic criteria for PCOS in different studies. It would appear that the presence of raised early follicular LH levels, the ultrasound diagnosis of PCOS, obesity, hyperinsulinaemia, and hyperandrogenaemia either singly or in combination are associated with an increased risk of miscarriage.

Multiple pregnancy

Early studies assessing pregnancy outcome in women with infertility, particularly after assisted conception treatment, showed that the increase in perinatal morbidity and mortality, as well as other adverse outcomes, was secondary to the increased rate of multiple pregnancy (Tan et al., 1992; Balen, MacDougall and Tan, 1993a; Tanbo and Åbyholm, 1996). The long-term psychological consequences of multiple pregnancy also appear to be detrimental to the children and to the family as a whole (Garel and Blondel, 1992).

Although many of the recent studies refer to IVF and the consequences of multiple embryo transfer, ovulation induction with clomiphene citrate and gonadotrophins also leads to an increase in the incidence of multiple pregnancy to about 15–30% (Balen et al., 1994; Tadokoro et al., 1997). Multiple pregnancy rates are obviously directly related to multiple ovulation and therefore to the number of mature follicles. Although many programmes would cancel treatment or convert the ovulation induction cycle to either IVF or GIFT if there were more than three mature follicles (Buckett et al., 1997), the comparison of multiple pregnancy rates between different studies can be difficult because different cancellation/conversion criteria are used.

Although there appears to be no increase in the risk of multiple pregnancy in women with PCOS who conceive spontaneously compared with that of the general population, there is conflicting evidence about the rates of multiple pregnancy following treatment when women with PCOS are compared with other women undergoing ovulation induction for other indications. When compared to women having ovulation induction for hypogonadotrophic hypogonadism, the rates of multiple pregnancy in women with PCOS are significantly increased (Balen et al.,

1994), but when compared to women having ovulation induction for unexplained infertility, the risks appear comparable (Tadokoro et al., 1997).

In conclusion, multiple pregnancy increases pregnancy loss and perinatal death, and leads to other adverse pregnancy outcomes. While there appears to be no increase in the rate of multiple pregnancy in women with PCOS who conceive spontaneously, there is certainly an increased rate following all ovulation induction or superovulation treatments.

Ovarian hyperstimulation syndrome

Ovarian hyperstimulation syndrome is the most serious complication that affects women undergoing induction of ovulation and superovulation for assisted conception therapy. The cardinal features of the syndrome which contribute to its morbidity are marked ovarian enlargement and acute third space sequestration of fluid, mainly intra-abdominal ascites. Direct action of the excessive exogenous gonadotrophins accounts for the ovarian enlargement, but no studies have identified the cause of the fluid shift, although the human chorionic gonadotrophin (hCG) given for ovulation and the rising hCG of early pregnancy (particularly in multiple pregnancy) are implicated in the severity of the syndrome. The fluid shift can cause respiratory distress secondary to a splinting effect of the abdominal ascites on the diaphragm, or directly as a result of pleural effusion or even pulmonary oedema. The resultant haemoconcentraion can also lead to renal failure, stroke and even death. Management remains supportive and the syndrome is ultimately self-limiting.

Women with any of the diagnostic features of PCOS, including those with a pretreatment ultrasound diagnosis of PCO only, are at increased risk of ovarian overresponse and therefore of developing OHSS (MacDougall et al., 1993; Wada et al., 1993).

While it is unlikely that OHSS directly affects pregnancy outcome, if the condition is severe and not managed appropriately, the maternal consequences can be disastrous. So far, increased intervention with dopamine and intravascular volume expanders (Morris et al., 1995) or with repeated paracentesis (Chen et al., 1998) has not shown any adverse effect on the pregnancy.

Ectopic pregnancy

Although there have been case reports of ovarian and tubal ectopic pregnancies in women with PCOS and in those who have had ovarian hyperstimulation following treatment with clomiphene citrate (Cataldo, 1992; Thakur and El-Manabawey, 1996), long-term, large studies have shown no increased risk of ectopic pregnancy either in PCOS alone or following treatment with clomiphene citrate (Naether et al., 1994; Dickey and Holtkamp, 1996).

Gestational diabetes

Gestational diabetes usually affects 5–10% of pregnancies, although there are significant differences between different populations. Although the perinatal outcome in pregnancies complicated by gestational diabetes continues to improve, probably as a result of better screening, diagnosis, and glycaemic control (Coustan, Berkovitch and Hobbins, 1980), the perinatal mortality and morbidity are still higher in these pregnancies (Cowett, 1988). Although the frequency of stillbirth is reduced secondary to better screening for gestational diabetes during pregnancy and therefore better glycaemic control, macrosomia, with its resultant birth injury and asphyxia, and respiratory distress syndrome continue to pose a problem.

Long-term follow-up of women with PCOS who had been treated previously with ovarian wedge resection has shown these women to be at increased risk of developing maturity-onset diabetes, independent of obesity (Dahlgren et al., 1992). As pregnancy has a diabetogenic effect, all women who are at risk of maturity-onset diabetes, by virtue of a positive family history or obesity, are also at risk of developing gestational diabetes.

The incidence of gestational diabetes amongst infertile women with PCOS, who either conceive spontaneously or with ovulation induction treatment, has been shown to be as high as 13%, and the incidence of impaired glucose challenge tests is as high as 32% (Urman et al., 1997). Although obesity itself is an independent risk factor for gestational diabetes and impaired glucose tolerance, there seems to be no difference in the incidence between obese and lean PCOS patients. The hyperinsulinaemia and insulin resistance associated with PCOS, regardless of whether the women are obese or lean, may be responsible for these pregnancy complications by altering insulin sensitivity in early pregnancy in these women (Paradisi et al., 1998).

Whereas most women with gestational diabetes experience uneventful pregnancy and delivery, women with severe, late or undiagnosed gestational diabetes have poorer outcomes (Cowett, 1988). Women with PCOS who become pregnant, either following treatment or spontaneously, should be made aware of their increased risk and screened for gestational diabetes during pregnancy.

Pregnancy-induced hypertension

While many names have been used to describe the different hypertensive disorders of pregnancy, in the USA the National High Blood Pressure Education Program recommend the original classification of Hughes (1972), rather than the more complex classifications of the World Health Organization (World Health Organization Study Group, 1987) or the International Society for the Study of Hypertension in Pregnancy (Davey and MacGillivray, 1988). This classification defines pregnancy-induced hypertension as hypertension that develops as a consequence of pregnancy and regresses postpartum. It further subdivides pregnancy-induced hypertension into hypertension without proteinuria, which can also be called transient hypertension, pre-eclampsia, which can be mild or severe, and eclampsia.

The fetal effects of pregnancy-induced hypertension are intra-uterine growth restriction, a higher rate of abruptio placentae, and prematurity secondary to early intervention for maternal indications. These are thought to be the major contributing factors that lead to an increase in perinatal mortality in these pregnancies. Pre-eclampsia is associated with a much higher perinatal mortality and, in particular, preterm delivery. It is still a significant cause of maternal morbidity and mortality (Scott and Owen, 1996).

Several studies of women with PCOS have shown a higher incidence of pregnancy-induced hypertension (Diamant, Rimon and Evron, 1982; Urman et al., 1997; de Vries, Dekker and Schoemaker, 1998). Although this appears to be independent of obesity and gestational diabetes, the increased insulin resistance and hyperinsulinaemia may nevertheless have a role in the pathogenesis of these pregnancy complications. Hypertension has been shown to develop in insulin-resistant patients (Baron, 1994), and this is a predisposing factor for pregnancy-induced hypertension. The action of insulin on the endothelium leading to nitric oxide synthesis and release may also be implicated in the development of pre-eclampsia (Buhimschi et al., 1995).

In the same way that women with PCOS must be made aware of their increased risk of gestational diabetes, they should also be informed of their increased risk of pregnancy-induced hypertension. They should, therefore, be screened and monitored regularly and closely. The severity of these complications is likely to be worse with higher-order gestations.

Haemorrhage

There have been no reports of an increased incidence of antepartum haemorrhage, unless complicated by pregnancy-induced hypertension. Similarly, there is no increase in the incidence of placenta praevia associated with PCOS, unless complicated by multiple pregnancy.

Medical treatment of polycystic ovary syndrome

The medical treatment of PCOS primarily involves induction of ovulation for an-ovulatory women trying to become pregnant, and the correction of the androgenic effects of hyperandrogenaemia in women not wishing to become pregnant. More recently, the successful correction of the PCOS-associated hyperinsulinaemia with oral hypoglycaemic agents leading to amelioration of symptoms has been reported (Velazquez et al., 1994). With reference to pregnancy outcome, assessment of medical treatment has concerned early pregnancy loss rather than the later pregnancy complications.

Choice of ovulation induction agent

Clomiphene citrate has been shown to be embryotoxic and to affect adversely pregnancy ourcome in animal studies (Dziadek, 1993). These effects and the anti-oestrogenic effect of clomiphene citrate on the endometrium have led some to conclude that the risk of early pregnancy loss can be reduced (to normal levels) if tamoxifen, human menopausal gonadotrophin (hMG) or FSH is used instead. Studies assessing hMG or FSH for ovulation induction in women with PCOS have shown conflicting results, with both normal rates of miscarriage (Tadokoro et al., 1997) and an increased rate of miscarriage being reported (Wang and Gemzell, 1980). However, when clomiphene citrate and hMG were compared prospectively, there was no difference in the miscarriage rates (Manganiello et al., 1997).

Pituitary desensitization

As discussed earlier, there remains some controversy about the role of GnRH agon-ists leading to pituitary desensitization for the treatment of PCOS, both with respect to ovarian response to gonadotrophins and also to the risk of miscarriage (Abdalla et al., 1990; Dor et al., 1992; Balen et al., 1993c; Clifford et al., 1996).

The use of GnRH agonists does not reduce the tendency of women with PCOS to multifollicular development and therefore multiple pregnancy (Charbonnel et al., 1987; Homburg et al., 1990). When GnRH agonists were initially incorporated into ovarian stimulation regimens, it was suggested that their use may reduce the incidence of OHSS, particularly because women with hypogonadotrophic amenor-rhoea rarely develop OHSS. However, treatment with GnRH agonists has, in fact, been shown to be associated with a significantly increased prevalence of severe OHSS (MacDougall, Tan and Jacobs, 1992). This may reflect the higher pregnancy rates associated with their use in PCOS patients undergoing IVF or GIFT.

Whereas the use of GnRH agonists in superovulation for assisted conception treatment is very widespread, their routine use in ovulation induction for women with PCOS cannot be recommended. Whether there is a role for the newer GnRH antagonists remains to be seen.

Progesterone support

Several early studies suggested that progesterone support commenced in the luteal phase for women with PCOS undergoing ovulation induction may decrease miscarriage rates (Check et al., 1987). However, larger prospective studies evaluating the efficacy of progesterone support, both in women with PCOS and in those with recurrent miscarriage, in the absence of a demonstrated luteal phase defect or the use of GnRH agonist, suggest that progesterone support is not indicated (Li, 1998).

Other treatments

Oral hypoglycaemic agents, such as metformin (Velazquez et al., 1994; Morin-Papunen et al., 1998), have been used for the treatment of PCOS with some resolution of symptoms. However, it remains uncertain whether there is any effect on either early or late pregnancy complications associated with PCOS. Centrally acting agents which interfere with opioid metabolism have also been used with some success in patients with PCOS (Cagnacci et al., 1994; Paoletti et al., 1996), but, like the hypoglycaemic agents, no data are available concerning pregnancy outcome. Whether these newer treatments can improve the insulin-mediated complications remains to be seen.

Surgical treatment of polycystic ovary syndrome

Ovarian wedge resection was initially performed to obtain specimens for histological analysis, but, following this invasive surgical procedure, spontaneous ovulation was frequently observed to return (Stein and Cohen, 1939). However, the high incidence of postoperative adhesions and the development of pharmacological agents to induce ovulation led to its demise. Advances in laparoscopic surgery during the 1980s, however, have resulted in a resurgence of interest in the surgical treatment of PCOS. Many techniques have been described, including multiple biopsies (Campo et al., 1983), laparoscopic scissors (Campo et al., 1993), electrocautery (Gjonnaess, 1984), and laser (Huber, Hosmann and Spona, 1988).

There are fewer data regarding pregnancy outcome when compared with standard ovulation induction treatment; however, the miscarriage rate in women who conceive spontaneously following the surgical treatment of PCOS has been reported at about 15%, which is lower than that in women with PCOS who conceive after ovulation induction (Fox, Bhal and James, 1995; Campo, 1998). The incidences of multiple pregnancy and ectopic pregnancy are also low, at about 2% and 1.5% respectively. These results suggest that the surgical treatment of PCOS reduces the chances of early pregnancy loss to the levels experienced by the pregnant population as a whole. Nevertheless, cautious interpretation of these findings is needed – the available data are generally retrospective, and, since not all women respond to the surgical treatment of PCOS, those who conceive following this treatment may represent a subset of PCOS patients.

The reduction in the rate of multiple pregnancy will, however, improve the pregnancy outcome in these patients.

The effect of surgical treatment on the later pregnancy complications associated with PCOS has not been evaluated. As the improvement in endocrine profiles following surgical treatment can be long-lasting, there may be a reduction in the risk of gestational diabetes and pregnancy-induced hypertension.

In conclusion, the surgical treatment of PCOS is an effective alternative to the use of exogenous gonadotrophins in women with clomiphene-resistant PCOS. Early pregnancy loss and multiple pregnancy rates appear similar to those of the general population, although further long-term studies need to be performed to confirm these outcomes and determine the long-term consequences of the treatment, including any on the ovary itself.

Conclusion

Most women with PCOS will conceive spontaneously or achieve pregnancy following treatment. Of those who become pregnant, the vast majority will have an uncomplicated pregnancy and a live birth. However, women with all forms of PCOS are at increased risk of early pregnancy loss when compared with the general population and of having multiple pregnancy should conception follow treatment. There is also an increased risk of gestational diabetes and pregnancy-induced hypertension. These increased risks lead to a higher chance of a poorer outcome of pregnancy in these women.

Surgical treatment of PCOS and weight loss in obese women with PCOS may reduce the risk of early pregnancy loss, although any longer-term benefits of these treatments with respect to later pregnancy complications remain unknown.

REFERENCES

Abdalla, H.I., Ahuja, K.K., Leonard, T. et al. (1990). Comparative trial of luteinizing hormone releasing hormone analogue/HMG and clomiphene citrate/HMG in an assisted conception programme. *Fertility and Sterility* **53**, 473–8.

Abdel Gadir, A., Khatim, M.S., Mowafi, R.S. et al. (1992). Implications of ultrasonically diagnosed polycystic ovaries. I. Correlations with basal hormonal profiles. *Human Reproduction* **4**, 453–7.

Adams, J., Polson, D.W. and Franks, S. (1986). Prevalence of polycystic ovaries in women with anovulation and idiopathic hirsuitism. *British Medical Journal* **239**, 355–9.

Aksoy, S., Celikkanat, H., Senoz, S. and Gokmen, O. (1996). The prognostic value of serum estradiol, progesterone, testosterone and free testosterone levels in detecting abortions. *European Journal of Obstetrics, Gynaecology and Reproductive Biology* **67**, 5–8.

Balen, A.H., MacDougall, J. and Tan, S.L. (1993a). The influence on the number of embryos transferred during in vitro fertilization on pregnancy outcome. *Human Reproduction* **8**, 1324–8.

Balen, A.H., Tan, S.L. and Jacobs, H.S. (1993b). Hypersecretion of luteinizing hormone – a significant cause of subfertility and miscarriage. *British Journal of Obstetrics and Gynaecology* **100**, 1082–9.

Balen, A.H., Tan, S.L., MacDougall, J. and Jacobs, H.S. (1993c). Miscarriage rates following in vitro fertilization are increased in women with polycystic ovaries and reduced by pituitary desensitization. *Human Reproduction* **8**, 959–64.

Balen, A.H., Braat, D.D.M., West, C., Patel, A. and Jacobs, H.S. (1994). Cumulative conception and live birth rates after the treatment of anovulatory infertility: safety and efficacy of ovulation induction in 200 patients. *Human Reproduction* **9**, 1563–70.

Baron, A. (1994). Haemodynamic actions of insulin. *American Journal of Physiology* **267**, E187–E202.

Bonney, R.C. and Franks, S. (1990). The endocrinology of implantation and early pregnancy. *Ballière's Clinical Endocrinology and Metabolism* **4**, 207–31.

Buckett, W.M., Luckas, M.J.M., Gazvani, M.R., Aird, I.A. and Kingsland, C.R. (1997). Conversion of intra-uterine insemination to gamete intra-fallopian transfer. *Journal of Gynecological Technology* **3**, 163–6.

Buhimschi, I., Yallampalli, C., Chwalisz, K. and Garfield, R.E. (1995). Preeclampsia-like conditions produced by nitric oxide inhibition: effect of L-arginine, D-arginine, and steroid hormones. *Human Reproduction* **10**, 2723–30.

Cagnacci, A., Soldani, R., Paoletti, A.M., Falqui, A. and Melis, G.B. (1994). Prolonged opioid blockade with naltrexone and luteinizing hormone modifications in women with polycystic ovary syndrome. *Fertility and Sterility* **62**, 269–72.

Campo, S. (1998). Ovulatory cycles, pregnancy outcome and complications after surgical treatment of polycystic ovary syndrome. *Obstetric and Gynecology Survey* **53**, 297–308.

Campo, S., Felli, A., Lamanna, M.A., Barini, A. and Garcea, N. (1993). Endocrine changes and clinical outcome after laparoscopic ovarian wedge resection in women with polycystic ovaries. *Human Reproduction* **8**, 359–63.

Campo, S., Garcea, N., Caruso, A. and Siccardi, P. (1983). Effect of celioscopic ovarian wedge resection in patients with polycystic ovaries. *Gynecological and Obstetric Investigation* **15**, 213–22.

Cataldo, N.A. (1992). Ovarian pregnancy in polycystic ovary syndrome: a case report. *International Journal of Fertility* **37**, 144–5.

Charbonnel, B., Krempf, M., Blanchard, P., Dano, F. and Delage, C. (1987). Induction of ovulation in polycystic ovary syndrome with a combination of LHRH analog and exogenous gonadotrophin. *Fertility and Sterility* **47**, 920–4.

Check, J.H., Chase, J.S., Wu, C.H. et al. (1987). The efficacy of progesterone in achieving success-ful pregnancy. I. Prophylactic use during luteal phase in anovulatory women. *International Journal of Fertility* **32**, 135–8.

Chen, C.D., Yang, J.H., Chao, K.H. et al. (1998) Effects of repeated abdominal paracentesis on uterine and intraovarian haemodynamics and pregnancy outcome in severe ovarian hyper-stimulation syndrome. *Human Reproduction* **13**, 2077–81.

Clark, A.M., Thornley, B., Tomlinson, L., Galletley, C. and Norman, R.J. (1998). Weight loss in obese infertile women results in improvement in reproductive outcome for all forms of fertil-ity treatment. *Human Reproduction* **13**, 1502–5.

Clifford, K., Rai, R., Watson, H., Franks, S. and Regan, L. (1996). Does suppressing luteinizing hormone secretion reduce the miscarriage rate? Results of a randomised controlled trial. *British Medical Journal* **312**, 1508–11.

Conway, G.S., Honour, J.W. and Jacobs, H.S. (1989). Heterogenicity of the polycystic ovary syn-drome: Clinical, endocrine and ultrasound features in 556 patients. *Clinical Endocrinology* **30**, 459–70.

Coustan, D.R., Berkovitch, R.L. and Hobbins, J.C. (1980). Tight metabolic control of overt dia-betes in pregnancy. *American Journal of Medicine* **68**, 845–52.

Cowett, R.M. (1988). The metabolic sequelae in the infant of a diabetic mother. In *Controversies in Diabetes and Pregnancy*, ed. L. Jovanovic, pp. 149–71. Berlin: Springer-Verlag.

Dahlgren, E., Johansson, S., Lindstedt, G. et al. (1992). Women with polycystic ovary syndrome wedge resected in 1956 to 1965: a long term follow up focusing on natural history and circu-lating hormones. *Fertility and Sterility* **57**, 505–13.

Davey, D.A. and MacGillivray, I. (1988). The classification and definition of the hypertensive dis-orders of pregnancy. *American Journal of Obstetrics and Gynecology* **158**, 892–8

de Vries, M.J., Dekker, G.A. and Schoemaker, J. (1998). Higher risk of pre-eclampsia in the poly-cystic ovary syndrome. A case control study. *European Journal of Obstetrics, Gynaecology and Reproductive Biology* **76**, 91–5.

DeVane, G.W., Czekala, N.M., Judd, H.L. and Yen, S.S. (1975). Circulating gonadotropins, estro-gens, and androgens in polycystic ovarian disease. *American Journal of Obstetrics and Gynecology* **121**, 496–500.

Diamant, Y., Rimon, E. and Evron, S. (1982). High incidence of preeclampsic toxaemia in patients with polycystic ovarian disease. *European Journal of Obstetrics, Gynaecology and Reproductive Biology* **14**, 199–200.

Dickey, R.P. and Holtkamp, D.E. (1996). Development, pharmacology and clinical experience with clomiphene citrate. *Human Reproduction Update* **2**, 483–506.

Dor, J., Ben-Shlomo, I., Levran, D. et al. (1992). The relative success of gonadotrophin-releasing hormone analogue, clomiphene citrate, and gonadotrophin in 1099 cycles of in vitro fertiliza-tion. *Fertility and Sterility* **58**, 986–90.

Dziadek, M. (1993). Preovulatory administration of clomiphene citrate to mice causes fetal growth retardation and neural tube defects (exencephaly) by an indirect maternal effect. *Teratology* **47**, 263–73.

FIVNAT (1995). Pregnancies and births resulting from in vitro fertilization: French National Registry, analysis of data 1986–1990. *Fertility and Sterility* **64**, 746–56.

Fox, R., Bhal, P. and James, M. (1995). Laparoscopic approaches to ovulation induction: an analysis of published data. *Gynaecological Endoscopy* **4**, 87–93.

Garel, M. and Blondel, B. (1992). Assessment at one year of the psychological consequences of having triplets. *Human Reproduction* **7**, 729–35.

Gjonnaess, H. (1984). The polycystic ovarian syndrome treated by ovarian electrocautery through the laparoscope. *Fertility and Sterility* **41**, 20–5.

Hamilton-Fairley, D., Kiddy, D., Watson, H., Paterson, C. and Franks, S. (1992). Association of moderate obesity with a poor pregnancy outcome in women with polycystic ovary syndrome treated with low-dose gonadotrophin. *British Journal of Obstetrics and Gynaecology* **99**, 128–31.

Hardy, K., Robinson, F.M., Paraschos, T. et al. (1995). Normal development and metabolic activity or preimplantation embryos in vitro from patients with polycystic ovaries. *Human Reproduction* **10**, 2125–35.

Homburg, R., Armar, N.A., Eshel, J., Adams, J. and Jacobs, H.S. (1988). Influence of serum luteinizing hormone concentrations on ovulation, conception, and early pregnancy loss in polycystic ovary syndrome. *British Medical Journal* **297**, 1024–6.

Homburg, R., Eshel, A., Kilborn, J., Adams, J. and Jacobs, H.S. (1990). Combined luteinizing hormone releasing hormone analogue and exogenous gonadotrophins for the treatment of infertility associated with polycystic ovaries. *Human Reproduction* **5**, 32–5.

Huber, J., Hosmann, J. and Spona, J. (1988). Polycystic ovary syndrome treated by laser through the laparoscope. *Lancet* **ii**, 215.

Hughes, E.C., ed. (1972). *Obstetric–Gynecologic Terminology*. Philadelphia: Davis.

Hull, M.G.R. (1987). Epidemiology of infertility and polycystic ovarian disease: endocrinological and demographic studies. *Gynecological Endocrinology* **1**, 235–45.

Li, T.C. (1998). Recurrent miscarriage: principles of management. *Human Reproduction* **13**, 478–82.

MacDougall, M.J., Tan, S.L., Balen, A.H. and Jacobs, H.S. (1993). A controlled study comparing patients with and without polycystic ovaries undergoing in vitro fertilization. *Human Reproduction* **8**, 233–7.

MacDougall, M.J., Tan, S.L. and Jacobs H.S. (1992). In vitro fertilisation and the ovarian hyperstimulation syndrome. *Human Reproduction* **7**, 597–600.

Manganiello, P.D., Stern, J.E., Stukel, T.A. et al. (1997). A comparison of clomiphene citrate and human menopausal gonadotropin for use in conjunction with intrauterine insemination. *Fertility and Sterility* **68**, 405–12.

Morin-Papunen, L.C., Koivunen, R.M., Ruokonen, A. and Martikainen, H.K. (1998). Metformin therapy improves the menstrual pattern with minimal endocrine and metabolic effects in women with polycystic ovary syndrome. *Fertility and Sterility* **69**, 691–6.

Morris, R.S., Miller, C., Jacobs, L. and Miller, K. (1995). Conservative management of ovarian hyperstimulation syndrome. *Journal of Reproductive Medicine* **40**, 711–14.

Naether, O.G.J., Baukloh, V., Fischer, R. and Kowalczyk, T. (1994). Long term follow up in 206 infertility patients with polycystic ovarian syndrome after laparoscopic electrocautery of the ovarian surface. *Human Reproduction* **9**, 2342–9.

Okon, M.A., Laird, S.M., Tuckerman, E.M. and Li, T.C. (1998). Serum androgen levels in women who have recurrent miscarriages and their corrleation with markers of endometrial function. *Fertility and Sterility* **69**, 682–90.

Paoletti, A.M., Cagnacci, A., Depau, G.F. et al. (1996). The chronic administration of cabergoline normalizes androgen secretion and improves menstrual cyclicity in women with polycystic ovary syndrome. *Fertility and Sterility* **66**, 527–32.

Paradisi, G., Fulghesu, A.M., Ferrazzani, S. et al. (1998). Endocrino-metabolic features in women with polycystic ovary syndrome during pregnancy. *Human Reproduction* **13**, 542–6.

Petersen, K., Hornnes, P.J., Ellingsen, S. et al. (1995). Perinatal outcome after in vitro fertilization. *Acta Obstetricia Gynecologica Scandinavica* **74**, 129–31.

Polson, D.W., Adams, J., Wadsworth, J. and Franks, S. (1988). Polycystic ovaries – a common finding in normal women. *Lancet* **i**, 870–2.

Regan, L., Owen, E.J. and Jacobs, H.S. (1990). Hypersecretion of luteinizing hormone, infertility and miscarriage. *Lancet* **336**, 1141–4.

Scott, A. and Owen, P. (1996). Recent advances in the aetiology and management of pre-eclampsia. *British Journal of Hospital Medicine* **55**, 476–8.

Stein, I.F. and Cohen, M.R. (1939). Surgical treatment of bilateral polycystic ovaries. *American Journal of Obstetrics and Gynecology* **38**, 465–80.

Stein, I.F. and Leventhal, M.L. (1935). Amenorrhea associated with bilateral polycystic ovaries. *American Journal of Obstetrics and Gynecology* **29**, 181–91.

Stirrat, G.M. (1990). Recurrent miscarriage I: Definition and epidemiology. *Lancet* **336**, 673–5.

Tadokoro, N., Vollenhoven, B., Clark, S. et al. (1997). Cumulative pregnancy rates in couples with anovulatory infertility compared with unexplained infertility in an ovulation induction programme. *Human Reproduction* **12**, 1939–44.

Takeuchi, T., Nishii, O., Okamura, T., Yaginuma, T. and Kawana, T. (1993). Free testosterone and abortion in early pregnancy. *International Journal of Gynaecology and Obstetrics* **43**, 151–6.

Tan, S.L. (1994). Simplifying in vitro fertilization therapy. *Current Opinion in Obstetrics and Gynecology* **6**, 111–14.

Tan, S.L., Doyle, P., Campbell, S. et al. (1992) Obstetric outcome of in vitro fertilization pregnancies compared with normally conceived pregnancies. *American Journal of Obstetrics and Gynecology* **167**, 778–84.

Tanbo, T. and Åbyholm, T. (1996). Obstetric and perinatal outcome in pregnancies after assisted reproduction. *Current Opinion in Obstetrics and Gynecology* **8**, 193–8.

Tanbo, T., Dale, P.O., Lunde, O., Mor, N. and Åbyholm, A. (1995). Obstetric outcome in singleton pregnancies after assisted reproduction. *Obstetrics and Gynecology* **86**, 188–92.

Thakur, R. and El-Menabawey, M. (1996). Combined intra-uterine and extra-uterine pregnancy associated with mild hyperstimulation syndrome after clomiphene ovulation induction. *Human Reproduction* **11**, 1583–4.

Tulppala, M., Stenman, U.H., Cacciatore, B. and Ylikorkala, O. (1993). Polycystic ovaries and levels of gonadotrophins and androgens in recurrent miscarriage: prospective study in 50 women. *British Journal of Obstetrics and Gynaecology* **100**, 348–52.

Urman, B., Sarac, E., Dogan, L. and Gurgan, T. (1997). Pregnancy in infertile PCOD patients. Complications and outcome. *Journal of Reproductive Medicine* **42**, 501–5.

Velazquez, E.M., Mendoza, S., Hamer, T., Sosa, F. and Glueck, C.J. (1994). Metformin therapy in polycystic ovary syndrome reduces hyperinsulinaemia, insulin resistance, hyperandrogenaemia, and systolic blood pressure while facilitating normal menses and pregnancy. *Metabolism* **43**, 647–54.

Wada, I., Matson, P.L., Troup, S.A. and Leiberman, B.A. (1993). Assisted conception using buserelin and human menopausal gonadotrophins in women with polycystic ovary syndrome. *British Journal of Obstetrics and Gynaecology* **100**, 365–9.

Wang, F.C., Gemzell, C. (1980). The use of human gonadotrophins for the induction of ovulation in women with polycystic ovarian disease. *Fertility and Sterility* **33**, 479–86.

Watson, H., Kiddy, D.S., Hamilton-Fairley, D. et al. (1993). Hypersecretion of luteinizing hormone and ovarian steroids in women with recurrent early miscarriage. *Human Reproduction* **8**, 829–33.

World Health Organization Study Group (1987). *The Hypertensive Disorders of Pregnancy.* WHO Technical Report Series No.758. Geneva: WHO.

Zaidi, J., Campbell S., Pittrof R. et al. (1995). Ovarian stromal blood flow in women with polycystic ovaries – a possible new marker for diagnosis? *Human Reproduction* **10**, 1992–6.

15

Should there be long-term monitoring of women with polycystic ovary syndrome?

Alison Venn and Julia Shelley

Introduction

There have been many suggestions in the literature that women with polycystic ovary syndrome (PCOS) are at increased risk of developing a number of chronic conditions, and that, consequently, their health should be monitored (Wild, 1995; Björntorp, 1996; Pettigrew and Hamilton-Fairley, 1997; Hopkinson et al., 1998). For monitoring of women with PCOS to be a worthwhile undertaking, there are a number of preconditions that must be met. First, women with polycystic ovaries (PCO) must indeed have an increased likelihood of adverse health outcomes as a result of, or in relation to, their PCO status. Second, there must be interventions available that are effective in preventing the adverse outcome from occurring. Finally, the monitoring and intervention must be shown to bestow more benefit than harm on the women being monitored.

This chapter addresses each of these issues. It first reviews the evidence for long-term adverse outcomes for women with PCOS, with emphasis on coronary heart disease, diabetes, and cancers of the breast and reproductive system. Then it addresses the issues of the possibility of successful intervention. Finally, it reviews the potential for benefit and the potential for harm in the long-term monitoring of women with PCOS, and discusses the research required to provide firmer recommendations in this area.

Evidence of long-term adverse outcomes

In describing the long-term follow-up of women with PCOS we refer to the condition as defined by the authors in each case. Differences in the way PCOS is defined and in the ways patients are selected for study can make comparisons between studies difficult and may account for some of the inconsistencies in the findings. The long-term health of women with PCO as defined by ultrasound and with few other presenting symptoms has not been studied.

Diabetes

Insulin resistance and resulting hyperinsulinaemia have been recognized features of PCOS for many years. It is now believed that insulin resistance is the underlying disorder of PCO/PCOS (Hopkinson et al., 1998). That women with PCOS may be at increased risk of developing non-insulin-dependent diabetes mellitus (NIDDM) is well recognized. In this section, the evidence regarding PCOS and NIDDM is presented. As well as being a concern in its own right, NIDDM is an established risk factor for cardiovascular disease. The relationship between PCO/PCOS and cardiovascular disease is addressed in the following section.

Evidence that women with PCOS are at increased risk of NIDDM is quite sparse. Two long-term follow-up studies have investigated whether women with PCOS have a greater risk of developing NIDDM than women without this condition, and both provide limited evidence of an excess of diabetes in women with PCOS.

Dahlgren et al. (1992) conducted a retrospective cohort study of 33 Swedish women who had evidence of PCO on ovarian histology from wedge resections or oophorectomy undertaken 22 to 31 years previously, and 132 controls age-matched to the women with PCOS at the time of the study in 1987. At that time, 15% of women with PCOS and 2.3% of the controls had diagnosed NIDDM, a statistically significant difference.

The study did not investigate any differences between the women other than their PCOS and diabetes status. Therefore, it was unable to determine whether PCOS alone is the cause of the difference in prevalence of diabetes between these two groups of women. In particular, there was no analysis of the relationship between body mass index (BMI) or waist-to-hip ratio (WHR) and diabetes in the PCOS and non-PCOS groups, although these measures of obesity are reported elsewhere in their paper.

In the only study of mortality in relation to PCOS status, Pierpoint et al. (1998) report the results of a study of 786 women with PCOS, diagnosed between 1930 and 1979 in the UK, who were followed up for an average of 30 years. Definite cases were defined by histological and clinical evidence, while evidence of histological PCOS or clinical PCOS or macroscopic evidence of ovarian dysfunction was regarded as possible PCOS.

Mortality from all causes for the group of women diagnosed with PCOS was no higher than the national rates for women of the same age (standardized mortality ratio [SMR] 0.90; 95% confidence interval [CI] 0.69–1.17). However, diabetes was mentioned as an underlying or contributing cause of death for six of the women with PCOS, although only 1.7 deaths would be expected based on national data (odds ratio 3.6; 95% CI 1.5–8.4; $p = 0.002$).

Pierpoint et al.'s study makes an important addition to our knowledge about PCOS and diabetes, but it has a number of limitations. In a study of this type it is not possible to consider other factors, such as BMI or other measures of obesity, that may contribute to or cause NIDDM. Even in a study of over 700 women with PCOS and an average of 30 years of follow-up, there are only six diabetes-related deaths recorded, and less than two expected.

Therefore, the extent to which NIDDM contributes to premature morbidity and mortality for women with PCOS remains unclear at present. It is unclear also whether PCOS itself, or the obesity that is a frequent attribute of the condition, or both, is the principal contributor to the observed excess of NIDDM among women with histologically proven PCOS. Further exploration of these questions will be necessary if monitoring and intervention are to be offered only to those women likely to experience long-term adverse consequences of this suite of physiological disruptions.

Cardiovascular disease

Clinicians have been concerned for some time about the possibility of an increase in cardiovascular disease in women with PCOS, due to the disturbances in insulin resistance and lipid profiles that often accompany this diagnosis. Studies have attempted to examine the relationship between PCO and cardiovascular disease in a number of different ways.

The majority of the research in this area has focused on risk factors for coronary heart disease, rather than on morbidity or mortality from coronary heart disease or other circulatory diseases. Findings from studies that have examined cardiovascular disease risk factors in relation to PCO are summarized below.

Lipids

Most studies that have attempted to investigate the relationship between coronary heart disease and PCO have examined the lipid profiles of women with PCO/PCOS and compared them to the lipid profiles of a group of women without PCO. The results of six studies that have taken this approach are summarized in Table 15.1.

There are three main groups among these studies: (1) those that compare women with clinically diagnosed PCOS with women without such a diagnosis (Mahabeer et al., 1990; Talbott et al., 1995, 1998); (2) those that compare women with PCO identified on ultrasound and clinical evidence of PCOS with women without PCOS (Conway et al., 1992; Norman et al., 1995); and (3) a recent study that compares twins discordant for PCO on ultrasound examination (Jahanfar et al., 1997).

Among the first group of studies comparing women with clinically diagnosed PCOS with those without such a diagnosis, there are actually only two distinct studies, as Talbott et al.'s papers of 1995 and 1998 both report results from essentially the same groups of women. There are a number of different comparisons reported in the three papers. Talbott et al.'s paper of 1995 compares their full

Table 15.1. Lipid profiles of women with polycystic ovaries/polycystic ovary syndrome in comparison to control women: a summary of six studies

Comparison	Reference	Number of cases	Number of controls	Total cholesterol	LDL cholesterol	HDL cholesterol	Triglyceride
Women with clinical PCOS compared with non-PCOS controls							
All PCOS vs all non-PCOS	Talbott et al. (1995)	206	206	↑	↑	↓	↑
All PCOS women <40 years vs all non-PCOS women <40 years	Talbott et al. (1998)	163	143	↑	↑	No difference	No difference
All PCOS women ≥40 years vs all non-PCOS women ≥40 years	Talbott et al. (1998)	66	87	No difference	No difference	No difference	↑
Lean women with PCOS vs lean controls	Mahabeer et al. (1990)	10	10	↑	↑	No difference	↑
Obese women with PCOS vs obese controls	Mahabeer et al. (1990)	10	10	↑	↑	↓	[↑]*
Women with features of PCOS detected clinically or by ultrasound							
Lean women with PCOS vs lean controls	Conway et al. (1992)	48	19	No difference	Not measured	↓	No difference
Obese women with PCOS vs lean controls	Conway et al. (1992)	54	19	No difference	Not measured	↓	↑
Women with PCOS or PCO vs non-PCOS/PCO controls	Norman et al. (1995)	97 PCOS, 21 PCO	26	No difference	No difference	↓	No difference
Women with PCO diagnosed on ultrasound							
Twins with discordant PCO status	Jahanfar et al. (1997)	11	11	No difference	Not measured	No difference	No difference

Note:

* Clinically significant increase that did not reach statistical significance due to small study size.

sample of women with PCOS with the full sample of controls, whereas their 1998 paper subdivides these groups by age and examines women under 40 years of age separately from those 40 years of age and over. Mahabeer et al. (1990) have selected two groups, each containing cases and controls, one non-obese group of cases and controls, and a second obese group of cases and controls. They have reported the two sets of comparisons in this paper.

Even though the studies report on a range of different comparisons, the findings are fairly consistent. They indicate poorer lipid profiles among the women with PCOS than among control women, regardless of the specific characteristics of the groups being examined. The largest, and arguably the best designed, of these studies, that by Talbott et al. (1995), reports adverse results among women with PCOS for all the lipids examined.

There are two notable exceptions to these general findings. High density lipoprotein (HDL) and triglyceride are now accepted as being the lipids of greatest importance to the development of coronary heart disease in women (Bush, Fried and Barrett-Connor, 1988; Jacobs et al., 1990), and yet it is for these two measures that the findings summarized in this chapter are least consistent. Of the five sets of results reported, only two indicate that women with PCOS have lower HDL levels than the control group. Although Talbott et al. (1995) found more adverse lipid measures in the PCOS group than in the non-PCOS control group, these findings were not replicated in either of the two age subgroups reported more recently. Only triglyceride levels differed between cases and controls in their later study.

Talbott et al.'s study of 1998 is the only one that investigates the association between lipid fractions and PCOS status in relation to age. Their finding that the differences in total cholesterol and low density lipoprotein (LDL) cholesterol evident in women under 40 years of age with and without PCOS are not evident in women 40 years and older raises some important questions for further research. Further studies to examine whether lipid levels in women with and without PCO/PCOS converge as women age and the implications of this for the long-term health of women with PCO/PCOS are needed.

There are only two studies in the second group identified above, those by Conway et al. (1992) and Norman et al. (1995). Conway et al. have defined two case groups, one lean and one obese, of women with PCO confirmed on ultrasound and with clinical signs of PCOS. Norman et al. (1995) compared 97 women with clinically diagnosed PCOS, 21 women with ultrasonically detected PCO but no clinical or endocrine characteristics of PCOS, and 26 women with neither PCOS nor PCO. The authors further subdivided the PCO and PCOS groups into those with regular (PCO, $n = 15$; PCOS, $n = 43$) and those with irregular cycles (PCO, $n = 6$; PCOS, $n = 54$). Their control group contained 19 lean women without PCO/PCOS.

Both studies report lower HDL levels for cases compared with controls. The obese women with PCOS in the study by Conway et al. also had higher triglyceride levels than the controls, but neither the lean case women nor Norman et al.'s case group exhibited triglyceride levels higher than their respective controls. There were no differences found between any of the groups of cases and controls for total cholesterol levels. Norman et al. found triglyceride levels to be statistically significantly higher in the group of women with PCO and irregular menstrual cycles than in any other group. However, as this group consisted of only six women, this may be a consequence of variability resulting from small numbers rather than a clinically significant finding.

The third group consists of only one study in which the lipid levels of pairs of twins, found to have discordant PCO status on ultrasound, were compared (Jahanfar et al., 1997). This is a very small study, comprising only 11 pairs of twins. As a result, the findings may reflect a real lack of difference in the lipid levels between the twins with and without PCO, or may just be the consequence of the lack of power in the study due to the small sample size.

In summary, the results of studies that have considered the relationship between PCO/PCOS and lipid levels are inconsistent. HDL levels are a possible exception, with the majority of studies finding lower HDL levels among women with PCO/PCOS than among controls, regardless of the selection criteria for either cases or controls.

The inconsistency of the findings regarding lipid profiles may have a number of causes. No two of these studies have used the same definition of cases and controls, and thus each study is reporting a different comparison. Sample definition and selection differ in two very important areas, the manner of diagnosis of PCO/PCOS status and the manner in which BMI is treated.

As BMI and lipid levels are closely related, the failure of many of these studies to take full account of possible differences in the distribution of BMI between case and control groups may be adding to imprecision in the results. The few comparisons between women of similar BMI with and without PCO/PCOS mean that the question of whether any observed differences in lipid profiles are related to the women's PCO/PCOS status or to their BMI remains unanswered.

With the exception of the studies by Talbott et al. (1995, 1998), the studies summarized above are very small. Small numbers are characterized by the type of variability that is evident here. Inconsistency may also result from the relatively poor reliability of single measures of the lipid fractions, given the variability of total cholesterol measures over time (Roeback et al., 1993).

It may be that these features of the research to date are clouding the picture with regard to lipid levels and PCO/PCOS, or it may be that there is, in fact, no difference in lipid profiles between women with and without PCO/PCOS. It is not possible to determine which of these is the more likely explanation on the evidence to date.

Hypertension

Very few studies have examined blood pressure levels among women with PCO/PCOS and compared them with a control group. Only one study has found higher diastolic blood pressure in women with PCOS than in a control group (Mahabeer et al., 1990). The same study is one of only two to have found higher systolic blood pressure in women with PCOS than in controls.

In Mahabeer et al.'s study, non-obese women with PCOS had higher diastolic and systolic blood pressures than non-obese controls, as did obese women with PCOS in comparison with obese controls. Conway et al. (1992) found higher systolic blood pressure in obese women with PCOS than in lean controls. Talbott et al. (1995, 1998) found higher systolic blood pressure in women with PCOS prior to taking account of differences in BMI, but not in a multivariate analysis that adjusted for differences in BMI. It may be that the results of Mahabeer et al.'s study reflect a disparity in BMI between cases and controls that remained regardless of the formation of obese and non-obese subgroups.

As McKeigue (1996) has highlighted, hypertension is predominantly a condition of older women rather than of the women of reproductive age who usually form the study groups in research on PCO/PCOS. In the Swedish follow-up study, Dahlgren et al. (1992) reported a prevalence of treated hypertension over three times as high among 40–59-year-old women with PCOS diagnosed 22 to 31 years earlier as among their non-PCOS control group. No adjustment has been made for BMI or other measures of obesity in this study.

Thus, further evidence is required to clarify whether PCO/PCOS has an influence on blood pressure per se, and/or whether the blood pressure of women with PCO/PCOS is higher than that of the general population of women due to the generally higher BMI of women with this condition.

Morbidity and mortality from cardiovascular disease

Regardless of the findings related to PCO/PCOS and risk factors for cardiovascular disease, it is important to consider whether morbidity and/or mortality from circulatory diseases are higher in women with PCO before deciding whether monitoring is likely to be worthwhile. We could locate only two studies that addressed these important questions.

Birdsall, Farquhar and White (1997) assessed the association between the extent of coronary artery disease and the presence or absence of PCO among 143 women undergoing coronary angiography. They found that women with PCO visible on ultrasonography had a greater number of arterial segments with more than 50% stenosis than did women without PCO (1.7 segments compared with 0.82).

The only long-term follow-up study of the relationship between PCO/PCOS and mortality is that by Pierpoint et al. (1998), described above. This large study, with a follow-up of an average of 30 years, found that mortality from all causes for the group of women diagnosed with PCOS was no higher than the national rates for women of the same age.

Of the total of 59 deaths, 15 were from circulatory diseases (SMR 0.83; 95% CI 0.46–1.37). Deaths from ischaemic heart disease (13 deaths) were no more frequent than in the population as a whole (SMR 1.40; 95% CI 0.75–2.40). However, there was a significantly *reduced* rate of death from other circulatory diseases (SMR 0.23; 95% CI 0.03–0.85) based on two deaths among women diagnosed with PCOS.

In summary, there is very little evidence that women with PCO/PCOS are at increased risk of cardiovascular disease independent of NIDDM, and there is some limited evidence that they have a lower rate of some forms of cardiovascular disease than do women without this diagnosis. In noting that there were fewer deaths from circulatory disease (excluding ischaemic heart disease) than expected, Pierpoint et al. (1998) speculated that the action of unopposed oestrogen in anovulatory cycles might protect women with PCOS from circulatory disease, despite the presence of other cardiovascular disease risk factors.

The study of Talbott et al. (1998) may provide some clues to the apparent discrepancy between the evidence provided by studies of cardiovascular disease risk factors, especially lipid fractions, and that provided by Pierpoint et al.'s study. The majority of the studies examining cardiovascular disease risk factors and PCOS status have done so in relatively young women. It is possible that the risk factor profiles of women without PCO/PCOS become more like those of women with this diagnosis as they age. Women's lipid levels have been shown to change in adverse directions with increasing age (Shelley et al., 1998). Cardiovascular disease is primarily a disease of ageing, and women's risk factor status as they approach older age may be the more important determinant of later morbidity and mortality. It remains for this hypothesis to be further investigated.

Cancer

Our understanding of cancer risk in women with PCOS comes from studies of women who have had anovulatory infertility, menstrual irregularity or oestrogen replacement therapy, as well from studies of women with clinically defined PCOS. The association between exposure to unopposed oestrogens and an increased risk of endometrial cancer has been well established (Parrazini et al., 1991), particularly through studies of the effects of oestrogen replacement therapy in menopausal and postmenopausal women. The association with PCOS has been reported in young women in several clinical series (Jafari, Jafaheri and Ruiz, 1978). In a relatively small case-control study of 176 women with endometrial cancer, Dahlgren et al. (1991) found significant associations with hirsutism, increased BMI and hypertension in women who were aged under and over 45. Most recently, an Israeli follow-up study of 2496 infertile women observed a significantly higher than expected incidence of endometrial cancer, particularly in women with normal oestrogen production but progesterone deficiency (Modan et al., 1998). During the follow-up period, 13 cases of endometrial cancer were observed, compared with 1.4 cases expected from age-standardized general population rates, giving a standardized incidence ratio (SIR) of 9.4 (95% CI 5.0–16.0). An increased incidence of endometrial cancer was found in a follow-up study of 1270 women with chronic anovulation syndrome identified from medical records at the Mayo Clinic Minnesota, USA (Coulam, Annegers and Kranz, 1983). Five cases of endometrial cancer were observed, compared with 1.59 cases expected (SIR = 3.1; 95% CI 1.1–7.3).

Obesity has been shown consistently to be an important risk factor for endometrial cancer (Parazzini et al., 1991) and is therefore likely to contribute to cancer risk in overweight women with PCOS. The association has generally been explained in terms of increased levels of unopposed peripheral oestrogens, particularly in post-menopausal obese women. Diabetes and hypertension have been associated with an increased risk of endometrial cancer in some studies but, overall, the findings have been inconsistent and the relationship is not well defined.

The risk of breast cancer in women with PCOS appears to be no greater than for women in the general population. Although a non-significantly increased risk has been reported in two studies (Cowan et al., 1981; Coulam et al., 1983), most studies show no difference or a reduced incidence compared with the general population.

A large, prospective, cohort study of 34 835 women aged over 55 found that women with a self-reported history of PCOS ($n = 472$) were no more likely to develop breast cancer than women without such a history, giving a relative risk estimate of 1.0 (95% CI 0.6–1.9) after adjusting for a range of potential confounders (Anderson et al., 1997). The Israeli cohort study of cancer in 2496 infertile women (Modan et al., 1998) also found that the incidence of breast cancer in women with normal oestrogen production but progesterone deficiency was not significantly higher than expected (23 cases were observed, compared with 16.3 expected; SIR = 1.4; 95% CI 0.9–2.1).

No association was seen between breast cancer and self-reported PCOS in an Italian case-control study of 2569 women with breast cancer and 2588 hospital controls, which found an adjusted odds ratio of 0.8 (95% CI 0.4–2.8) (Parrazini et al., 1997). A USA case-control study of breast cancer based on 4730 cases and 4688 controls (Gammon and Thompson, 1991) found a significantly reduced risk of breast cancer in women who self-reported a history of physician diagnosed PCOS (adjusted odds ratio = 0.47, 95% CI 0.26–0.85). A significantly reduced risk of breast cancer in women with a self-reported history of ovulatory infertility, many of whom might be assumed to have had PCOS, was recently found in the Nurses Health Study II (Garland et al., 1998), with an adjusted relative risk of 0.41 (95%

CI 0.18–0.93). Women whose usual cycle length at age 18–22 was more than 39 days or too irregular for estimation of usual cycle length were also at a significantly decreased risk of breast cancer. These findings were interpreted as supporting the hypothesis that reduced exposure to ovulatory menstrual cycles is protective against breast cancer.

Ovarian cancer has been less well studied in women with PCOS than breast and endometrial cancer. Cohort studies that have examined ovarian cancer in infertile women with progesterone deficiency have shown no significant increase in risk (Brinton et al., 1989; Rossing et al., 1994; Modan et al., 1998). Few case-control studies of ovarian cancer have had sufficient data or statistical power to estimate the risk for women with PCOS. Schildkraut et al. (1996) used data from the Cancer and Steroid Hormone Study to look at the relationship between ovarian cancer and PCOS in 476 cases and 4081 controls. More cases than controls reported that they had been diagnosed with PCOS with an odds ratio of 2.5 (95% CI 1.1–5.9). Women with PCOS who had never used oral contraceptives and who were in the lowest quartile of BMI at age 18 appeared to have the highest risk. In a large Danish case-control study, Mosgaard et al. (1997) showed no association between invasive ovarian cancer and a history of hyperandrogenism. Ovarian cancer was not associated with a history of irregular periods in a large Australian case-control study (Purdie et al., 1995).

The studies describing cancer risk in women with PCOS have suffered important limitations, particularly low statistical power and imprecise or proxy measures of a history of PCOS. In some studies, only women with infertility and PCOS have been included, and they are likely to have had treatment with clomiphene citrate or gonadotrophins to induce ovulation. The question of whether fertility drugs are associated with an increased risk of breast or gynaecological cancer has been reviewed elsewhere (Venn and Healy, 1997). Currently, the evidence suggests no increase in breast or endometrial cancer associated with fertility drugs, but the findings on ovarian cancer risk have been inconsistent.

The need for more long-term follow-up studies

Although there has been much discussion of the risk of cardiovascular disease, diabetes and endometrial cancer in women with PCOS, few studies have examined the long-term incidence of these outcomes in women with PCOS. The British study of mortality in women with PCOS (Pierpoint et al., 1998) is the only cohort study to date with long-term follow-up. We know very little about the incidence of non-fatal cardiovascular disease events and NIDDM. Findings from the mortality study, which did not show a higher death rate from cardiovascular disease, highlight the need for caution in predicting the long-term health of women with this complex disorder.

In future studies there is a need for clear definitions and measurements of PCO and PCOS to determine which women are at greatest risk of long-term health problems. The effects of PCO/PCOS and obesity on long-term health need to be separated. Large prospective cohort studies would offer the best opportunity to answer these questions, but would not generate results in the short term. It is likely that there would be difficulties in identifying a representative sample of women with PCO diagnosed by ultrasound and few other presenting symptoms. Studies aiming to determine the prevalence of ultrasound-detected PCO in the general female population have had response rates of less than 25% (Clayton et al., 1992; Farquhar et al., 1994) and have therefore been prone to selection bias. Retrospective cohort studies of the long-term health of women with PCO/PCOS will give more immediate answers, but will have to rely on past assessments of PCOS status. Cohort studies of either type will need to include a large number of women, which might only be achieved through the collaborative efforts of several centres.

Monitoring: can morbidity and mortality be reduced?

In order to answer the question about whether there should be long-term monitoring of women with PCOS, we need to consider the known risks of long-term health problems and the effectiveness of any interventions that might be offered to reduce morbidity and/or mortality.

Although it is not yet clear whether the predicted risks of health problems in women with PCOS actually translate into significant excess long-term morbidity and/or mortality, it has been suggested that women with PCOS could reduce their risk of NIDDM and cardiovascular disease through weight reduction and exercise, and that the use of medications that reduce insulin resistance might also be warranted (Guzick, 1998; Hopkinson et al., 1998).

Some studies have demonstrated the benefits of weight reduction and exercise programmes for infertile women with PCOS (Clarke et al., 1998; Norman and Clarke, 1998). It seems that a relatively modest reduction in weight may be associated with increased insulin sensitivity and improved fertility. Weight reduction and exercise programmes in the setting of an infertility clinic probably owe some of their success to ongoing support from clinic staff and other affected women, and the relatively short-term goal of achieving a pregnancy. Many women will be highly motivated.

If advice about diet and exercise is to be a major component of the long-term monitoring of women with PCOS, then there needs to be consideration of the effectiveness of that advice. Advice to lose weight may be given quickly and easily during a clinical consultation, but women may find it very difficult to achieve and maintain the recommended weight loss. It is likely that, for some women, well-intentioned advice could lead to anxiety and a sense of failure when weight loss proves to be difficult. Many overweight women have a long history of unsuccessful attempts to lose weight.

A high prevalence of bulimia nervosa in women with PCOS has been reported by McCluskey et al. (1991, 1992). Morgan (1999) has highlighted the need for disordered eating to be stabilized before weight reduction is attempted, and the potential for unsupervised dieting, with cycles of binge eating and purging, to exacerbate symptoms of PCOS.

Recent reviews of current and future treatments for PCOS (Hopkinson et al., 1998; Legro, 1998) have discussed the role of the insulin-sensitizing agents, metformin and troglitazone, in the treatment of women with PCOS. Although initial short-term results have shown some promise in improving the endocrine profile and in restoring regular menstrual cycles and ovulation, their role in the long-term therapy of women with PCOS has yet to be determined. Hopkinson et al. noted that troglitazone has been removed from the market because of adverse effects on hepatic function.

Because of the public health importance of cardiovascular disease and NIDDM, there has been much discussion of the value of weight reduction and exercise as methods of primary prevention of morbidity and mortality in the general population. Randomized, controlled trials are currently underway to determine the effectiveness of different interventions, including weight reduction, exercise and/or pharmacological agents (Linday, 1997; Pan et al., 1997; Azen et al., 1998).

In general, methods of weight loss and weight control have been shown to be effective in the short term, but longer-term follow-up shows that people tend to regain weight (Wadden, 1993). Multiple risk factor interventions, including counselling, education and pharmacological agents, have been shown to be largely ineffective in reducing morbidity and mortality from cardiovascular disease in a systematic review of completed studies (Ebrahim and Smith, 1997). There is mixed evidence about the effectiveness of lifestyle advice offered by general practitioners, particularly in relation to advice about diet and exercise (Ashenden, Silagy and Weller, 1997).

Although the results of trials will help to establish the value of primary prevention programmes for NIDDM and cardiovascular disease in the general population, studies will be needed to determine their effectiveness in women with PCOS, given the specific disorders that underlie their condition. Measures of general health status and quality of life are being used more frequently in studies designed to test the effectiveness of health interventions, and could be useful in future evaluations of interventions with women with PCOS. A quality-of-life questionnaire designed for women with PCOS has been described by Cronin et al. (1998). The short form 36 general health status questionnaire (SF-36) has been found to be valuable when used before and after the implementation of a range of health interventions, including the treatment of menorrhagia (Garratt et al., 1993).

Whereas weight loss and exercise may prove to be valuable interventions for overweight women with PCOS, the options for lean women are more limited. It is not clear whether the incidence of NIDDM and cardiovascular disease in women with PCO and without clinical signs of PCOS differs from that of the general population. Studies are needed to determine whether interventions are warranted and effective.

The prospects for the primary prevention of breast, ovarian and uterine cancer are poor because so few of the identified risk factors are modifiable (Kelsey and Whittemore, 1994). Cancer screening programmes reduce morbidity and mortality through early detection of the disease. Although breast cancer screening is now widely available, there are no effective population screening programmes for endometrial or ovarian cancer. Women can be monitored for endometrial hyperplasia, but as yet there is no reliable means of detecting preclinical or early ovarian cancer.

The epidemiological evidence to date does not support a significantly increased risk of breast cancer in women with PCOS. It is appropriate, therefore, for women with PCOS to follow the breast screening recommendations for women in the general population.

In conclusion, to answer the question of whether there should be long-term monitoring of women with PCOS, we need more accurate estimates of the incidence of adverse health outcomes and ways to identify the women with PCO and PCOS who are most at risk. The hope for long-term monitoring of women with PCOS would be to offer effective interventions that reduce morbidity and mortality. The results of randomized trials of primary prevention strategies to reduce NIDDM and cardiovascular disease in the general population will have important implications for women with PCOS, but will not necessarily be generalizable. Evidence of their effectiveness in women with PCO/PCOS will also be necessary. Interventions and advice aimed at reducing long-term health problems in women with PCOS should be mindful of the potential to do harm and should be directed to those who will derive most benefit.

REFERENCES

Anderson, K.E., Sellers, T.A., Chen, P-L. et al. (1997). Association of Stein–Leventhal syndrome with the incidence of postmenopausal breast carcinoma in a large prospective study of women in Iowa. *Cancer* 79, 494–9.

Ashenden, R., Silagy, C. and Weller, D. (1997). A systematic review of the effectiveness of promoting lifestyle change in general practice. *Family Practice* 14, 160–75.

Azen, S.P., Peters, R.K., Berkowitz, K. et al. (1998). TRIPOD (TRoglitazone In the Prevention Of Diabetes): a randomized, placebo controlled trial of troglitazone in women with prior gestational diabetes mellitus. *Controlled Clinical Trials* **19**, 217–31.

Birdsall, M.A., Farquhar, C.M. and White, H.D. (1997). Association between polycystic ovaries and extent of coronary artery disease in women having cardiac catheterization. *Annals of Internal Medicine* **126**, 32–5.

Björntorp, P. (1996). The android woman – a risky condition. *Journal of Internal Medicine* **239**, 105–10.

Brinton, L.A., Melton, J., Malkasian, G.D., Bond, A. and Hoover, R. (1989). Cancer risk after evaluation for infertility. *American Journal of Epidemiology* **129**, 712–22.

Bush, T., Fried, L. and Barrett-Connor, E. (1988). Cholesterol, lipoproteins and coronary heart disease in women. *Clinical Chemistry* **34**, B60–B70.

Clarke, A.M., Thornley, B., Tomlinson, L., Galletley, C. and Norman, R.J. (1998). Weight loss in obese infertile women results in improvement in reproductive outcome for all forms of fertility treatment. *Human Reproduction* **13**, 1502–5.

Clayton, R.N., Ogden, V., Hodgkinson, J. et al. (1992). How common are polycystic ovaries in normal women and what is their significance for the fertility of the population? *Clinical Endocrinology* **37**, 127–34.

Conway, S.G., Agrawal, R., Betteridge, D.J. and Jacobs, H.S. (1992). Risk factors for coronary artery disease in lean and obese women with the polycystic ovary syndrome. *Clinical Endocrinology* **37**, 119–25.

Coulam, C.B., Annegers, J.F. and Kranz, J.S. (1983). Chronic anovulation syndrome and associated neoplasia. *Obstetrics and Gynecology* **61**, 403–7.

Cowan, L.D., Gordis, L., Tonascia, J.A. and Jones, G.S. (1981). Breast cancer incidence in women with a history of progesterone deficiency. *American Journal of Epidemiology* **114**, 209–17.

Cronin, L., Guyatt, G., Griffith, L. et al. (1998). Development of a health-related quality-of-life questionnaire (PCOSQ) for women with polycystic ovary syndrome (PCOS). *Journal of Clinical Endocrinology and Metabolism* **83**, 1976–87.

Dahlgren, E., Friberg, L.-G., Johansson, S. et al. (1991). Endometrial carcinoma; ovarian dysfunction – a risk factor in young women. *European Journal of Obstetrics, Gynaecology and Reproductive Biology* **41**, 143–50.

Dahlgren, E., Johansson, S., Lindstedt, G. et al. (1992). Women with polycystic ovary syndrome wedge resected in 1956 to 1965: a long-term follow-up focusing on natural history and circulating hormones. *Fertility and Sterility* **57**, 505–13.

Ebrahim, S. and Smith, G.D. (1997). Systematic review of randomised controlled trials of multiple risk factor interventions for preventing coronary heart disease. *British Medical Journal* **314**, 1666–74.

Farquhar, C.M., Birdsall, M., Manning, P., Mitchell, J.M. and France, J.T. (1994). The prevalence of polycystic ovaries on ultrasound scanning in a population of randomly selected women. *Australian and New Zealand Journal of Obstetrics and Gynaecology* **34**, 67–72.

Gammon M.D. and Thompson, W.D. (1991). Polycystic ovaries and the risk of breast cancer. *American Journal of Epidemiology* **134**, 818–24.

Garland, M., Hunter, D.J., Colditz, G.A. et al. (1998). Menstrual cycle characteristics and history of ovulatory infertility in relation to breast cancer risk in a large cohort of US women. *American Journal of Epidemiology* 147, 636–43.

Garratt, A.M., Ruta, D.A., Abdalla, M.I., Buckingham, J.K. and Russell, I.T. (1993). The SF36 health survey questionnaire: an outcome measure suitable for routine use within the NHS? *British Medical Journal* 306, 1440–4.

Guzick, D. (1998). Polycystic ovary syndrome: symptomatology, pathophysiology, and epidemiology. *American Journal of Obstetrics and Gynecology*, 179, S89–93.

Hopkinson, Z.E.C., Sattar, N., Fleming, R. and Greer, I.A. (1998). Polycystic ovarian syndrome: the metabolic syndrome comes to gynaecology. *British Medical Journal* 317, 329–32.

Jacobs, D.R., Mebane, I.L., Bangdiwala, S.I., Criqui, M.H. and Tyroler, H.A. for the Lipid Research Clinics Program (1990). High density lipoprotein cholesterol as a predictor of cardiovascular disease mortality in men and women: the follow-up of the Lipid Research Clinics prevalence study. *American Journal of Epidemiology* 131, 32–47.

Jafari, K., Jafaheri, G. and Ruiz, G. (1978). Endometrial adenocarcinoma in Stein–Leventhal syndrome. *Obstetrics and Gynecology* 51, 97–100.

Jahanfar, S., Eden, J.A., Nguyen, T., Wang, X.L. and Wilcken, D.E. (1997). A twin study of polycystic ovary syndrome and lipids. *Gynecological Endocrinology* 11, 111–17.

Kelsey, J.L. and Whittemore, A.S. (1994). Epidemiology and primary prevention of cancers of the breast, endometrium and ovary. A brief overview. *Annals of Epidemiology* 4, 89–95.

Legro, R.S. (1998). Polycystic ovary syndrome: current and future treatment paradigms. *American Journal of Obstetrics and Gynecology* 179, S101–8.

Linday, L.A. (1997). Trivalent chromium and the diabetes prevention program. *Medical Hypotheses* 49, 47–9.

McCluskey, S., Evans, C., Lacey, J.H., Pearce, J.M. and Jacobs, H. (1991). Polycystic ovary syndrome and bulimia. *Fertility and Sterility* 55, 287–91.

McCluskey, S.E., Lacey, J.H. and Pearce, J.M. (1992). Binge-eating and polycystic ovaries. *Lancet* 340, 723.

McKeigue, P. (1996). Cardiovascular disease and diabetes in women with polycystic ovary syndrome. *Ballière's Clinical Endocrinology and Metabolism* 10, 311–18.

Mahabeer, S., Naidoo, C., Norman, R.J., Reddi, K. and Joubert, S.M. (1990). Metabolic profiles and lipoprotein lipid concentrations in non-obese and obese patients with polycystic ovarian disease. *Hormones and Metabolism Research* 22, 537–40.

Modan, B., Ron, E., Lerner-Geva, L. et al. (1998). Cancer incidence in a cohort of infertile women. *American Journal of Epidemiology* 147, 1038–42.

Morgan, J.F. (1999). Bulimic eating patterns should be stabilised in polycystic ovarian syndrome (letter). *British Medical Journal* 318, 328.

Mosgaard, B.J., Lidegaard, O., Kjaer, S.K., Schou, G. and Andersen, A.N. (1997). Infertility, fertility drugs, and invasive ovarian cancer: a case-control study. *Fertility and Sterility* 67, 1005–12.

Norman, R.J. and Clarke, A.M. (1998). Obesity and reproductive disorders: a review. *Reproduction, Fertility and Development* 10, 55–63.

Norman, R.J., Hague, W.M., Masters, S.C. and Wang, X.J. (1995). Subjects with polycystic ovaries without hyperandrogenaemia exhibit similar disturbances in insulin and lipid profiles as those with polycystic ovary syndrome. *Human Reproduction* 10, 2258–61.

Pan, X.R., Li, G.W., Hu, Y.H. et al. (1997). Effects of diet and exercise in preventing NIDDM in people with inpaired glucose tolerance. The Da Qing IGT and diabetes study. *Diabetes Care* 20, 537–44.

Parazzini, F., La Vecchia, C., Bocciolone, L. and Franceschi, S. (1991). The epidemiology of endometrial cancer. *Gynecologic Oncology* 41, 1–16.

Parazzini, F., La Vecchia, C., Franceschi, S. et al. (1997). Association of Stein–Leventhal syndrome with the incidence of postmenopausal breast carcinoma in a large prospective study of women in Iowa (letter). *Cancer* 80, 1360–2.

Pierpoint, T., McKeigue, P.M., Isaacs, A.J., Wild, S.H. and Jacobs, H.S. (1998). Mortality of women with polycystic ovary syndrome at long-term follow up. *Journal of Clinical Epidemiology* 51, 581–6.

Pettigrew, R. and Hamilton-Fairley, D. (1997). Obesity and female reproductive function. *British Medical Bulletin* 53, 341–58.

Purdie, D., Green, A., Bain, C. et al. (1995). Reproductive and other factors and risk of epithelial ovarian cancer: an Australian case-control study. *International Journal of Cancer* 62, 678–84.

Roeback, J.R., Cook, J.R., Guess, H.A. and Heyse, J.F. (1993). Time-dependent variability in repeated measurements of cholesterol levels: clinical implications for risk misclassification and intervention monitoring. *Journal of Clinical Epidemiology* 46, 1159–71.

Rossing, M.A., Daling, J.R., Weiss, N.S., Moore, D.E. and Self, S.G. (1994). Ovarian tumors in a cohort of infertile women. *The New England Journal of Medicine* 331, 771–6.

Schildkraut, J.M., Schwingl. P.J., Bastos, E., Evanoff, A. and Hughes, C. (1996). Epithelial ovarian cancer risk among women with polycystic ovary syndrome. *Obstetrics and Gynecology* 88, 554–9.

Shelley, J.M., Green, A., Smith, A.M.A. et al. (1998). Relationship of endogenous sex hormones to lipids and blood pressure in mid-aged women. *Annals of Epidemiology* 8, 39–45.

Talbott, E., Clerici, A., Berga, S.L. et al. (1998). Adverse lipid and coronary heart disease risk profiles in young women with polycystic ovary syndrome: results of a case-control study. *Journal of Clinical Epidemiology* 51, 415–22.

Talbott, E., Guzick, D., Clerici, A. et al. (1995). Coronary heart disease risk factors in women with polycystic ovary syndrome. *Arteriosclerosis, Thrombosis and Vascular Biology* 15, 821–6.

Venn, A.J. and Healy, D.L. (1997). Fertility drugs and cancer. *Reproductive Medicine Review* 6, 185–98.

Wadden, T.A. (1993). Treatment of obesity by moderate and severe caloric restriction. Results of clinical research trials. *Annals of Internal Medicine* 119, 688–93.

Wild, R.A. (1995). Obesity, lipids, cardiovascular risk, and androgen excess. *American Journal of Medicine* 98, 27S–32S.

Index

Note: page numbers in *italics* refer to figures and tables.